Chronic Respiratory Diseases: Updates on Pathophysiology, Symptoms, Diagnosis and Treatment

Chronic Respiratory Diseases: Updates on Pathophysiology, Symptoms, Diagnosis and Treatment

Guest Editors

Marcin Kurowski
Laura Malinauskienė
Corrado Pelaia

MDPI

Basel • Beijing • Wuhan • Barcelona • Belgrade • Novi Sad • Cluj • Manchester

Guest Editors
Marcin Kurowski
Department of Immunology and Allergy
Medical University of Lodz
Lodz
Poland

Laura Malinauskienė
Department of Pulmonology and Allergology
Vilnius University Hospital Santaros Klinikos
Vilnius
Lithuania

Corrado Pelaia
Department of Medical and Surgical Sciences
University "Magna Græcia" of Catanzaro
Catanzaro
Italy

Editorial Office
MDPI AG
Grosspeteranlage 5
4052 Basel, Switzerland

This is a reprint of the Special Issue, published open access by the journal *Medicina* (ISSN 1648-9144), freely accessible at: https://www.mdpi.com/journal/medicina/special_issues/Z4QF0Q94M3.

For citation purposes, cite each article independently as indicated on the article page online and as indicated below:

Lastname, A.A.; Lastname, B.B. Article Title. *Journal Name* **Year**, *Volume Number*, Page Range.

ISBN 978-3-7258-8341-7 (Hbk)
ISBN 978-3-7258-8342-4 (PDF)
https://doi.org/10.3390/books978-3-7258-8342-4

Contents

About the Editors

Marcin Kurowski

Marcin Kurowski is an Associate Professor at the Department of Immunology and Allergy of the Medical University of Łódź, Poland. His research and clinical interests encompass asthma, in particular exercise-induced asthma and the management of severe asthma with biological treatment; hereditary and acquired angioedema; urticaria; food allergies and hypersensitivity; and allergic rhinitis. He has been involved in multiple research projects, and in international collaborations within GA^2LEN, UCARE and ACARE collaborative networks. He has also been an active member of the European Academy of Allergy and Clinical Immunology (EAACI), the European Respiratory Society (ERS), the Polish Society of Allergology, and the Polish Society of Lung Diseases. He has been involved in several initiatives within these societies and serves as Board Member of the EAACI Asthma Section, and Chairperson of the "Allergy, Asthma and Sports" Working Group within the EAACI. Currently, he chairs the "Allergy, Asthma and Sports" Section of the Polish Society of Allergology and is a member of the Editorial Boards of various allergy journals, including the *Polish Journal of Allergology*, *Frontiers in Allergy*, *BMC Immunology*, *BMC Pulmonary Medicine*, *European Journal of Medical Research*, and *Biologics*.

Laura Malinauskienė

Laura Malinauskienė is Professor at the Institute of Clinical Medicine, Clinic of Chest Diseases, Immunology and Allergology, Vilnius University, Lithuania. Her clinical and research interests focus on allergology and clinical immunology, with particular emphasis on contact allergy, allergic contact dermatitis, textile dye and cosmetic allergens, heavy metal sensitization, venom allergy, molecular allergy diagnostics, immunodeficiency, urticaria, severe asthma, and the long-term consequences of COVID-19 pneumonia. Her research activity has spanned national and international projects on contact allergy, as well as cosmetics, propolis, textile dyes and metals, the development and validation of diagnostic systems for Hymenoptera venom allergy, and the development of an artificial intelligence-based individualized allergy diagnostic tool. She collaborates with research groups at Lund University, Gothenburg University, the European Academy of Dermatology and Venereology Contact Dermatitis Task Force, and GA^2LEN UCARE. She is the President of the Lithuanian Society of Allergologists and Clinical Immunologists. She has authored numerous peer-reviewed publications, contributed to European contact allergy research, supervised doctoral and student research, and received the 2024 Lithuanian Science Prize in Medical and Health Sciences for work on food and chemical allergy.

Corrado Pelaia

Corrado Pelaia is Associate Professor of Respiratory Medicine at the Department of Medical and Surgical Sciences, Magna Græcia University of Catanzaro, Italy, and a pulmonologist at the Respiratory Unit of the "Renato Dulbecco" University Hospital of Catanzaro. His clinical and research interests focus on the pathophysiology of respiratory diseases, severe asthma, biological therapies, chronic airway diseases, and pulmonary mechanical ventilation. His translational research activity includes clinical and laboratory-based projects aimed at improving the diagnostic and therapeutic management of patients with respiratory disorders, with particular attention to proteomic and peptidomic analyses of induced sputum, blood, and other biological samples. He completed specialist training in Respiratory Diseases at Magna Græcia University of Catanzaro and served as a Research Fellow at the Nuffield Department of Clinical Medicine, University of Oxford. He has authored numerous peer-reviewed international publications and has achieved a strong citation record in the field of respiratory medicine.

Preface

We hereby present the Reprint of the Special Issue of the *Medicina* journal titled "Chronic Respiratory Diseases: Updates on Pathophysiology, Symptoms, Diagnosis and Treatment". This Reprint is intended to comprehensively collect and share current views, opinions, and scientific research results in respiratory medicine. Common and overlapping areas, potentially attractive to both pneumonologists and allergists, are an additional focus of this collection of reviews and original articles. Currently, medical practice tends to evolve, in certain aspects, from a highly specialized to an interdisciplinary approach. We believe that this Special Issue Reprint addresses the frequently expressed desire for interdisciplinary knowledge sharing and will be considered a valuable source of knowledge for medical practitioners seeking a broader perspective. Equally, we hope that the readers will find a reflection of, and maybe a solution to, the challenges they may encounter in their practice.

Marcin Kurowski, Laura Malinauskienė, and Corrado Pelaia
Guest Editors

medicina

MDPI

Editorial

Chronic Respiratory Diseases: The Stories You Don't Want to Miss

Marcin Kurowski [1,*], Laura Malinauskienė [2,*] and Corrado Pelaia [3,*]

[1] Department of Immunology and Allergy, Medical University of Lodz, 90-419 Lodz, Poland
[2] Department of Pulmonology and Allergology, Vilnius University Hospital Santaros Klinikos, Santariskiu 2, LT-08661 Vilnius, Lithuania
[3] Department of Health Sciences, University "Magna Græcia" of Catanzaro, 88100 Catanzaro, Italy
* Correspondence: marcin.kurowski@umed.lodz.pl (M.K.); laura.malinauskiene@santa.lt (L.M.); pelaia.corrado@gmail.com (C.P.)

Chronic respiratory disease is rarely boring. One day it is cilia that do not move; the next, it is an herbal tea that turns out to be an allergen, a life-saving drug that bites back, or lungs that will not quite forget a virus. This Special Issue of *Medicina* titled "Chronic Respiratory Diseases: Updates on Pathophysiology, Symptoms, Diagnosis and Treatment" brings these very different clinical stories under one roof and shows how closely they are connected by infection, immunity, and treatment.

The case report by Packi et al. [1] reminds us that even in patients with a well-defined chronic respiratory disorder, diagnostic thinking must remain wide open. A young woman with Kartagener syndrome and primary ciliary dyskinesia (PCD) developed persistent pleural effusion and eosinophilic pneumonia, initially treated as a bacterial process. Only after careful re-evaluation, recognition of marked eosinophilia, and targeted serology was pulmonary toxocariasis due to *Toxocara canis* confirmed, and the patient subsequently responded to albendazole.

This "first in the literature" co-occurrence of PCD and pulmonary toxocariasis highlights two key messages. First, structural or functional defects of mucociliary clearance profoundly reshape the lung's infectious landscape, allowing usually trivial or transient pathogens—including parasites—to persist and trigger severe inflammation. Second, in any patient with chronic respiratory disease who does not improve on standard therapy, clinicians must resist anchoring bias and actively search for atypical causes, including parasitic infections, drug reactions, and autoimmune phenomena.

Preda and co-authors take us to the opposite end of the spectrum—from rare parasites to very common weeds [2]. Their review of IgE-mediated allergy to Asteraceae weed pollen and herbal medicinal products shows just how far-reaching ragweed, mugwort, and their relatives can be in everyday practice. They walk the reader through sensitization patterns; cross-reactivity with chamomile, marigold, echinacea, and milk thistle; and the sometimes dramatic reactions linked to "natural" remedies and bee products. The message is practical: structured diagnostics (skin tests, molecular allergology, challenge where needed) and good history-taking around herbal use are not optional extras, but part of modern respiratory and allergy care.

The theme of iatrogenic risk is taken up from a different angle by Mereškevičienė and Danila [3], who systematically review adverse effects of both first- and second-line antituberculosis drugs. As tuberculosis remains one of the leading infectious killers worldwide, multidrug and extensively drug-resistant strains necessitate prolonged multidrug

 https://doi.org/10.3390/medicina62040746

regimens that are often toxic. The review synthesizes data on gastrointestinal, hepatic, neurological, cardiac, renal, and cutaneous reactions, identifies risk factors such as age, alcohol use, comorbidities, and acetylator status, and summarizes management strategies—from laboratory monitoring to dose adjustment, pyridoxine supplementation, and, inevitably, in some cases, treatment discontinuation.

Two points stand out. First, even the "old" drugs—isoniazid, rifampicin, pyrazinamide, ethambutol—still have safety profiles that are incompletely characterized in diverse real-world populations, underscoring the need for continued pharmacovigilance. Second, while new agents such as bedaquiline, delamanid, and pretomanid expand therapeutic options, they also introduce new patterns of toxicity and drug–drug interactions. Balancing a microbiological cure against the risk of serious adverse events is at the core of modern TB care, and this review offers a valuable, pragmatic guide for clinicians navigating that balance.

In another contribution to this Special Issue, Strumilienė et al. [4] provide a longitudinal window into what happens after the acute fight is over in severe and critical COVID-19. In a prospective cohort of 85 patients who were followed for 12 months after hospital discharge, they document gradual but incomplete recovery of spirometric parameters and diffusion capacity, with a substantial proportion of patients retaining restrictive patterns and impaired DLCO at one year. High-resolution CT scans reveal that while inflammatory changes diminish, profibrotic and fibrotic abnormalities remain strikingly prevalent.

Perhaps most intriguingly, the authors couple these structural and functional data with detailed immunophenotyping. They show sustained alterations in lymphocyte subsets, including reductions in CD3+, CD8+, and activated CD3HLA-DR+ cells, and identify associations between specific T-cell populations expressing CCR2 (CD192) and lung function indices—higher CD4+/CD28+/CD192+ counts correlate with worse total lung capacity, whereas higher CD8+/CD28+/CD192+ levels correlate with better outcomes. These findings reinforce the concept that long COVID is not merely "slow healing" but reflects ongoing immune dysregulation that can shape the trajectory of pulmonary repair and fibrosis.

What do these four contributions tell us when we read them side by side? First, they indicate that chronic respiratory diseases today sit at a crossroads where genetics, environment, infection, and treatment constantly intersect. Second, they make us think beyond classic bacteria and viruses and encourage us to question the safety of "natural" products in sensitized patients, respect the toxic potential of essential drugs, and follow our patients well beyond the acute phase of illness.

For clinicians, there is something immediately usable in each paper: a reminder to re-evaluate stubborn pneumonia, a framework for approaching "herbal" allergy, a structured approach to monitoring for TB drug toxicity, and concrete reasons to set up long-term follow-up for survivors of severe COVID-19. For researchers, these articles highlight priorities ranging from rare host–pathogen interactions to pharmacovigilance and immune mechanisms of repair.

A review by Janić et al. [5] takes the reader into the area of respiratory disease comorbidities. The glucagon-like peptide-1 (GLP-1) and glucose-dependent insulinotropic polypeptide/GLP-1 (GIP/GLP-1) receptor agonists have already gained wide recognition in several indications, including glucose control in type 2 diabetes and weight loss in people with and without diabetes. Janić et al. provide a comprehensive account of their potential influence on metabolic changes in the context of chronic obstructive pulmonary disease (COPD), asthma, pneumonia, obstructive sleep apnea, pulmonary hypertension, lung cancer, and lung transplantation. Given the known possible contribution of systemic inflammation associated with metabolic dysregulation to the development and progression

https://doi.org/10.3390/medicina62040746

of airway inflammatory conditions, this review is a must-read for all clinicians who are interested in updating their knowledge on systemic inflammation in respiratory disease.

Two articles in this Special Issue of *Medicina* address the role of sensitization to airborne allergens in the development of respiratory disease. A review by Klain et al. [6] highlights the role of *Alternaria* allergens in the development of respiratory allergy symptoms. In addition, the paper covers multiple aspects of allergen-specific immunotherapy for *Alternaria* allergy and provides insights into possible cross-reactivity between Alternaria allergens and those from other sources. Since mold allergy is an emergent and important, yet sometimes underestimated mechanism underlying respiratory allergy symptoms, this review is an important contribution to increasing awareness of mold spore allergy among allergy and respiratory practitioners. An original article by Majkowska-Wojciechowska and colleagues [7] explores patterns of reactivity to inhalant allergens in a central Polish population sample comprising over 1700 subjects. In the studied population, IgE sensitization to perennial allergens was significantly associated with asthma, whereas sensitization to seasonal airborne allergens, such as grass, rye, hazel, and alder pollen, was associated with the development of the symptoms of allergic rhinitis.

Last but not least, this Special Issue also contains articles addressing clinically important issues relating to cystic fibrosis (CF) [8], bronchiectasis [9], and respiratory failure in patients with chronic obstructive pulmonary disease (COPD) [8]. That last paper, by Ozdemir et al. [8], importantly identifies a higher comorbidity burden in females with COPD, along with heart failure and heart failure risk factors being more prominent in female COPD patients. A systematic review on the use of azithromycin in the management of CF in pediatric patients with or without concomitant *P. aeruginosa*, provided by Hassan Al-Shehri and Dana Albassam from Riyadh, Saudi Arabia [9], revealed widely beneficial effects of azithromycin in pediatric CF patients, leading to lung function improvement and considerable reduction in the number of exacerbations requiring antibiotic treatment. These effects of azithromycin contribute significantly to the improved efficacy of pediatric CF management and justify its use in pediatric CF. Finally, the research article by Janković and colleagues [10], from Belgrade, Serbia, explores differences in clinical characteristics, presentation, severity, or distribution in focal and multifocal bronchiectasis, as well as their prognostic implications. The bottom line of their article is that the presence of multifocal bronchiectasis may serve as a biomarker of disease severity and poor outcomes.

The wide range of topics addressed by the contributors to this Special Issue evidently reflects the heterogeneity of clinical challenges that most pulmonologists and allergists face almost every day when managing patients with respiratory conditions. Addressing these challenges may be facilitated by guidelines and recommendations issued by international scientific groups with regard to asthma [11], COPD [12], tuberculosis [13], COVID-19 [14], cystic fibrosis [15], bronchiectasis [16], and primary ciliary dyskinesia [17] within comparable frames.

IgE-dependent allergen sensitization is an important factor in the development of type 2 inflammation in allergic respiratory diseases, such as asthma and allergic rhinitis. Recent advances in molecular biology and component-resolved diagnostics (CRD) of allergy have improved the accuracy of identifying the culprit allergenic proteins and enabled more detailed recommendations based on the sensitization profile [18]. This is particularly applicable to the identification of possible cross-reactivity between airborne and food allergens, which may be vital for preventing anaphylactic reactions [19–27]. Molecular identification of sensitizing allergen components is also a valuable tool for a detailed assessment of inhalant allergy [28–32] and facilitates decisions regarding allergen-specific immunotherapy, increasing the possibility of successful outcomes [33–37].

 https://doi.org/10.3390/medicina62040746

Last but not least, a wide and optimistic perspective in respiratory disease management opens up with the implementation of biological treatment. Biologics are increasingly becoming the mainstay of treatment for severe asthma [38–41] and chronic rhinosinusitis with nasal polyps [42–44], while recent developments in biologics for COPD [45–47] raise hopes for substantial benefits for patients with other respiratory conditions as well.

If you look after lungs—in the clinic, in intensive care, in a TB ward, or in an allergy lab—this Special Issue is an invitation to pause, take a breath, and read further. Each article presents a different story, but together, they sketch a single, evolving picture of what it means to live with and treat chronic respiratory disease today. We hope to have convinced you to read the articles in the Special Issue that we have had the pleasure and honor of co-editing.

Author Contributions: Conceptualization, M.K., L.M., and C.P.; writing—original draft preparation M.K., L.M., and C.P.; writing—review and editing, M.K., L.M., and C.P. All authors have read and agreed to the published version of the manuscript.

Funding: This research received no external funding.

Institutional Review Board Statement: Not applicable.

Informed Consent Statement: Not applicable.

Conflicts of Interest: The authors declare no conflicts of interest.

References

1. Packi, K.; Fugiel, W.; Gołąbek, V.; Rudek, A.; Śliwińska, A. Eosinophilic Pneumonia Triggered by Toxocara Canis in a Patient with Primary Ciliary Dyskinesia: A Clinical Case Report. *Medicina* **2024**, *60*, 1874. [CrossRef] [PubMed]
2. Preda, M.; Smolinska, S.; Popescu, F.-D. Diagnostic Workup in IgE-Mediated Allergy to Asteraceae Weed Pollen and Herbal Medicine Products in Europe. *Medicina* **2024**, *60*, 1494. [CrossRef]
3. Mereškevičienė, R.; Danila, E. The Adverse Effects of Tuberculosis Treatment: A Comprehensive Literature Review. *Medicina* **2025**, *61*, 911. [CrossRef]
4. Strumiliene, E.; Urbonienė, J.; Jurgauskiene, L.; Zeleckiene, I.; Bliudzius, R.; Malinauskiene, L.; Zablockiene, B.; Samuilis, A.; Jancoriene, L. Long-Term Pulmonary Sequelae and Immunological Markers in Patients Recovering from Severe and Critical COVID-19 Pneumonia: A Comprehensive Follow-Up Study. *Medicina* **2024**, *60*, 1954. [CrossRef]
5. Janić, M.; Škrgat, S.; Harlander, M.; Lunder, M.; Janež, A.; Pantea Stoian, A.; El-Tanani, M.; Maggio, V.; Rizzo, M. Potential Use of GLP-1 and GIP/GLP-1 Receptor Agonists for Respiratory Disorders: Where Are We At? *Medicina* **2024**, *60*, 2030. [CrossRef]
6. Klain, A.; Giovannini, M.; Arasi, S.; Barni, S.; Castagnoli, R.; Caminiti, L.; Gelsomino, M.; Liotti, L.; Mastrorilli, C.; Mori, F.; et al. Alternaria Allergy and Asthma in Children. *Medicina* **2025**, *61*, 1639. [CrossRef]
7. Majkowska-Wojciechowska, B.; Kulma, M.; Kurowski, M. Aeroallergen IgE-Reactivity Patterns and Respiratory Allergy in Children and Adults: A Retrospective Study in 1711 Patients from the Central Poland Urban Area. *Medicina* **2025**, *61*, 1676. [CrossRef]
8. Ozdemir, T.; Yıldız, M.; Arı, M.; Arı, E.; Eraslan Doğanay, G.; Cırık, M.Ö.; Doğancı, M.; Özdilekcan, Ç.; Kızılgöz, D.; Şipit, Y.T. Gender-Based Differences in COPD Patients with Type 2 Respiratory Failure—Impact on Clinical Practice. *Medicina* **2025**, *61*, 587. [CrossRef]
9. Al-shehri, H.; Albassam, D. Efficacy of Long-Term Use of Azithromycin in the Management of Cystic Fibrosis in Pediatric Patients with or Without Pseudomonas Aeruginosa: A Systematic Review and Meta-Analysis Article. *Medicina* **2025**, *61*, 653. [CrossRef] [PubMed]
10. Jankovic, J.; Jandric, A.; Djurdjevic, N.; Vukosavljevic, D.; Bojic, Z.; Zecevic, A.; Stjepanovic, M. Phenotype and Clinicoradiological Differences in Multifocal and Focal Bronchiectasis. *Medicina* **2024**, *60*, 795. [CrossRef] [PubMed]
11. Global Initiative for Asthma. Global Strategy for Asthma Management and Prevention, 2025. Updated 15 November 2025. Available online: https://www.Ginasthma.Org (accessed on 3 March 2026).
12. Global Initiative for Chronic Obstructive Lung Disease. Global Strategy for Prevention, Diagnosis and Management of COPD (2025 Report). 2025. Available online: https://Goldcopd.Org/2025-Gold-Report/ (accessed on 3 March 2026).
13. Saukkonen, J.J.; Duarte, R.; Munsiff, S.S.; Winston, C.A.; Mammen, M.J.; Abubakar, I.; Acuña-Villaorduña, C.; Barry, P.M.; Bastos, M.L.; Carr, W.; et al. Updates on the Treatment of Drug-Susceptible and Drug-Resistant Tuberculosis: An Official ATS/CDC/ERS/IDSA Clinical Practice Guideline. *Am. J. Respir. Crit. Care Med.* **2025**, *211*, 15–33. [CrossRef]

 https://doi.org/10.3390/medicina62040746

14. Roche, N.; Crichton, M.L.; Goeminne, P.C.; Cao, B.; Humbert, M.; Shteinberg, M.; Antoniou, K.M.; Ulrik, C.S.; Parks, H.; Wang, C.; et al. Update June 2022: Management of Hospitalised Adults with Coronavirus Disease 2019 (COVID-19): A European Respiratory Society Living Guideline. *Eur. Respir. J.* **2022**, *60*, 2200803. [CrossRef] [PubMed]
15. Huang, Y.; Zhang, J.; Zhang, M.; Kong, X.; Wang, Z.; Zhang, Y.; Zou, Z.; Zong, Z.; Guo, J.; Liu, Q.; et al. Evaluation of Clinical Practice Guidelines on Treatment of Cystic Fibrosis: A Systematic Review. *J. Cyst. Fibros.* **2025**, *24*, 446–456. [CrossRef]
16. Polverino, E.; Goeminne, P.C.; McDonnell, M.J.; Aliberti, S.; Marshall, S.E.; Loebinger, M.R.; Murris, M.; Cantón, R.; Torres, A.; Dimakou, K.; et al. European Respiratory Society Guidelines for the Management of Adult Bronchiectasis. *Eur. Respir. J.* **2017**, *50*, 1700629. [CrossRef]
17. Shoemark, A.; Goutaki, M.; Kinghorn, B.; Ardura-Garcia, C.; Baz-Redón, N.; Chilvers, M.; Davis, S.D.; De Brandt, J.; Dell, S.; Dhar, R.; et al. European Respiratory Society and American Thoracic Society Guidelines for the Diagnosis of Primary Ciliary Dyskinesia. *Eur. Respir. J.* **2025**, *66*, 2500745. [CrossRef]
18. Dramburg, S.; Hilger, C.; Santos, A.F.; de Las Vecillas, L.; Aalberse, R.C.; Acevedo, N.; Aglas, L.; Altmann, F.; Arruda, K.L.; Asero, R.; et al. EAACI Molecular Allergology User's Guide 2.0. *Pediatr. Allergy Immunol.* **2023**, *34*, e13854. [CrossRef]
19. Kato, Y.; Morikawa, T.; Fujieda, S. Comprehensive Review of Pollen-Food Allergy Syndrome: Pathogenesis, Epidemiology, and Treatment Approaches. *Allergol. Int.* **2025**, *74*, 42–50. [CrossRef] [PubMed]
20. Wawrzeńczyk, A.; Napiórkowska-Baran, K.; Lis, K.; Tykwińska, M.; Szota, M.; Treichel, P.; Durślewicz, J.; Bartuzi, Z. Food Allergen Component Sensitization Patterns in Eosinophilic Esophagitis: Insights from a Retrospective Comparative Study. *Foods* **2026**, *15*, 748. [CrossRef] [PubMed]
21. Pukalyak, S.; Gromek, W.; Tomczak, A.; Markut-Miotła, E.; Woźniak, M.; Wysokiński, M.; Smolinska, S.; Majsiak, E. Wheat Allergy in the Era of Precision Medicine: From Novel Molecular Markers to New Therapeutic Perspectives. *Int. J. Mol. Sci.* **2026**, *27*, 1717. [CrossRef] [PubMed]
22. Ossowska, A.; De Jager, A.T.; Abdul Cader, K.; Sanchez, D. Multiple Nut Allergies and Anaphylaxis Risk in Children: A Narrative Review. *Allergies* **2025**, *5*, 43. [CrossRef]
23. Luo, W.; Zheng, X.; Zhang, J.; Li, A.; Wu, J.; Ma, J.; Zhao, Y.; Sun, X.; Wei, C.; Ren, H.; et al. Component-Resolved Diagnostics Study on Nut Sensitization and Cross-Reactivity in China. *Respir. Med.* **2025**, *248*, 108365. [CrossRef]
24. Torres-Arroyo, A.; Suárez-Gutiérrez, M.; Iglesias-Amaya, A.; López-Durán, A.; Díaz-García, L.; Reyes-Vivas, H.; Mendoza-Hernández, D. Immunoblotting Analysis of Fruit Proteins in Mexican Pediatric Patients Suggests the Existence of New Allergens. *Diseases* **2025**, *13*, 284. [CrossRef]
25. Turkalj, M.; Banić, I.; Fressl Juroš, G. Component-Resolved and Multiplex-Specific IgE Diagnostics: Utility in Anaphylaxis and Beyond. *Children* **2025**, *12*, 933. [CrossRef]
26. Majsiak, E.; Traczyk, I.; Cabaj, M.; Pukalyak, S.; Samoliński, B.K. Planetary Diet and Hidden Risk: The Significance of Foodallergies in Vulnerable Populations. *Alergol. Pol.—Pol. J. Allergol.* **2026**, *13*, 12–20. [CrossRef]
27. Rymarczyk, B.; Jura-Szołtys, E.; Gluck, J.; Gawlik, R. Does a Healthy Diet Always Mean a Safe Diet? Food Allergy as an Obstacle to a Healthy Lifestyle. *Alergol. Pol.—Pol. J. Allergol.* **2025**, *12*, 91–97. [CrossRef]
28. Didžiokaitė, G.; Kuznecovaitė, A.; Biliūtė, G.; Kvedarienė, V. Gender and Age-Related Trends in Inhalant Allergen Sensitization in Lithuania: A Cross-Sectional Study. *Int. J. Mol. Sci.* **2025**, *26*, 9719. [CrossRef]
29. Gheorghita, L.-M.; Preda, M.; Marghidan, C.-S.; Lazar, M.-I.; Papacocea, I.-R.; Smolinska, S.; Popescu, F.-D. Molecular Biomarkers in IgE Immunoassays Used for Grass Pollen Allergy Diagnosis in European Clinical Settings. *Int. J. Mol. Sci.* **2026**, *27*, 1393. [CrossRef] [PubMed]
30. Yasniuk, M.; Rodinkova, V.; Mokin, V.; Kryzhanovskyi, Y.; Kryvopustova, M.; Kish, R.; Yuriev, S. Atmospheric Pollen Monitoring and Bayesian Network Analysis Identify Bet v 1 and Cross-Reactive Cry j 1 as Dominant Tree Allergens in Ukraine. *Atmosphere* **2026**, *17*, 128. [CrossRef]
31. Lam, K.; Au, E.; Ip, W.K.; Tam, J.K.; Leung, P.S.C. Inhalant Mediated Allergy: Immunobiology, Clinical Manifestations and Diagnosis. *Clin. Rev. Allergy Immunol.* **2025**, *68*, 43. [CrossRef] [PubMed]
32. Schoos, A.-M.M.; Nwaru, B.I.; Borres, M.P. Component-Resolved Diagnostics in Pet Allergy: Current Perspectives and Future Directions. *J. Allergy Clin. Immunol.* **2021**, *147*, 1164–1173. [CrossRef]
33. Blank, S.; Bilò, M.B.; Ollert, M. Component-resolved Diagnostics to Direct in Venom Immunotherapy: Important Steps towards Precision Medicine. *Clin. Exp. Allergy* **2018**, *48*, 354–364. [CrossRef]
34. Sakalauskaite, S.; Pilkyte, L.; Gasiuniene, E.; Gradauskiene, B. Prospective Evaluation of Specific IgE Profile and Quality-of-Life During Allergen-Specific Immunotherapy with House Dust Mite: A Pilot Study. *Medicina* **2025**, *62*, 9. [CrossRef]
35. Hatzler, L.; Panetta, V.; Lau, S.; Wagner, P.; Bergmann, R.L.; Illi, S.; Bergmann, K.E.; Keil, T.; Hofmaier, S.; Rohrbach, A.; et al. Molecular Spreading and Predictive Value of Preclinical IgE Response to Phleum Pratense in Children with Hay Fever. *J. Allergy Clin. Immunol.* **2012**, *130*, 894–901.e5. [CrossRef] [PubMed]
36. Kupczyk, M. Component Resolved Diagnostics in Allocation to Specific Immunotherapy. *Alergol. Pol.—Pol. J. Allergol.* **2019**, *6*, 146–151. [CrossRef]

 https://doi.org/10.3390/medicina62040746

37. Izmailovich, M.; Semenova, Y.; Abdushukurova, G.; Mukhamejanova, A.; Dyussupova, A.; Faizova, R.; Gazaliyeva, M.; Akhvlediani, L.; Glushkova, N.; Kalmakhanov, S.; et al. Molecular Aspects of Allergen-Specific Immunotherapy in Patients with Seasonal Allergic Rhinitis. *Cells* **2023**, *12*, 383. [CrossRef]
38. Varricchi, G.; Poto, R.; Lommatzsch, M.; Brusselle, G.; Braido, F.; Virchow, J.C.; Canonica, G.W. Biologics and Airway Remodeling in Asthma: Early, Late, and Potential Preventive Effects. *Allergy* **2025**, *80*, 408–422. [CrossRef] [PubMed]
39. Suzuki, T.; Tajiri, T.; Ozawa, Y.; Amakusa, Y.; Ito, K.; Mori, Y.; Fukumitsu, K.; Fukuda, S.; Kanemitsu, Y.; Uemura, T.; et al. Clinical Remission and Its Predictors After 12 Months of Biologic Therapy in Severe Asthma. *Biologics* **2026**, *6*, 4. [CrossRef]
40. Rattu, A.; Dixey, P.; Charles, D.; Brightling, C.; Chung, K.F.; Bossios, A.; Bourdin, A.; Djukanovic, R.; Dahlén, S.; Fleming, L.; et al. Predictors of Response to Biologics for Severe Asthma: A Systematic Review and Meta-Analysis. *Allergy* **2026**, *81*, 24–55. [CrossRef]
41. Lipworth, B.J.; Greig, R.; Chan, R.; Kuo, C.R.; Jackson, C. Head-To-Head Comparison of Biologic Efficacy in Asthma: What Have We Learned? *Allergy* **2025**, *80*, 1226–1241. [CrossRef]
42. Hellings, P.W.; Alobid, I.; Anselmo-Lima, W.T.; Bernal-Sprekelsen, M.; Bjermer, L.; Caulley, L.; Chaker, A.; Constantinidis, J.; Conti, D.M.; De Corso, E.; et al. EUFOREA/EPOS2020 Statement on the Clinical Considerations for Chronic Rhinosinusitis with Nasal Polyps Care. *Allergy* **2024**, *79*, 1123–1133. [CrossRef]
43. Xian, M.; Yan, B.; Song, X.; Chen, J.; Tang, J.; Jiang, Y.; Wan, L.; Liu, W.; Xue, J.; Cao, Z.; et al. Chinese Position Paper on Biologic Therapy for Chronic Rhinosinusitis with Nasal Polyps. *Allergy* **2025**, *80*, 1208–1225. [CrossRef] [PubMed]
44. Cai, S.; Xu, S.; Zhao, Y.; Zhang, L. Efficacy and Safety of Biologics for Chronic Rhinosinusitis With Nasal Polyps: A Meta-Analysis of Real-World Evidence. *Allergy* **2025**, *80*, 1256–1270. [CrossRef] [PubMed]
45. Ferri, S.; Paoletti, G.; Pelaia, C.; Heffler, E.; Canonica, G.W.; Puggioni, F. COPD and Biologic Treatment: State of the Art. *Curr. Opin. Allergy Clin. Immunol.* **2023**, *23*, 309–318. [CrossRef] [PubMed]
46. Romano, C.; Cozzolino, D.; Corona, M.E.; Aitella, E. Efficacy and Safety of Dupilumab Across Different Th2-Type-Mediated Diseases: A Real-Life Preliminary Experience. *Biologics* **2025**, *5*, 3. [CrossRef]
47. Young, J.; Spisany, T.; Guidry, C.M.; Hong, J.; Le, J.; El Rassi, E.; Boylan, P.M. Dupilumab for Chronic Obstructive Pulmonary Disease: A Systematic Review. *Biologics* **2025**, *5*, 5. [CrossRef]

https://doi.org/10.3390/medicina62040746

medicina

MDPI

Article

Phenotype and Clinicoradiological Differences in Multifocal and Focal Bronchiectasis

Jelena Jankovic [1,2], Aleksandar Jandric [1], Natasa Djurdjevic [1,2], Dragan Vukosavljevic [1], Zlatan Bojic [1], Andrej Zecevic [1] and Mihailo Stjepanovic [1,2,*]

[1] Clinic for Pulmonology, University Clinical Center of Serbia, 11000 Belgrade, Serbia; jjelena1984@gmail.com (J.J.); jandricalexander@gmail.com (A.J.); natalidjurdjevic@yahoo.com (N.D.); gan_dra@live.com (D.V.); bojic.zlatan@gmail.com (Z.B.); zecevic92andrej@gmail.com (A.Z.)

[2] Medical Faculty, University of Belgrade, 11000 Belgrade, Serbia

* Correspondence: mihailostjepanovic@gmail.com

Abstract: *Introduction:* Bronchiectasis is a chronic progressive respiratory disease characterized by permanent dilatation of the bronchi. It is a complex condition with numerous different etiologies, co-morbidities, and a heterogeneous presentation. As we know, there is a lack of studies that describe the differences and compare the characteristics between focal and multifocal bronchiectasis. The aim of this study is to identify differences in clinical characteristics presentation, severity or distribution in focal and multifocal bronchiectasis, and prognostic implications. *Methods:* 126 patients with computed tomography (CT)-verified bronchiectasis were enrolled. Baseline characteristics that included age, sex, smoking history, and respiratory symptoms were recorded, with special attention paid to hemoptysis appearance, body mass index, and comorbidities. The type of bronchiectasis determined by CT scan and the modified Reiff scores indicating radiological severity were recorded. Patients were divided in two groups (I is focal and II is multifocal). *Results:* There were no statistically significant differences in age, smoking status, comorbidity, and BMI between the two groups. Multifocality was associated with a significantly higher proportion of females (p = 0.014), the rate of hemoptysis (p = 0.023), and the number of hospitalizations, but not of exacerbations and prevalence of immunodeficiency (p = 0.049). Significantly, a high number of subjects with multifocality had bronchiectasis of moderate severity, and post-infective and asthma-associated phenotypes were the dominant in this group. Unexpectedly, the cystic and varicose radiological phenotype (which need more time to develop) were more dominant in the focal group. The cylindrical phenotype was equally observed in the multifocal and focal groups. *Conclusions:* Our study suggests that multifocality is not related to age, number of exacerbations, or radiological phenotype, but it seems to be associated with the clinical post-infective phenotype, immunodeficiency, frequent hospitalizations, and severity. Thus, the presence of multifocal bronchiectasis may act as a biomarker of severity and poor outcomes in these patients.

Keywords: bronchiectasis; phenotype; chest CT scan; hemoptysis; multifocal

1. Introduction

Bronchiectasis is a chronic progressive respiratory disease characterized by permanent damage and dilatation of the bronchi [1]. Bronchiectasis can be considered a syndrome and a common endpoint of various diseases, but it can also occur as a single radiological appearance that may or may not be associated with various diseases [2]. It is a complex condition with numerous different etiologies (infective, deficiency of alpha 1 antitrypsin, immunodeficiency, cystic fibrosis, and tuberculosis), co-morbidities (asthma and chronic obstructive pulmonary disease), and a heterogeneous presentation associated with respiratory symptoms and recurrent respiratory infections because of reduced mucus clearance, which favors mucus impaction [3]. The most common symptoms are cough, sputum production, hemoptysis, and fatigue. This clinical presentation is a consequence of the production of inflammatory mediators that lead to the destruction of elastin, affecting the muscular and cartilaginous part of the bronchus [4]. When local defense mechanisms are impaired, inflammation progresses, resulting in fibrosis and dilation of the bronchial wall and hyperinflation. This leads to a progressive decrease in pulmonary function parameters, which results in irreversible bronchodilation [5].

Previous epidemiological studies have largely considered bronchiectasis a rare disease, but the prevalence of bronchiectasis is increasing worldwide. It is now the third most common of all respiratory diseases [6]. A trend of increasing prevalence of bronchiectasis has been observed, with a rate of up to 566 per 100,000 persons [6,7]. Due to improved understanding and awareness, bronchiectasis with different clinical presentations is increasingly being reported. For a long time, bronchiectasis was an incidental radiological finding on chest computed tomography (CT) scans. Chest CT scans are now the gold standard in establishing the diagnosis of bronchiectasis, along with its staging, localization (in one or more lobes), and complications [8,9]. Radiological criteria for existing bronchiectasis include a broncho–arterial ratio of more than one, lack of bronchial tapering, or indirect signs such as peri-bronchial thickening, pulmonary nodules, mucus plugging, mosaicism, or air-trapping [1,9]. Thoracic scan imaging can establish the distribution pattern of bronchiectasis, supporting the severity assessment and long-term follow-up monitoring of its structural abnormalities and progression.

The first classification of bronchiectasis is cystic fibrosis (CF)-related bronchiectasis or non-CF-related bronchiectasis. The Reid classification includes three main types of radiological phenotype of bronchiectasis: cylindrical, varicose, and cystic [10]. This classification describes cylindrical bronchiectasis as the mildest form of bronchiectasis with uniform caliber where there is a loss of tapering of the bronchus and dilatation of the bronchial lumen. As bronchiectasis progresses, it develops into varicose form bronchiectasis with irregularities in the bronchial wall and a distorted and significant shortening of the number of identifiable airway branches along with further dilatation. The most severe grade is cystic bronchiectasis with progressive saccular dilatation of the bronchial lumen terminating in a large cystic structure, often with increased air–fluid levels [10,11].

The distribution of bronchiectasis may also reflect the specific etiology. CT scans allow differentiation between focal (involving only one lobe) and diffuse or multifocal (involving two or more lobes) bronchiectasis [12]. Diffuse bronchiectasis develops most often in patients with genetic disorders, immunodeficiency, chronic diseases, or anatomical defects that affect the airways. Focal bronchiectasis develops as a result of untreated pneumonia or obstructions (due to foreign bodies or tumors) where the large airway is obstructed resulting in an inability to clear secretions and leading to a cycle of infection, inflammation, and airway wall damage. Multifocal bronchiectasis occurs when an underlying disorder triggers inflammation in the small- and medium-sized airways [13]. As for tumors, bronchiectasis multifocality surgical treatment is difficult. According to the European Respiratory Society (ERS) guidelines for the management of adult bronchiectasis, surgical treatment should not be considered until the maximum effect from all therapeutic options has been achieved [14]. For this reason, it is important to be aware of the characteristics and potential for multifocal bronchiectasis. The disease profile, prognosis, and outcome of treatment of bronchiectasis are different for each patient.

There is a lack of studies describing the differences and comparing the characteristics of focal and multifocal bronchiectasis. The aim of this study was to elucidate the differences in the clinical characteristics and presentation, severity, and radiological phenotype of focal and multifocal bronchiectasis.

2. Materials and Methods

2.1. Study Group and Data Collection

In this retrospective study, 126 patients with bronchiectasis who were treated at the Clinic for Pulmonology, University Clinical Center of Serbia, between 2020 and 2023 were included. This study was approved by the Local Committee in Belgrade and all the subjects gave signed informed consent, based on the principles of the International Declaration of Helsinki.

The baseline characteristics of all participants, including age, sex, smoking history, respiratory symptoms (particularly hemoptysis appearance), weight, height, body mass index (BMI), and self-reported comorbidities (asthma, chronic obstructive pulmonary disease, diabetes mellitus, arterial hypertension, atrial fibrillation, rheumatic diseases, immunodeficiency, and others) were obtained from their electronic medical records. Exacerbations and hospitalizations were obtained by patients' self-reports and validated through electronic medical records. Standard management in our center includes blood cell count; spirometry functional tests; detection of immunological factors; and sputum culture. The inclusion criteria were an age of over 18 years, a diagnosis of non-cystic fibrosis bronchiectasis via a computed tomography (CT) scan, and clinical symptoms consistent with bronchiectasis.

The exclusion criteria were cystic fibrosis, active tuberculosis (TB), and active malignancy.

2.2. Radiological Assessment

One chest radiologist evaluated the CT findings, the type of bronchiectasis, and the number of lobes affected by bronchiectasis. The CT findings were used to divide the participants into the focal (involving one lobe) and multifocal (involving two or more lobes) groups. The three radiological types of bronchiectasis are cylindrical, varicose, and cystic (Figure 1) [10]. The modified Reiff scores indicating the radiological severity of bronchiectasis were calculated [15]. This score takes into account the number of lobes involved (considering the lingual as a separate lobe) and the dilatation degree (cylindrical = 1, varicose = 2, and cystic = 3), to give a score between 1 and 18. The CT scoring system was as follows: mild bronchiectasis, 0–6; moderate, 7–12; and severe bronchiectasis, 13–18 [16]. The CT findings were evaluated by radiologist with more than 15 years of experience in the field, who worked at the Center for Radiology and Magnetic Resonance, University Clinical Center of Serbia.

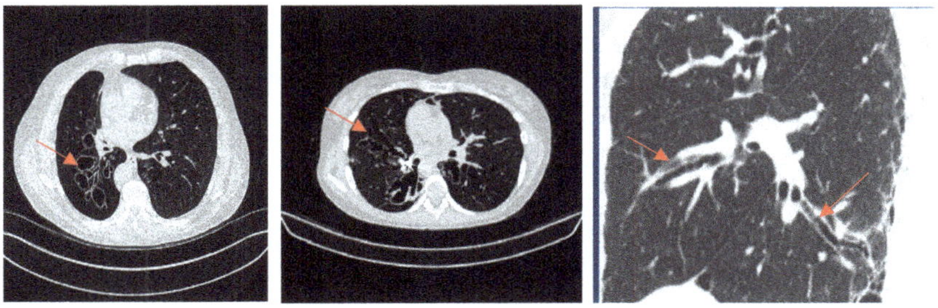

Figure 1. Three radiological types of bronchiectasis: (**a**) cystic, (**b**) varicose, and (**c**) cylindrical.

2.3. Statistical Analysis

The analyses were performed in SPSS Statistics for Windows, version 21.0 (Chicago, IL, USA). A p value < 0.05 was significant. Mean and standard deviation values were used for continuous variables and were compared using the t-test for independent samples. The Chi-squared test was used to compare categorical variables, and the data were presented as numbers with a percentage. A one-way ANOVA was used to compare the mild, moderate, and severe sub-scores of the modified Reiff score. The results are presented as graphics and tables.

3. Results

This study was a retrospective study of 126 patients with confirmed bronchiectasis, treated at the Clinic for Pulmonology, University Clinical Center of Serbia, for the period from 2019 to 2023. The mean age of the patients was 62.1 years. Nearly two-thirds of the patients were females, and the same percentage is found in the multifocal group. Nearly the same percentage of patients were non-smokers and former or current smokers. More than 80% of the patients in both groups had one or more comorbidities, the most frequent were obstructive diseases (asthma and COPD), with no statistically significant differences between groups. Other comorbidities, found in less than 10% of all patients, were diabetes mellitus, atrial fibrillation, nasal polyposis, and gastroesophageal reflux disease. Chronic rhinosinusitis was the most frequent comorbidity in the multifocal group ($p = 0.006$). Immunodeficiency was statistically more frequent in focal group ($p = 0.049$). In the focal group, patients were overweight and had higher values of BMI than in those of the multifocal group (26.3 vs. 23.2). But there were no statistically significant differences. The demographic characteristics are presented in Table 1.

Table 1. Demographic characteristics between the two groups.

	Focal	Multifocal	*p*
N (%)	50 (39.7)	76 (60.3)	
Age years	62.8 ± 7.1	61.4 ± 6.4	0.762
Gender N (%) m/f	17 (34)/41 (66)	36 (47.4)/40 (52.6)	0.014
Smoking N (%) no/yes	23 (46)/27 (54)	41 (53.9)/35 (46.1)	0.065
BMI	26.3	23.3	0.062
Immunodeficiency N (%)	8 (16)	10 (13.1)	0.049
Comorbidity N (%)	46 (92)	63 (82.9)	0.121
Chronic rhinosinusitis	12 (24)	17 (46)	0.006
COPD	17 (34)	29 (38)	0.119
Asthma	15 (30)	22 (28.9)	0.237

Bronchiectasis was confirmed by chest CT scan. In 78 (61.9%) of the patients the cylindrical type was diagnosed. Varicose was diagnosed in 14 (11.1%), and cystic in 24 (19%). More than one type of bronchiectasis was observed in 48 subjects (38.1%). But there was difference in predominance in types between two groups: cystic (26 vs. 19.7%) and varicose (14 vs. 13.4%) in focal group, opposite then cylindrical (60 vs. 66.7%) in multifocal group. The prevalence of multifocality and focality with regards to specific radiological phenotypes of bronchiectasis is presented in Figure 2.

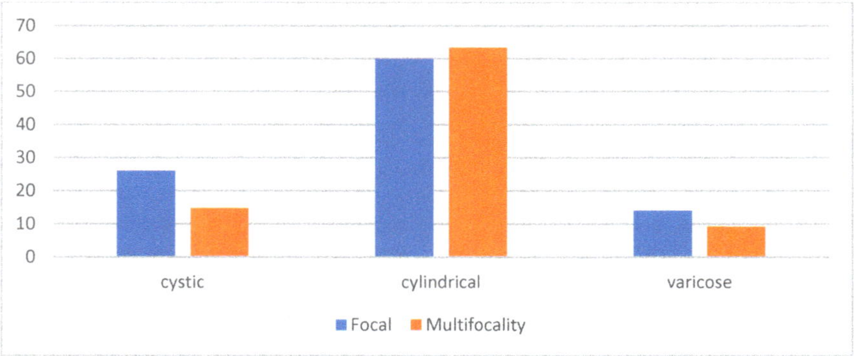

Figure 2. Prevalence of multifocality (orange) and focal (blue) in regard to specific radiological phenotypes of bronchiectasis.

Multifocality was associated with a significantly higher proportion of the female sex ($p = 0.014$), rate of hemoptysis ($p = 0.023$), the number of hospitalizations, and the prevalence of immunodeficiency ($p = 0.049$).

All patients had typical respiratory symptoms such as fatigue, cough, and expectoration, but there was a difference in the frequency of hemoptysis with predominance in the multifocal group ($p = 0.023$). There were no statistically significant differences in the use of long-term oxygen treatment (LTOT) and the number of exacerbations in one year between the two groups. Patients with multifocal disease had a higher number of hospitalizations in one year (average of three or more). The clinical characteristics of the two groups are presented in Table 2.

Table 2. Clinical characteristics between two groups.

	Focal	Multifocal	*p*
N (%)	50 (39.7)	76 (60.3)	
Hemoptysis	8 (16)	15 (19.7)	0.023
≥2 hospitalizations in 1 year N (%)	3 (12)	17 (22.4)	0.011
LTOT N (%)	5 (10)	8 (10.5)	0.665
≥2 exacerbations in 1 year N (%)	11 (22)	18 (23.7)	0.073

According to the modified the Reiff score, 103 patients had mild bronchiectasis (81.8%), 10 patients had moderate bronchiectasis (7.9%), and 13 patients had severe bronchiectasis (10.3%). Only eight (6.3%) patients had multifocality on one side (left or right); the majority had it on both sides. Significantly, a higher number of cases with moderate severity was observed in the subjects with multifocality. Post-infective and asthma-associated phenotypes were dominant in the multifocal group of patients.

Unexpectedly, the cystic radiological phenotype was more dominant in the focal group, and the cylindrical and varicose phenotypes were close to equal in both groups. The rate of cystic type (26% vs. 19.7%, $p = 0.007$) was significantly higher in patients with a focal pattern compared to patients with multifocality. The radiological presentation and phenotype differences between the two groups are presented in Table 3.

Table 3. Radiological presentation and phenotypes differences between the two groups.

	Focal	Multifocal	*p*
Type N(%)			
Cystic	13 (26)	15 (19.7)	0.007
Cylindrical	30 (60)	50 (66.7)	0.126
Varicose	7 (14)	11 (13.4)	0.331
Localization N (%)			
Left	25 (50)	2 (2.6)	0.974
Right	25 (50)	6 (7.9)	0.893
Bilateral	N\A	68 (89.5)	
Severity N(%)			
Mild	49 (98)	54 (71.1)	0.017
Moderate	1 (2)	9 (11.8)	0.009
Severe	0	13 (17.1)	0.003
Clinical phenotype	Post-infective	Post-infective Asthma	

4. Discussion

Multifocality is defined as the presence of multiple distinct disease foci and may have an impact on the management of the primary lesion and influence treatment decisions [17]. Multifocality mostly refers to tumors (breast and thyroid gland), but other lesions and changes, if not localized, can be classified using this term. Multifocal or diffuse bronchiectasis affect many areas of the lungs, with various different pathophysiological presentations [13].

We confirmed multifocality if bronchiectasis occurred in two or more lobes on the same or opposite side. Only 8 of 126 patients had multifocality on one side (left or right lung), the majority had bronchiectasis on both sides, predominantly in the lower lobes. This means that the underlying disease did not develop unilaterally; the aspiration of contents was usually on one side and tended to be more dominant on the right side due to the anatomical position of the right main bronchus [18]. The clinical post-infectious phenotype is a consequence of repeated infections and pneumonia and is also associated with asthma, which is relevant to the both-side theory. The association with asthma—considering the pathophysiology and mechanism of asthma—and the changes in the airways—which cannot occur in only one lung—explain the multifocal finding of bronchiectasis in this phenotype [19,20]. Bronchiectasis is the most frequent asthma-associated comorbidity according to the literature and GINA guidelines [20]. These two diseases have same etio-pathogenesis and common causes (such as gastroesophageal reflux disease, chronic rhinosinusitis, and allergic patterns) [19,21]. The concomitant presence of asthma and bronchiectasis (as a comorbidity or overlapping) is characterized by more severe respiratory symptoms, frequent exacerbations, functional decline, and worse outcomes [19–21]. In our study, rinosinusitis was significantly more frequent in multifocal bronchiectasis, which was also the most frequent clinical phenotype associated with asthma. Eosinophils are dominant inflammatory cells in asthma and rinosinusitis, causing inflammation and worsening of disease or remodeling. Failure to recognize asthma-associated bronchiectasis is often responsible for the worsening of symptoms and frequent exacerbations, along with greater disease severity. Bronchiectasis must be recognized and the most appropriate therapeutic approach selected in order to prevent poor outcomes [21]. In our study group, the patients with the asthma clinical phenotype had rhinosinusitis more frequently; the best treatment for this group is corticosteroids. The post-infective phenotype, depending on the frequency and localization of the infection itself, depends on whether a focal or diffuse form of bronchiectasis develops and was present in both groups [9]. The pathophysiology of focal bronchiectasis is usually the result of a local event, such as pneumonia [22]. This explains the most frequent post-infective phenotype in focal presentations.

There were no differences in the frequency of the cylindrical radiological phenotype in the two groups. This is in line with the literature, which indicates that this is a dominant phenotype. The data also supported its presence in obstructive diseases and post-infectious phenotypes and its predominance in the lower lobes in these disorders [22,23]. Based on the radiological type and involvement of lobes and according to the modified Reiff score in our study, a significantly higher number of patients with moderate severity had multifocality. This may have been the reason for the statistically higher frequency of hospitalizations in this group of patients. We can conclude that the post-infectious phenotype, in moderate and severe form, frequent bilateral representation of the lower lobes, and LTOT use are related to the number of hospitalizations in patients with multifocal bronchiectasis.

Chronic respiratory failure is serious complication of bronchiectasis. According to previous studies, up to 40% of patients with bronchiectasis require LTOT at home because of asthma or chronic obstructive pulmonary disease (COPD). Bronchiectasis is present in 29–50% of COPD patients [24]. COPD was the main comorbidity in our study population. COPD and bronchiectasis can be related in three ways. COPD can lead to the development of bronchiectasis through airway inflammation and repeated bacterial infections [25]. Bronchiectasis in a non-smoker leads to a fixed airway obstruction and can progress to COPD [25,26]. Finally, COPD and bronchiectasis can be two independent and coexisting diseases [26]. Respiratory insufficiency was present in 13 of our patients with LTOT, and nearly 80% of them had history of COPD or pulmonary fibrosis. There was no difference between the groups in the use of LTOT because most of them were patients who had already been prescribed oxygen therapy at home. In both groups, there were patients with advanced COPD or fibrosis without a difference in the prevalence of these two diseases in both groups.

The main respiratory symptoms in patients with bronchiectasis are cough, sputum expectoration, and breathlessness [27]. All of our patients had typical respiratory symptoms, although we focused on the frequency of hemoptysis in our study group. Hemoptysis was dominant in the multifocal group. This was typically not life-threatening hemoptysis; there was a need for embolization in two cases. Bronchiectasis is a frequent cause of hemoptysis, which can range from mild to massive hemoptysis [28]. In previous studies, hemoptysis occurred in 22–25% of bronchiectasis patients [29]. In a similar study performed in Germany, hemoptysis was a diagnosed in 15% of hospitalized patients with bronchiectasis [30]. Our result of 18.3% is in accordance with the literature. Male sex, smoking history (former or current), the lower right lobe, $\geq$2 involved lobes, cylindrical bronchiectasis, and COPD comorbidity were more likely to be associated with hemoptysis in our study population. Our study demonstrated that bronchiectasis patients with hemoptysis had less severe bronchiectasis (the Reiff score for all but two patients was six or lower). This is in accordance with a study by Seo and colleagues who also showed that bronchiectasis with hemoptysis had a lower bronchiectasis severity and short-term mortality [31]. The explanation for those results and ours—with lower severity scores—may be that the hemoptysis phenotype is not associated with severe bronchiectasis but with specific etiology and radiological findings. In our case, this is so with the cylindrical type, but in Seo's study, this is so with the cystic type. If we are talking about etiology, in the abovementioned study, hemoptysis was associated with the infective phenotype (tuberculosis and mycetoma); also, in our both groups, the main clinical phenotype is post-infective.

Bronchiectasis can occur at any age, but the highest prevalence is in older women [32]. Only a few studies have described sex differences in patients with bronchiectasis. Women have a different lung physiology: their lungs are smaller, and they have smaller conducting airways, with pseudostratified ciliated epithelial tissue with mucus-secreting properties. Continuous chronic inflammation can potentially contribute to greater lung tissue damage and worse disease severity [32,33]. Female sex was dominant in our bronchiectasis study population and was also more frequent in the focal group than the multifocal group.

This study had several limitations. First, as with any retrospective study, our data were dependent on the availability of medical history and records. This was a single-center study, so geographical differences could not be assessed. A large, multicenter study is needed. The amount of expectorated blood was determined from the medical records, so there may have been some limitations in assessing hemoptysis severity. Finally, not all patients had their BMI measured.

5. Conclusions

The results of our research indicated that, compared with a focal presentation, multifocality should be regarded as a significant prognostic factor for clinically severe disease, especially in patients with immunodeficiency, frequent hospitalizations, and hemoptysis, which can sometimes be life-threatening and is associated with a decreased quality of life. Our data also suggested that the presence of multifocality is associated with clinical post-infective and asthma related phenotypes. Identification of distinct phenotypes and the spread of the disease will lead to greater insight into the characteristics, treatment, and outcomes of bronchiectasis, as bronchiectasis is often underreported and underdiagnosed. Appropriate management to reduce the disease burden associated with poor quality of life is needed in patients with bronchiectasis.

Author Contributions: All authors contributed to the study conception and design. Data collection and analysis were performed by J.J., A.J., N.D. and D.V. Study concept and design: J.J. All authors commented on previous versions of the manuscript. Critical revision and editing of manuscript: M.S. Data and statistical analysis: Z.B. and A.Z. All authors contributed significantly to the study design and read and approved the final manuscript. All authors have read and agreed to the published version of the manuscript.

Funding: This research received no external funding.

Institutional Review Board Statement: This study was approved by the Institutional Review Board (protocol code 841/2 11.03.2023.).

Informed Consent Statement: Informed consent was obtained from all subjects involved in this study.

Data Availability Statement: The data that support the findings of this study are available from the corresponding author (M.S.) upon reasonable request.

Conflicts of Interest: The authors declare no conflicts of interest.

References

1. Contarini, M.; Finch, S.; Chalmers, J.D. Bronchiectasis: A case-based approach to investigation and management. *Eur. Respir. Rev.* **2018**, *27*, 180016. [CrossRef]
2. Amati, F.; Simonetta, E.; Pilocane, T.; Gramegna, A.; Goeminne, P.; Oriano, M.; Pascual-Guardia, S.; Mantero, M.; Voza, A.; Santambrogio, M.; et al. Diagnosis and Initial Investigation of Bronchiectasis. *Semin. Respir. Crit. Care Med.* **2021**, *42*, 513–524. [CrossRef] [PubMed]
3. Pasteur, M.C.; Bilton, D.; Hill, A.T. British Thoracic Society guideline for non-CF bronchiectasis. *Thorax* **2010**, *65* (Suppl. S1), i1–i58. [CrossRef] [PubMed]
4. European Respiratory Society. Bronchiectasis. Chapter 15. In *European Lung White Book*; European Respiratory Society: Lausanne, Switzerland, 2018. Available online: https://www.erswhitebook.org/chapters/bronchiectasis (accessed on 1 April 2024).
5. Martinez-García, M.A.; Oscullo, G.; Posadas, T.; Zaldivar, E.; Villa, C.; Dobarganes, Y.; de la Rosa, D. Pseudomonas aeruginosa and lung function decline in patients with bronchiectasis. *Clin. Microbiol. Infect.* **2021**, *27*, 428–434. [CrossRef] [PubMed]
6. Aliberti, S.; Sotgiu, G.; Lapi, F.; Gramegna, A.; Cricelli, C.; Blasi, F. Prevalence and incidence of bronchiectasis in Italy. *BMC Pulm. Med.* **2020**, *20*, 15. [CrossRef] [PubMed]
7. Quint, J.K.; Millett, E.R.; Joshi, M.; Navaratnam, V.; Thomas, S.L.; Hurst, J.R.; Smeeth, L.; Brown, J.S. Changes in the incidence, prevalence and mortality of bronchiectasis in the UK from 2004 to 2013: A population-based cohort study. *Eur. Respir. J.* **2016**, *47*, 186–193. [CrossRef] [PubMed]
8. Visser, S.K.; Bye, P.; Morgan, L. Management of bronchiectasis in adults. *Med. J. Aust.* **2018**, *209*, 177–183. [CrossRef] [PubMed]
9. Fraser, C.S.; José, R.J. Insights into Personalised Medicine in Bronchiectasis. *J. Pers. Med.* **2023**, *13*, 133. [CrossRef] [PubMed]
10. Reid, L.M. Reduction in bronchial subdivision in bronchiectasis. *Thorax* **1950**, *5*, 233–247. [CrossRef] [PubMed]
11. Grippi, M.A.; Elias, J.A.; Fishman, J.A.; Kotloff, R.M.; Pack, A.I.; Senior, R.M.; Kaiser, L.R. *Fishman's Pulmonary Disease and Disorders*, 3rd ed.; McGraw-Hill: New York, NY, USA, 1998; pp. 2045–2070.
12. Martin, C.; Regard, L.; Chassagnon, G.; Burgel, P.R. Diagnostic étiologique d'une dilatation des bronches [Bronchiectasis in adults: Etiological diagnosis]. *Rev. Pneumol. Clin.* **2018**, *74*, 292–298. [CrossRef] [PubMed]
13. Cole, P.J. Inflammation: A two-edged sword—The model of bronchiectasis. *Eur. J. Respir. Dis. Suppl.* **1986**, *147*, 6–15. [PubMed]
14. Buscot, M.; Pottier, H.; Marquette, C.H.; Leroy, S. Phenotyping Adults with Non-Cystic Fibrosis Bronchiectasis: A 10-Year Cohort Study in a French Regional University Hospital Center. *Respiration* **2016**, *92*, 1–8. [CrossRef] [PubMed]
15. Reiff, D.B.; Wells, A.U.; Carr, D.H.; Cole, P.J.; Hansell, D.M. CT findings in bronchiectasis: Limited value in distinguishing between idiopathic and specific types. *AJR Am. J. Roentgenol.* **1995**, *165*, 261–267. [CrossRef] [PubMed]
16. Gupta, A.; Verma, U.P.; Verma, A.K.; Chaudhary, S.C.; Lal, N.; Singh, N.; Shrivastava, A.; Kant, S. A retrospective correlative profiling of lung functions, microbiological, radiological, periodontal, hematological parameters in noncystic fibrosis bronchiectasis patients of North India. *Natl. J. Maxillofac. Surg.* **2022**, *13*, 44–53. [PubMed]
17. Haffner, M.C.; Zwart, W.; Roudier, M.P.; True, L.D.; Nelson, W.G.; Epstein, J.I.; De Marzo, A.M.; Nelson, P.S.; Yegnasubramanian, S. Genomic and phenotypic heterogeneity in prostate cancer. *Nat. Rev. Urol.* **2021**, *18*, 79–92. [CrossRef] [PubMed]
18. Chang, A.B.; Fortescue, R.; Grimwood, K.; Alexopoulou, E.; Bell, L.; Boyd, J.; Bush, A.; Chalmers, J.D.; Hill, A.T.; Karadag, B.; et al. European Respiratory Society guidelines for the management of children and adolescents with bronchiectasis. *Eur. Respir. J.* **2021**, *26*, 2002990. [CrossRef] [PubMed]
19. Mao, B.; Yang, J.W.; Lu, H.W.; Xu, J.F. Asthma and bronchiectasis exacerbation. *Eur. Respir. J.* **2016**, *47*, 1680–1686. [CrossRef]
20. Global Initiative for Asthma. Global Strategy for Asthma Management and Prevention. 2023. Available online: https://www.ginasthma.org (accessed on 1 April 2024).
21. Crimi, C.; Ferri, S.; Campisi, R.; Crimi, N. The Link between Asthma and Bronchiectasis: State of the Art. *Respiration* **2020**, *99*, 463–476. [CrossRef] [PubMed]
22. Tiddens, H.A.W.M.; Meerburg, J.J.; van der Eerden, M.M.; Ciet, P. The radiological diagnosis of bronchiectasis: What's in a name? *Eur. Respir. Rev.* **2020**, *29*, 190120. [CrossRef] [PubMed]
23. Milliron, B.; Henry, T.S.; Veeraraghavan, S.; Little, B.P. Bronchiectasis: Mechanisms and imaging clues of associated common and uncommon diseases. *Radiographics* **2015**, *35*, 1011–1030. [CrossRef] [PubMed]
24. Habesoglu, M.A.; Ugurlu, A.O.; Eyuboglu, F.O. Clinical, radiologic, and functional evaluation of 304 patients with bronchiectasis. *Ann Thorac Med.* **2011**, *6*, 131–136. [CrossRef] [PubMed]

25. Athanazio, R. Airway disease: Similarities and differences between asthma, COPD and bronchiectasis. *Clinics* **2012**, *67*, 1335–1343. [CrossRef] [PubMed]
26. Blasi, F.; Chalmers, J.D.; Aliberti, S. COPD and bronchiectasis: Phenotype, endotype or co-morbidity? *COPD* **2014**, *11*, 603–604. [CrossRef] [PubMed]
27. Gao, Y.H.; Abo Leyah, H.; Finch, S.; Lonergan, M.; Aliberti, S.; De Soyza, A.; Fardon, T.C.; Tino, G.; Chalmers, J.D. Relationship between Symptoms, Exacerbations, and Treatment Response in Bronchiectasis. *Am. J. Respir. Crit. Care Med.* **2020**, *15*, 1499–1507. [CrossRef]
28. Mondoni, M.; Carlucci, P.; Job, S.; Parazzini, E.M.; Cipolla, G.; Pagani, M.; Tursi, F.; Negri, L.; Fois, A.; Canu, S.; et al. Observational, multicentre study on the epidemiology of haemoptysis. *Eur. Respir. J.* **2018**, *51*, 1701813. [CrossRef] [PubMed]
29. Aksamit, T.R.; O'Donnell, A.E.; Barker, A.; Olivier, K.N.; Winthrop, K.L.; Daniels, M.L.A.; Johnson, M.; Eden, E.; Griffith, D.; Knowles, M.; et al. Adult Patients With Bronchiectasis: A First Look at the US Bronchiectasis Research Registry. *Chest* **2017**, *151*, 982–992. [CrossRef] [PubMed]
30. Ringshausen, F.C.; de Roux, A.; Pletz, M.W.; Hämäläinen, N.; Welte, T.; Rademacher, J. Bronchiectasis-associated hospitalizations in Germany, 2005-2011: A population-based study of disease burden and trends. *PLoS ONE* **2013**, *8*, e71109. [CrossRef] [PubMed]
31. Seo, H.; Cha, S.I.; Park, J.; Lim, J.K.; Park, J.E.; Choi, S.H.; Lee, Y.H.; Yoo, S.S.; Lee, S.Y.; Lee, J.; et al. Hemoptysis as the presenting manifestation of bronchiectasis-associated hospitalization in Korea. *J. Thorac. Dis.* **2023**, *15*, 3636–3645. [CrossRef] [PubMed]
32. Vidaillac, C.; Yong, V.F.L.; Jaggi, T.K.; Soh, M.M.; Chotirmall, S.H. Gender differences in bronchiectasis: A real issue? *Breathe* **2018**, *14*, 108–121. [CrossRef] [PubMed]
33. Casimir, G.J.; Lefevre, N.; Corazza, F.; Duchateau, J. Sex and inflammation in respiratory diseases: A clinical viewpoint. *Biol. Sex Differ.* **2013**, *4*, 16. [CrossRef]

medicina

MDPI

Review

Diagnostic Workup in IgE-Mediated Allergy to Asteraceae Weed Pollen and Herbal Medicine Products in Europe

Mariana Preda [1], Sylwia Smolinska [2] and Florin-Dan Popescu [1,*]

[1] Faculty of Medicine, Department of Allergology "Nicolae Malaxa" Clinical Hospital, "Carol Davila" University of Medicine and Pharmacy, 022441 Bucharest, Romania; mariana.preda@umfcd.ro
[2] Faculty of Medicine, Department of Clinical Immunology, Wroclaw Medical University, 51-616 Wroclaw, Poland; sylwia.smolinska@umw.edu.pl
* Correspondence: florindanpopescu@gmail.com

Abstract: Anemophilous weeds from the Asteraceae family are highly allergenic and represent a significant source of aeroallergens in late summer and autumn. Ragweed and mugwort pollen allergies have become a significant health burden in Europe. Some people with respiratory allergies to weed pollen may also suffer hypersensitivity reactions to herbal medicines obtained from certain cross-reactive plants in the Compositae family, such as chamomile, marigold, and purple coneflower. General physicians, ear, nose, and throat (ENT) specialists, and pulmonologists need to be familiar with the diagnostic tests used by allergists in clinical practice to support accurate diagnosis in such patients. Allergists must also be aware of the suggestions of the European Medicines Agency (EMA)'s Herbal Medicinal Products Committee and the broad spectrum of herbal therapies to educate their patients about potential risks.

Keywords: allergy diagnosis; Asteraceae pollen; herbal products

1. Introduction

The Asteraceae family, also known as Compositae, consists of over 25,000 species worldwide and is known for its wide variety of flowering plants in Europe. Some highly allergenic species, such as ragweed and mugwort, are anemophilous (wind-pollinated) weeds that produce large amounts of airborne pollen, which can be significant sources of aeroallergens in late summer and fall, especially in regions where these weeds are abundant but also outside the local pollination areas due to atmospheric long-distance transport. Currently, more than 15 million people in Europe have clinically significant sensitization to ragweed pollen alone, and the worst projections suggest that sensitization to this weed pollen will more than double by 2060 [1–4]. However, most Asteraceae species are entomophilous, and their composite flower heads are particularly effective at facilitating insect pollination. Some patients with weed pollen respiratory allergy may face risks of IgE-mediated hypersensitivity adverse reactions when consuming apitherapeutic products, such as artisanal honey and bee pollen as a food supplement, because such edible products may contain many pollen grains from some Asteraceae plants, like dandelion and sunflower, which can cross-react with those from allergenic anemophilous weeds. Similar risks exist with herbal products derived from the aerial parts and flowers of Compositae plants, such as camomile, marigold, and purple coneflower, used for their phytotherapeutic compounds [5–8].

2. IgE-Mediated Allergy to Asteraceae Weed Pollen

The most important Asteraceae pollen grains responsible for late summer-autumn seasonal respiratory allergies in Europe are produced by common/short ragweed (*Ambrosia artemisiifolia*) and common mugwort (*Artemisia vulgaris*), weeds with ruderal and segetal distribution. In the nineteenth century, common ragweed was accidentally introduced in

Europe as a seed contaminant. *Ambrosia artemisiifolia* (NCBI: txid4212) has a heterotypic synonym *Ambrosia paniculata*, while *Ambrosia artemisiifolia* var. *elatior* (NCBI: txid4215) has the homotypic synonym *Ambrosia elatior*. Other invasive *Ambrosia* species in Europe are western ragweed (*Ambrosia psilostachya*) and giant ragweed (*Ambrosia trifida*). Besides the largely distributed common mugwort, other species grow in Europe and are represented by white mugwort (*Artemisia alba*), Chinese mugwort (*Artemisia verlotiorum*), common wormwood (*Artemisia absinthium*), and sweet wormwood (*Artemisia annua*), all with recognized ethnobotanical tradition. Sunflower (*Helianthus annuus*) is primarily grown for commercial use, while uncultivated wild plants may be considered weeds. *Artemisia* spp. belong to the Anthemideae tribe in the Asteroideae subfamily, part of the Asteraceae family, while *Helianthus* and *Ambrosia* spp. belong to the Heliantheae tribe of the same subfamily and family [1,2,9,10].

The clinical spectrum of IgE-mediated allergies to Asteraceae weed pollen varies from seasonal rhinitis/rhinoconjunctivitis to severe asthma. Because ragweed and mugwort pollen have a high degree of allergenic cross-reactivity, and in many parts of Europe, the distribution and pollination of mugwort and ragweed overlap, an accurate allergy diagnosis may be challenging [1,11].

Ragweed and mugwort pollen aeroallergens have molecular components represented by defensin-like proteins linked to polyproline-rich region (defensin-polyproline-linked proteins) Art v 1 and Amb a 4, pectate lyases Amb a 1 and Art v 6, cysteine protease Amb a 11, enolase Amb a 12, superoxide dismutase Amb t 13, triosephosphate isomerase Amb t 18, type 1 non-specific lipid transfer proteins (nsLTPs) Art v 3 and Amb a 6, pathogenesis-related protein PR-1 Art v 2, plastocyanines Amb a 3 and Amb a 7, group 5 allergens Amb a 5, Amb p 5 and Amb t 5, polcalcins Art v 5, Amb a 9 and Amb a 10, profilins Art v 4, Amb a 8 and Amb t 8 [12]. It should be emphasized that some ragweed pollen molecules have protease activity that can degrade tight junction proteins in the airway epithelial cells, thus facilitating allergenicity [13]. In addition, mugwort pollen is a significant vector for airborne endotoxin lipopolysaccharides, essential factors for inflammatory responses and allergic sensitization. Such endotoxins also adhere to ragweed pollen [14].

It is also relevant to highlight that cross-reactivity between Asteraceae aeroallergens and some food allergens in patients with weed pollen allergy may be associated with IgE-mediated hypersensitivity symptoms ranging from oral allergy syndrome to severe anaphylaxis. Many pollen-food syndromes and associations were described, such as celery-mugwort-spice syndrome and mugwort-peach, mugwort-mustard, and ragweed-melon-banana associations. Cross-reactive allergen components may be defensin-like proteins, nsLTPs, profilins, and high-molecular-weight allergens [6,15]. Interestingly, there are only several non-food exposure sources of nsLTP allergens, such as *Platanus acerifolia*, *Cannabis sativa*, *Ambrosia artemisiifolia*, and *Artemisia vulgaris*, and only some pollen grains, such as those from mugwort and plane tree, are potentially playing a major role in sensitization to food nsLTPs [16].

3. IgE-Mediated Allergy to Asteraceae Herbal Medicine Products (HMPs)

Herbal medicine, with thousands of years of tradition, is still increasingly popular in Europe as a complementary and alternative medicine. The European Directive 2004/24/EC provides the basis for using HMPs in the EU. Their safety profile should be evaluated based on existing data from clinical studies, pre-clinical studies, and case reports [17]. A critical part of the general population, as well as allergic patients, use unconventional remedies, including herbal products [18,19]. Sometimes, HMPs can cause unexpected (type B) adverse events, such as allergic/hypersensitivity reactions and dose-dependent pharmacological/toxic (type A) adverse effects. Herb-drug interactions are also possible. For example, there have been reports that green tea extract can reduce the levels of fexofenadine by inhibiting the organic anion-transporting polypeptide OATP1A2-mediated intestinal absorption and that quercetin, a compound found in *Achillea millefolium*, decreases the levels and effects of fexofenadine and loratadine by inhibiting P-glycoprotein (MDR1) efflux transporter. Fortunately, such drug interactions are considered to be minor [20–22].

Allergic patients must be aware that 'natural' does not necessarily mean 'safe'. The spectrum of hypersensitivity reactions to Asteraceae HMPs is large, both life-threatening systemic immediate type 1 ones, such as anaphylaxis, and cutaneous delayed type 4 adverse reactions, such as allergic contact dermatitis, being possible [5,20,23,24].

IgE-mediated (type 1) hypersensitivity reactions to Asteraceae HMPs may occur due to new sensitization to the herbs or, more commonly, cross-reactivity due to pre-existing IgE-mediated sensitization to weed pollen. Allergenic cross-reactivity is specified for *Chamomilla*, *Echinacea*, and other Asteraceae plants. Immediate adverse reactions to HMPs can manifest as oral allergy syndrome, urticaria, angioedema, conjunctivitis, asthma exacerbation, and even anaphylaxis [23,25,26]. According to a World Health Organization (WHO) global database, the number of reports on allergy-like reactions increased along with the use of HMPs. Commonly suspected Asteraceae plants associated with immediate reactions are *Echinacea purpurea*, along with *Matricaria recutita* and *Calendula officinalis* [27].

To effectively educate patients, it is essential to include information about Asteraceae weeds and the plants used in HMPs with cross-reactive allergenic potential, alongside conducting a proper allergy assessment.

3.1. HMPs from Plants Belonging to the Anthemideae Tribe in the Asteroideae Subfamily

Matricaria chamomilla/*Chamomilla recutita* (chamomile, also known as German chamomile, also spelled camomile) and *Chamaemelum nobile*/*Anthemis nobilis* (Roman chamomile), entomophilous herbaceous plants native to Southern Europe, are two Asteraceae representatives frequently used as HMPs. The flowers for medicinal use are obtained from cultivated or wild plants. Herbal products containing *Matricaria* flowers are usually administered as herbal infusions, more rarely as camomile enemas. The mugwort-camomile association consists of primary respiratory IgE sensitization to *Artemisia vulgaris* pollen and secondary allergic symptoms, from allergic contact conjunctivitis to anaphylaxis, in patients exposed to herbal infusion of camomile flowers. Anaphylactic reactions caused by camomile are rare, with only a few well-documented reports, but the incidence of mugwort-camomile association is considered underestimated. Some patients with allergic rhinitis to mugwort pollen may present allergic reactions to camomile, but most patients with camomile allergy are IgE-sensitized to *Artemisia* pollen. The possible cross-reactive component in this association is Art v 1 defensin, while a Bet v 1 homolog and high-molecular-weight allergens may also have a role, but not the profilin pan-allergens [6,25,28,29].

Patients who are allergic to HMPs containing camomile flos (Latin: flower) should be assessed for IgE sensitization to mugwort pollen and the allergy risks for other HMPs, honey, and bee pollen products (HBPs) consumption. Camomile may cross-react with other HMPs Asteraceae family plants, including echinacea, feverfew, and milk thistle. According to the Herbal Medicinal Products Committee (HMPC) of the EMA, *Matricaria* flower HMPs must not be used by those allergic to Asteraceae plants. Moreover, honey samples may contain pollen grains from sunflower, camomile, and yarrow [30–32].

Tanacetum parthenium/*Chrysanthemum parthenium*, known as feverfew, native to the Balkans, has yellow flowers resembling camomile, and its aerial parts are included as raw material in the European Pharmacopoeia. They may cross-react with echinacea, camomile, and milk thistle. IgE sensitization to *Tanacetum parthenium* flowers was reported in the case of mugwort pollinosis associated with anaphylaxis after drinking camomile infusion for the first time. Therefore, according to EMA's HMPC, feverfew should not be used in patients with hypersensitivity/allergy to Asteraceae family plants [33–35].

Achillea millefolium, also known as the yarrow, is a well-known and widely distributed Asteraceae species, frequently used in HMPs as dried inflorescences for infusions. Its pollen is highly allergenic, and patients with mugwort allergic rhinoconjunctivitis may develop occupational asthma from exposure to dried yarrow flowers. According to EMA's HMPC, yarrow flower HMPs are contraindicated in patients with known allergies to Asteraceae plants, including matricaria or marigold flowers [36,37].

Artemisia absinthium, or wormwood, may also cause IgE sensitization in patients with seasonal allergic rhinitis, and its leafy flowering tops may be used as HMP. Although no side effects have been reported, wormwood should not be taken by patients who are allergic to plants of the Asteraceae family [38,39].

3.2. HMPs from Plants Belonging to the Heliantheae Tribe in the Asteroideae Subfamily

Echinacea purpurea and *Echinacea angustifolia*, purple coneflowers native to North America, are two of the most well-known Asteraceae species worldwide used as HMPs due to their potential beneficial effects. *Echinacea pallida* is also utilized as HMP [40]. The flowering aerial parts of *Echinacea* spp. are available as HMPs for oral administration and can cause allergic reactions. It is clinically helpful to note that immediate pharyngeal irritation by echinacein, an isobutyl amide constituent, may cause marked local tingling and increased salivation. Relevant cases of IgE-mediated hypersensitivity reactions include urticaria, angioedema, bronchospasm, and anaphylaxis, reported even upon first known exposure. Patients allergic to *Ambrosia artemisiifolia* pollen seem more likely to present IgE sensitization to *Echinacea*, but the risk of clinically significant adverse events appears relatively low [19,26,41–43]. Current advice from the European Drug Safety is to caution against purple coneflower HMPs use in atopic and asthmatic patients. Due to allergic cross-reactivity risk, ragweed-allergic patients should avoid taking *Echinacea* HMPs. These should likewise not be used in patients who are hypersensitive/allergic to any plant of the Asteraceae family, according to the EMA's HMPC [44,45].

Helianthus annuus, known as sunflower, has an important position as the world's vegetable oilseed. Although historically, it was ethnomedicinally significant, presently, it is rarely used as herbal medicine in Europe. Instead, ingestion of HMPs in combination with HBPs is more common. In patients with Asteraceae anemophilous pollen allergy, especially with IgE sensitization to mugwort, HBPs were reported to induce allergic reactions due to cross-reactivity between pollen of wind-pollinated weeds and other Asteraceae insect-pollinated plants, such as sunflower and dandelion [5,46]. Moreover, in the mugwort-sunflower association, the clinical picture may include oral allergy syndrome or even anaphylaxis to ingestion of commercially peeled sunflower seeds contaminated with pollen. A similar risk in some patients sensitized to mugwort pollen is also possibly associated with the ingestion of unpeeled sunflower seeds not cleaned enough or herbal remedies with sunflower petals. Pollen grains originate from the unripe flower heads mixed during harvest with the ripe ones [6,47].

Xanthium strumarium (common cocklebur) and *Xanthium spinosum* (Bathurst burr or spiny cocklebur) are other Asteraceae plants used in herbal remedies in Europe, including as infusions with aerial parts. The pollen grains of cocklebur and ragweed are similar in appearance. Despite their close botanical proximity, only some published data found cross-reactivity between cocklebur and short ragweed, while others did not [48–50].

3.3. HMPs from Plants from Calenduleae and Astereae Tribes in the Asteroideae Subfamily

Calendula officinalis, also known as common marigold or pot marigold, is a widely cultivated plant from the Calenduleae tribe. Its flower preparations, which may be obtained by drying and comminuting, are usually used for infusions. Reported allergic adverse reactions include severe anaphylaxis after gargling with an infusion of *Calendula* and contact angioedema to pot marigold infusion in a patient with fall seasonal allergic rhinoconjunctivitis sensitized to mugwort and ragweed allergens. According to EMA's HMPC, *Calendula* flower medicines should not be used in patients allergic to Asteraceae family plants [51–53].

Solidago virgaurea, known as European goldenrod, is a herbaceous weedy plant from the Astereae tribe, widespread across most of Europe. It is also grown as a garden flower and a familiar medicinal plant. Although it is primarily insect-pollinated, significant anemophily may occur. However, whether goldenrod is an important cause of allergic rhinitis has been debated. Cross-reactivity between goldenrod and ragweed is considered minor, but it was suggested between *Solidago*, *Matricaria*, and *Chrysanthemum* species. Goldenrod also exhibits cross-reactivity with sunflower pollen, albeit not as significant as mugwort. According to the EMA's HMPC, HMPs with *Solidago virgaurea* are not indicated in patients with known hypersensitivity to Asteraceae family plants [25,54,55].

3.4. HMPs from Plants Belonging to the Cichorioideae and Carduoideae Subfamilies

Taraxacum officinale, known as dandelion, is a prevalent weed from the Cichorioideae subfamily and a popular folk medicine plant. Its comminuted herbal substance is used as an herbal infusion for oral use. Cross-allergenicity of pollen from dandelion with *Artemisia vulgaris* and *Chrysanthemum* × *morifolium* (*Dendranthema grandiflorum*) is reported. *Taraxacum* and *Chrysanthemum* spp. are frequently cosensitized with mugwort in the general population with respiratory allergies. Although these two species reveal extensive cross-allergenicity with mugwort, monosensitizations are also possible [56–58].

Silybum marianum, known as milk thistle, is a versatile Carduoideae subfamily plant adapted to different conditions worldwide. Its fruits ("seeds") are a reliable source of silymarin, a mixture of flavonolignans, mainly silybin. Milk thistle may prompt an allergic reaction in patients with hypersensibility to Compositae plants, such as ragweed, marigolds, and chrysanthemums. The EMA's HMPC mentions that milk thistle HMPs should not be used in patients with hypersensibility/allergy to Asteraceae family plants [58,59].

4. In Vivo Diagnosis Tests for IgE-Mediated Allergy

Considering the need for an accurate diagnosis of respiratory allergies with sensitization to weed pollen and the assessment of associated risks related to the use of HMPs, the allergy diagnostic workup for such patients, both in vivo and in vitro diagnosis tests, must be presented.

4.1. Allergy Skin Tests

Skin testing with commercial allergen extracts and non-standardized native materials represents the first-line in vivo diagnostic tool for assessing immediate type 1 hypersensitivity in clinical practice.

Epidermal skin prick testing (SPT) is an essential diagnostic tool indicated if Asteraceae IgE-mediated sensitization and allergy are suspected. The SPT provides objective confirmation of IgE sensitization, whereas the clinical relevance should always be interpreted from the perspective of detailed personal history and disease manifestations. The SPT with commercial extracts may exceptionally induce systemic reactions. Intradermal tests with Asteraceae pollen or herbal extracts are not recommended because the clinical value is not known and are less safe to perform. Skin scratch testing is also not recommended because it is difficult to interpret due to varying quantities of allergen exposure and mechanical skin irritation, with a higher risk of adverse allergic reactions [60–63]. The SPT is minimally invasive and inexpensive. Results are immediately available and reproducible when carried out by trained health professionals. The recommended method of SPT includes the appropriate use of allergen extracts, positive and negative controls, and interpretation of the tests after 15 min of application. Tests are usually applied to the volar aspect of the forearm according to European guidelines [60,61]. The positive control is histamine dihydrochloride 10 mg/mL (54.3 mmol/L), equivalent to 6.14 mg/mL histamine base, and the negative control is a saline solution, with phenol 0.5% or glycerine 50%, and no active ingredient [64].

In Europe, the SPT panel with aeroallergen extracts includes the most important Asteraceae weed pollen from short ragweed (*Ambrosia artemisiifolia*) and mugwort (*Artemisia vulgaris*), as presented in Table 1 [65–69].

Table 1. Examples of Asteraceae weed pollen allergen extracts used as individual diagnostic allergens for SPT in the EU.

Skin Prick Test Allergen Solutions *	Potency/Concentration **	Marketing Authorization ***
Mugwort Soluprick® SQ 312	10 HEP/mL	ALK-Abelló
Ragweed (*Ambrosia*) Soluprick® N 302	1:100 *w/v* (10 mg/mL)	ALK-Abelló
Dandelion prick test solution 143	50,000 BU/mL	Allergopharma
Mugwort prick test solution 106	50,000 SBU/mL	Allergopharma
Ragweed prick test solution 154	50,000 BU/mL	Allergopharma
Dandelion prick test solution	10,000 DU/mL	Bencard Allergy
Mugwort prick test solution	10,000 DU/mL ODC	Bencard Allergy
Ragweed prick test solution	10,000 DU/mL	Bencard Allergy
Mugwort prick test solution	30 HEP/mL	Leti Pharma
Mugwort pollen prick test solution	10,000 AU/mL	HAL Allergy
Ragweed (*Ambrosia*) pollen prick test solution	10,000 AU/mL	HAL Allergy
Mugwort (*Artemisia vulgaris*) Alyostal®	100 IR/mL	Stallergenes
Ragweed (*Ambrosia elatior*) Alyostal®	100 IR/mL	Stallergenes

Note: * weed pollen allergen products authorized in Germany included in the database of the Paul-Ehrlich-Institut, with the exception of Alyostal prick solutions with pollen allergen extracts from common mugwort (*Artemisia vulgaris*) and short ragweed (*Ambrosia artemisiifolia* var. *elatior*) commercially available in other EU countries; other prick test solutions used in some EU countries include mugwort and ragweed prick tests Bial Aristegui/Roxall, and skin prick tests Lofarma with individual Asteraceae pollen extracts from mugwort, short ragweed, giant ragweed (*Ambrosia trifida*), wormwood (*Artemisia absinthium*), sunflower (*Helianthus annuus*). In the USA, there are commercially available additional Stallergenes Asteraceae pollen extracts for SPT besides those from short ragweed and mugwort, namely from giant ragweed (*Ambrosia trifida*), sagebrush (*Artemisia tridentata*), prairie sage (*Artemisia ludoviciana*), lanceleaf ragweed (*Ambrosia bidentata*), western ragweed (*Ambrosia psilostachya*), burrobrush (Ambrosia salsola), rabbit bush (*Ambrosia deltoidea*), false ragweed (*Ambrosia acanthicarpa*), dandelion (*Taraxacum officinale*) and sunflower. ** Potency/concentration of allergen preparations expressed in different proprietary units used by each allergen manufacturer: HEP = Histamine Equivalent in Prick testing; *w/v* = weight/volume; SBU = Standardized Biological Units, BU = Biological Units; DU = Diagnostic Units, ODC = Optimal Diagnostic Concentration; AU = Allergy Units; IR = Index of Reactivity; *** Marketing Authorization Holder name.

Differences in allergen potency and concentration of major allergens among commercial SPT reagents used for the Asteraceae weed pollen allergy have been reported [70]. There is a real need for the availability of a wider range of high-quality diagnostic allergens for in vivo diagnosis of IgE-mediated allergies, covering not only predominant but also less frequent allergen sources [71,72].

We indirectly assess the HBPs' allergic risks by SPT with *Helianthus annuus* pollen extract in patients presenting with Asteraceae anemophilous pollen allergy who were not significantly previously exposed to sunflower pollen in surroundings of farmlands with cultivated sunflowers or in agricultural occupational settings [5,46].

Different Asteraceae inflorescences utilized as HMPs may be used for SPT as pure floral liquid extracts, hot water flower infusions after cooling, or suspension of comminuted, dried inflorescences or powdered capitulum in sterile saline solution at room temperature. Native floral products used for SPT are obtained from infusion bags purchased in a local retail shop or brought by the patient from the herbal box used before the reaction.

A camomile extract 1:10 *w/v* used for SPT may be obtained from 2 g of dried comminuted or pulvis of *Matricaria chamomilla* flowers, defatted with acetone, and extracted in 20 mL of 0.01 mol/L of phosphate and 0.15 mol/L of NaCI (phosphate buffered saline). The mixture is then stirred for 24 h at 4 °C, centrifuged for 20 min, and passed through a paper filter with 0.22 µm pores. The SPTs begin with a 1:100,000 *w/v* concentration, then 1:10,000 *w/v*, 1:1000 *w/v* and 1:100 *w/v* camomile extracts. It is important to note that control nonatopic subjects consistently do not react to camomile infusion extract 1:10 *w/v* or 10% *w/v* solution [73,74].

Hot water camomile infusion for SPT may be used as a 3% *w/v* solution, equivalent to 30 mg/mL. Reports were published either with SPT with brewed commercial camomile infusion obtained by soaking 3 g flowers with 100 mL boiled water for 10 min cooled before testing [29] or with SPT with hot water camomile infusion prepared by pouring 3 g pure natural, ready-filled, dried camomile flowers into 250 mL of water at a rolling boil, allowed to infuse for 5 min and then to cool down to room temperature slowly [28,75]. The SPT may also be performed with a commercial oily extract of manzana camomile flowers 98.91% [76] or camomile commercial infusion 10 mg/mL prepared by mixing 1 g of dried flowers in 100 mL of sterile saline for 30 min [77]. *Calendula officinalis* flores 30 mg/mL pulvis suspension obtained by mixing dried pot marigold flowers in sterile saline may also be used for SPT [53]. SPTs with aqueous extracts from dried flowers of yarrow *Achillea millefolium*, aqueous *Echinacea* solutions, extracts prepared from *Echinacea* aerial parts in increasing concentrations, and glycerinated *Echinacea* extracts obtained from an HMP manufacturer were published [26,36,41]. Moreover, SPT with components of non-Asteraceae herbal medicines may be additionally needed if combined or complex herbal products are suspected [78].

An alternative in vivo diagnostic approach is the prick-prick test (PPT) with native allergens, which is practical and less resource-consuming [79]. The PPT with soaked flowers in normal saline may be performed. Central disk tubular florets and peripheral ray or ligulate florets may be used separately. A PPT was reported with non-heated central tubular florets, where most pollen adhered, and ligulate florets of feverfew inflorescence [35].

4.2. Allergen Provocation Tests

Allergen challenges are in vivo diagnostic tools offering reproducible data in patients with pollen allergy using standardized allergen extracts applied to the nasal or bronchial mucosa to induce symptoms according to European guidelines for the purpose of demonstrating the clinical relevance of IgE-mediated sensitization identified by SPT and in vitro immunoassays. The most frequently applied airway allergen provocation is the nasal allergen challenge (NAC). There is evidence of a relationship between positive nasal challenges and ocular reactions. The conjunctival allergen provocation test, which instills the allergen solution on the ocular surface, is less frequently used. Moreover, the bronchial allergen challenge (BAC) is usually considered a research tool only, and its reproducibility was not evaluated for weed pollen allergens. All these provocation tests are instrumental in confirming the allergy diagnosis if detailed clinical history, SPT, and specific IgE findings are inconclusive, considering the potential for systemic adverse reactions, especially with inhalation challenges [79–82]. Examples of Asteraceae weed pollen allergen extracts used as individual diagnostic allergens for NAC and BAC, commercially available in some European countries, are presented in Table 2 [25,36,67,83,84]. All in vivo allergy provocation tests require highly qualified staff and safety measurements [79,81,82].

Table 2. Examples of Asteraceae weed pollen allergen extracts used as individual diagnostic allergens for nasal and bronchial allergen provocation in some European countries.

Provocation Allergen Solution *	Potency **	Authorization ***
Dandelion provocation test solution for nasal spray	5000 BU/mL	Allergopharma
Mugwort provocation test solution for nasal spray	5000 SBU/mL	Allergopharma
Ragweed provocation test solution for nasal spray	5000 BU/mL	Allergopharma
Ragweed provocation test solution for nasal spray (Allergy Provo Spray)	10,000 AU/mL	HAL Allergy
Mugwort provocation test solution for nasal spray (Allergy Provo Spray)	10,000 AU/mL	HAL Allergy
Mugwort provocation test solution for nebulizer (Allergy Provo Test ****)	10,000 AU/mL	HAL Allergy
Mugwort provocation test (powder for solution) for nasal spray/nebulizer	30 HEP/mL	Leti Pharma

Note: * weed pollen allergen products authorized in Germany included in the database of the Paul-Ehrlich-Institut. ** Potency/concentration of allergen preparations expressed in different proprietary units: BU = Biological Units, SBU = Standardized Biological Units; AU = Allergy Units; HEP = Histamine Equivalent units. *** Marketing Authorization Holder name. **** May also be used for conjunctival provocation; BAC was performed in individual cases with aqueous extracts of camomile *Matricaria chamomilla* and yarrow *Achillea millefolium* (1.25 mg/mL).

The NAC is a valuable diagnostic and research tool for evaluating the response of the nasal mucosa to aeroallergens with high sensitivity and specificity. It is the gold standard in the diagnosis of local allergic rhinitis. It can be used to diagnose seasonal allergic rhinitis, especially to detect clinically relevant allergens in polysensitized patients or those with discrepancies between clinical history, SPT, and specific IgE results. NAC also offers valuable information in evaluating asthmatic patients since 85% of patients reveal identical responses at the nasal and bronchial mucosa upon allergen provocation. The advantage of NAC is that it is a much safer procedure than BAC [85,86].

Allergen exposure chambers (AECs) are modern specialized medical installations designed for patients' standardized and reproducible allergen challenges. They mimic real-world natural exposure to aeroallergens while allowing for precise control over the allergen concentration and other environmental variables. Until recently, one study has been published using a ragweed AEC model to assess immunotherapy preparation [87–89].

Oral provocation tests with Asteraceae HMPs liquid preparation are performed in clinical practice only after a carefully assessed risk/benefit ratio.

A labial provocation test was carried out by applying one drop of undiluted camomile infusion on the lip, obtained from 3 g flowers with 100 mL boiled water for 10 min, and cooled before testing. An open oral challenge may follow starting at 1:100,000–1,000,000 dilution of herbal infusion prepared as usual and increased 10-fold to full strength at 15–20 min intervals, using a 5 mL volume. If there is no reaction after full strength, ad-lib drinking under observation may be suggested [9,63].

5. In Vitro Diagnosis Tests for IgE-Mediated Allergy

Immunoassays for specific IgE are the most widely used in vitro tests for IgE-mediated allergy to Asteraceae weed pollen and HMPs. BAT is an emerging additional method.

5.1. Serum Specific IgE (ssIgE)

The measurement of ssIgE antibodies against natural allergen extracts and molecular components, either well-defined highly purified natural or recombinant molecules, is an essential complementary in vitro tool to diagnose IgE-mediated sensitization to Asteraceae pollen, especially in subjects who cannot undergo SPT, such as those with dermographism or who are taking H1 antihistamines or other medications that interfere with the proper interpretation of results [61]. Either ssIgE or SPT are acceptable for diagnosing respiratory allergies and guiding allergen immunotherapy [90].

Immunoassays used to detect ssIgE to allergen extracts and components are either singleplex, multiparameter, or multiplex assays, depending on the number of allergen extracts and molecular components used [91].

The radioallergosorbent test (RAST) was the first generation isotopic singleplex immunoassay that used allergens covalently coupled to an allergosorbent filter paper solid phase, radioiodinated polyclonal anti-IgE, and bound radioactivity quantification by gamma counter. The ssIgE were detected by this method in a case of anaphylaxis to *Echinacea* sp. Such ssIgE in asymptomatic atopic subjects never exposed to oral HMPs or ornamental *Echinacea* suggests cross-reactivity between structurally related allergens in *Echinacea* and other Asteraceae pollen grains [91,92].

Current commercial singleplex, nonisotopic, more sensitive in vitro methods for ssIgE to many natural extracts and molecular components use either solid-phase coupled allergens (i.e., fluorescence enzyme immunoassay) or liquid-phase allergens (i.e., chemiluminescence immunoassay). Asteraceae pollen whole allergens as native extracts (Table 3) are obtained from the pollen grains of many entomophilous weeds and primarily anemophilous plants used as HMPs [91,93–95]. When compared with multiplex technology, the advantages of singleplex assays for allergen ssIgE testing with allergenic molecules/components include increased sensitivity at low ssIgE levels [91].

Table 3. Examples of Asteraceae pollen individual diagnostic allergens in singleplex IgE immunoassays.

Asteraceae Allergen	Latin Name, Protein Group	Code	Singleplex Method	
Asteraceae pollen whole allergens (native extracts)				
Common ragweed	*Ambrosia artemisiifolia* (*A. elatior*)	w1	ImmunoCAP® FEIA	Immulite® CLIA
Western ragweed	*Ambrosia psilostachya*	w2	ImmunoCAP® FEIA	Immulite® CLIA
Giant ragweed	*Ambrosia trifida*	w3	ImmunoCAP® FEIA	Immulite® CLIA
False ragweed	*Ambrosia acanthicarpa*	w4	ImmunoCAP® FEIA	Immulite® CLIA
Wormwood	*Artemisia absinthium*	w5	ImmunoCAP® FEIA	Immulite® CLIA
Mugwort	*Artemisia vulgaris*	w6	ImmunoCAP® FEIA	Immulite® CLIA
Marguerite/Ox-eye daisy	*Chrysanthemum leucanthemum*	w7	ImmunoCAP® FEIA	Immulite® CLIA
Dandelion	*Taraxacum vulgare*	w8	ImmunoCAP® FEIA	Immulite® CLIA
Cocklebur	*Xanthium strumarium/commune*	w13	ImmunoCAP® FEIA	Immulite® CLIA
Rough marshelder	*Iva annua/ciliata*	w16	ImmunoCAP® FEIA	Immulite® CLIA
Rabbit bush	*Ambrosia deltoidea*	w36		Immulite® CLIA
Common sagebrush	*Artemisia tridentata*	w43		Immulite® CLIA
Groundsel bush	*Baccharis halimifolia*	w67		Immulite® CLIA
Sunflower	*Helianthus annuus*	w204	ImmunoCAP® FEIA	
Camomile/chamomille	*Matricaria chamomilla*	w206	ImmunoCAP® FEIA	
Asteraceae weed pollen allergen components				
nAmb a 1 ragweed	pectate lyase *Ambrosia artemisiifolia*	w230	ImmunoCAP® FEIA	
nArt v 1 mugwort	DPLP *Artemisia vulgaris*	w231	ImmunoCAP® FEIA	Immulite® CLIA
nArt v 3 LTP mugwort	nsLTP type 1 *Artemisia vulgaris*	w233	ImmunoCAP® FEIA	

Note: FEIA = fluorescence enzyme immunoassay, CLIA = chemiluminescence immunoassay; DPLP = defensin-polyproline-linked protein (a defensin-like protein linked to polyproline-rich region), nsLTP = non-specific lipid transfer protein; n = natural purified, r = recombinant.

The fluorescence enzyme immunoassay (FEIA) with capsulated cellulose polymer solid-phase coupled allergens (ImmunoCAP®, Thermo Fisher Scientific Inc., Phadia AB, Uppsala, Sweden) is a currently used singleplex assay to measure ssIgE to Asteraceae pollen allergens. Allergens are covalently coupled in FEIA to a hydrophilic carrier polymer consisting of a cyanogen bromide-activated cellulose derivative with a large surface for protein binding. This method uses β-galactosidase-labeled anti-IgE monoclonal antibodies and 4-methylumbelliferyl-β-galactoside as fluorogenic substrate, fluorescence measurement being performed with a fluorocounter [91,96].

The enzyme-enhanced chemiluminescence immunoassay (CLIA) with liquid-phase allergens is another advanced singleplex detection method for ssIgE that exploits liquid-phase kinetics in a bead format (3gAllergy™ Immulite® 2000 and Immulite® 2000 XPi immunoassay; Siemens Healthcare Diagnostics Inc., Erlangen, Germany). Asteraceae allergens covalently bound to soluble biotinylated polylysine polymer in a fluid phase bind to streptavidin-coated polystyrene bead in the reaction tube (through a streptavidin-biotin interaction). This method uses alkaline phosphatase enzyme-labeled anti-IgE monoclonal antibodies and adamantyl 1,2-dioxetane aryl phosphate as chemiluminescent substrate, chemiluminescence being measured using a luminometer [91].

In the past, patients with ssIgE concentrations of 0.35 kU_A/L or higher were considered to have a positive result. However, more recently, ssIgE tests have been reported as analytical results, not based on positive or negative thresholds. Also, it was suggested that the lowest detectable limit for autoanalyzer-based IgE immunoassays should be 0.1 kU_A/L. Nevertheless, ssIgE levels between 0.1 and 0.35 kU_A/L should be carefully considered along with the clinical manifestations. It is essential to distinguish between IgE sensitization and allergy at all concentrations. Elevated ssIgE values alone, without characteristic symptoms, are insufficient for a definitive allergy diagnosis [97].

A multiparameter line blot immunoassay with allergens coating membrane strips in thin parallel lines as line blots (Euroline™; Euroimmun AG, Lübeck, Germany) may be used to measure simultaneously ssIgE against several allergen extracts, including common ragweed (w1) and mugwort (w6) pollen. This in vitro diagnosis method based on immunoblot technology uses alkaline phosphatase enzyme-labeled anti-IgE monoclonal antibodies and nitroblue tetrazolium chloride/5-bromo-4-chloro-3-indolylphosphate for colorimetric detection, with subsequent image acquisition and evaluation. If anti-CCD IgE antibodies are detected in serum reflected in a positive CCD marker band, the serum should be re-incubated in the assay with anti-CCD absorbent [91,98].

Multiplex ssIgE immunoassays enable the detection of the profile of IgE sensitizations against a wide array of allergens (more than one hundred from various sources). Asteraceae pollen allergens are present as native extracts and molecular components (Table 4) [93,94]. The microarray immunoassay on a preactivated amine-reactive polymer-coated glass slide as a solid phase for allergen components uses fluorophore-labeled anti-human IgE monoclonal antibodies (Immuno CAP® ISAC™, Thermo Fisher Scientific Inc., Phadia AB). The ELISA-based macroarray immunoassay uses nano-bead technology as a molecular allergy explorer (ALEX®, MacroArray Diagnostics, Vienna, Austria) with allergen extracts and molecular components spotted in a cartridge chip onto a nitrocellulose membrane, using anti-human IgE labeled with alkaline phosphatase. Its protocol integrates a potent CCD inhibitor during serum incubation, thus increasing the specificity of the test results [91,96].

Because pollen allergy is heterogeneous regarding clinical manifestations and sensitization profiles, including poly-sensitization, molecular customized in vitro IgE immunoassays can detect relevant sensitizations [99].

Table 4. Examples of Asteraceae pollen allergen extracts and components used in multiplex IgE immunoassays.

Asteraceae Allergen	Latin Name, Protein Group	Code	Singleplex Method
Asteraceae pollen whole allergens (native extracts)			
Common ragweed	*Ambrosia artemisiifolia* (*A. elatior*)	w1	ALEX2®
Mugwort	*Artemisia vulgaris*	w6	ALEX2®
Asteraceae weed pollen allergen components			
nAmb a 1 ragweed	pectate lyase *Ambrosia artemisiifolia*	w230	ImmunoCAP® ISAC™ E112i
rAmb a 1 ragweed	pectate lyase *Ambrosia artemisiifolia*	w230	ALEX2®
rAmb a 4 ragweed	plant defensin/DPLP *Ambrosia artemisiifolia*	w300	ALEX2®
nArt v 1 mugwort	plant defensin/DPLP *Artemisia vulgaris*	w231	ImmunoCAP® ISAC™ E112i
rArt v 1.0101 mugwort	plant defensin/DPLP *Artemisia vulgaris*	w231	ALEX2®
nArt v 3 LTP mugwort	non-specific LTP type 1 *Artemisia vulgaris*	w233	ImmunoCAP® ISAC™ E112i
rArt v 3.0201 LTP mugwort	non-specific LTP type 1 *Artemisia vulgaris*	w233	ALEX2®

Note: ALEX2® is the improved successor product of ALEX® = Allergy Xplorer ELISA-based macroarray immunoassay, ImmunoCAP® ISAC™ = Immuno Solid-Phase Allergen Chip microarray immunoassay; DPLP = defensin-polyproline-linked protein (defensin-like protein linked to polyproline-rich region), LTP = lipid transfer protein; n = natural purified, r = recombinant; Both multiplex immunoassays include pan-allergens from Timothy grass pollen: polcalcin marker rPhl p 7 and profilin marker rPhl p 12.

Asteraceae weed pollen allergen components used in singleplex immunoassays are ragweed pectate lyase Amb a 1, mugwort defensin-like protein Art v 1, and non-specific lipid transfer protein Art v 3 (Table 3).

A useful diagnostic marker for genuine IgE sensitization to *Ambrosia artemisiifolia* pollen is ssIgE to major allergen Amb a 1. This pectate lyase is responsible for more than 90% of the IgE responses in short ragweed pollen-allergic patients. Amb a 1.01 is its most allergenic isoform. Although it shows cross-reactivity with mugwort Art v 6 and sunflower Hel a 6, in areas of concomitant exposure to ragweed and mugwort with overlapping pollination seasons, Amb a 1 assists with the identification of the primary sensitizer [100,101]. The cysteine protease Amb a 11 is also considered a major ragweed pollen allergen with an IgE sensitization rate of up to almost 70%; however, sensitization studies in larger cohorts remain to be conducted [102,103].

Several less frequently recognized allergens are considered relevant, such as defensin Amb a 4, non-specific lipid transfer protein type 1 Amb a 6, and profilin Amb a 8, due to their ability to cross-react with other homologous allergens, such as Art v 1 (with Amb a 4), Art v 3 (with Amb a 6), and profilin pan-allergens from Timothy grass Phl p 12 and birch pollen Bet v 2 (with Amb a 8) [1,6,104].

Amb a 4 is a minor allergen from *Ambrosia* pollen present in multiplex macroarray immunoassay but with limited quantity in ragweed extracts. The IgE binding frequency to Amb a 4 is about 20% in ragweed-allergic patients and even higher in mugwort-cosensitized populations. Among weed pollen-allergic patients, positive IgE reactivity to Amb a 4 may be up to 40%, and it is typically associated with Art v 1 sensitization. DPLP Amb a 4 is an Art v 1 homolog protein with a defensin-like domain, but its proline-rich region differs from Art v 1, affecting the IgE binding. Thus, Amb a 4 has different degrees of cross-reactivity with the major mugwort pollen allergen Art v 1. Amb a 4 is also responsible for primary sensitization in some patients with high ragweed exposure [1,103,105].

Other *Ambrosia* pollen allergen components not yet included in commercial assays, such as plastocyanins Amb 3 and Amb a 7, polcalcins or calcium-binding proteins Amb a 9 and Amb a 10, and enolase Amb a 12, may also contribute to the molecular IgE sensitization profiles of patients with respiratory allergy to ragweed pollen [106].

A prominent diagnostic marker for genuine IgE sensitization to *Artemisia vulgaris* pollen is ssIgE to common mugwort major allergen Art v 1. This defensin-polyproline-linked protein, also named defensin-like protein linked to polyproline-rich region (DPLP), is recognized by more than 70% of mugwort-sensitized patient IgE antibodies. Native Art v 1 (nArt v 1) was revealed to have higher reactivity than the recombinant Art v 1 (rArt v 1) due to the involvement of carbohydrate-specific antibodies in epitope recognition. The wide-ranging carbohydrate structures (representing 30–40% of the nArt v 1) with C-terminal hydroxyprolines revealing different degrees of *O*-glycosylation are important in IgE recognition. Although rArt v 1 produced in *E. coli* lacks the posttranslational modifications present in nArt v 1, both share common epitopes recognized by human IgE antibodies. While nArt v 1 is a complex mixture of different isoallergens and glycosylation variants, rArt v 1.0101 is considered a relevant mugwort pollen isoallergen [1,103,105,107]. There is extensive cross-reactivity among the major allergens of different species of mugwort (more than 94% protein sequence identity). Pollen grains from Asteraceae plants botanically related, such as sunflower and wormwood, possess Art v 1 cross-reactive structures. Art v 1-like molecules are responsible for the cross-reactivity of mugwort with sunflower and camomile [107,108].

Art v 6 also plays a crucial role in mugwort pollen allergy, and the cross-reactivity between Art v 6 and Amb a 1 is frequent, bidirectional, and relevant. Double sensitization to ragweed and mugwort is common in many areas. Cross-reactivity is responsible for double sensitization in most cases. In some regions, if individuals sensitized to profilins and polcalcins are excluded, both IgE sensitization and allergy to mugwort pollen in the absence of ragweed sensitization are rare. A practical approach was suggested for patients with IgE sensitization to both mugwort and ragweed extracts reactive to Art v 1 to be prescribed mugwort immunotherapy, whereas those not reactive to Art v 1 to be prescribed ragweed immunotherapy because *Ambrosia* is probably the primary sensitizer [109].

The nsLTP Art v 3 is a marker allergen for complex sensitization profiles to mugwort pollen. Patients with allergic rhinitis to *Artemisia vulgaris*, living in areas with high mugwort pollen exposure, exhibit more complex sensitization profiles, including more frequent Art v 3 sensitization, which is associated with an increased prevalence of allergic asthma [1,108]. The relevant isoallergen rArt v 3.0201 possesses similar structural and immunological properties as nArt v 3, enabling batch-to-batch reproducibility for a high-quality diagnosis [110]. Moreover, this PR-14 protein is also a marker allergen for nsLTP pan-allergen sensitization. Art v 3 cross-reactivities with homologous peach Pru p 3 from hazelnut Cor a 8 and other nsLTPs are involved in some pollen-food syndromes, including mugwort-peach and Asteraceae-hazelnut associations [6,16,53,91].

Other cross-reactive allergen components, such as PR-1 protein Art v 2, profilin Art v 4, polcalcin Art v 5, may also contribute to the molecular IgE sensitization profiles in mugwort respiratory allergy [106,111]. Some authors suggested that using Art v 1 and Art v 4 could identify 91% of mugwort pollen-sensitized patients [112].

Because polysensitizations to different pollen sources are found in about 20% of pollen-allergic subjects, molecular diagnosis is needed to distinguish broad cross-reactivity due to pan-allergen profilins such as Bet v 2 or Phl p 12 and/or polcalcins such as Bet v 4 or Phl p 7, from primary IgE sensitizations to major marker allergens [113].

Moreover, group 1 and 4 allergen molecules of grass pollen are significant inducers of carbohydrate cross-reactive determinants (CCDs), moieties of glycoproteins that induce highly cross-reactive IgE antibodies. CCDs do not usually induce mast cell degranulation in vivo and, therefore, do not elicit positive reactions to SPT with allergen extracts or symptoms upon allergen exposure. However, the presence of CCDs may cause false-positive results in IgE immunoassays with CCD-containing natural allergen extracts from pollen, plant foods, and hymenopteran venoms. CCD inhibition improves the accuracy of in vitro detection of pollen allergen-specific IgE [1,114,115].

5.2. Specific IgE in Nasal Secretions (nssIgE)

Although some published research data suggested that nssIgE against aeroallergens seems to be a non-specific phenomenon since they can also be detected in nonallergic rhinitis and healthy subjects [116], several novel studies suggested using nssIgE as an additional local allergic rhinitis (LAR) diagnostic criterion [117]. A characteristic feature of LAR is the presence of nssIgE in 20–40% of subjects [118]. If the nasal cytological test reveals a prominent accumulation of eosinophils in nasal mucosa without detectable levels of ssIgE, local levels of nssIgE may be used to support the diagnosis of LAR as an alternative to NAC [97].

The nssIgE against mugwort pollen may be determined using FEIA with capsulated cellulose polymer solid-phase coupled allergens (ImmunoCAP®, Thermo Fisher Scientific Inc., Phadia AB, Uppsala, Sweden). Nasal secretions may be obtained using a sinus sponges pack in each nostril or bilateral nasal lavage performed with physiologic saline solution at room temperature. The detection limit is 0.35 kU_A/L. Measurements are performed at baseline and 15 min and 1 h after the NPTs [119,120].

5.3. Basophil Activation Test (BAT)

The Flow CAST (Cellular Allergy Stimulation Test) is a standardized BAT (Bühlmann Laboratories AG, Schönenbuch, Switzerland) may be used in clinical research and diagnostic labs for the quantitative assessment of in vitro basophil activation by common ragweed and mugwort allergens, by flow cytometry performed using the FACSCalibur® system (Becton-Dickinson Immunocytometry System, Heidelberg, Germany). The chemokine receptor CCR3 is used as an identification marker for basophils, while CD63 is used as a basophil activation marker, labeled with anti-CCR3-phycoerythrin and anti-CD63-fluorescein-isothiocyanate monoclonal antibodies, respectively. BAT is considered a functional ex vivo assay differentiating sensitization and relevant allergy. Basophil allergen threshold sensitivity (CD-sens) has been shown to correlate with NAC and BAC threshold sensitivity [96,121,122]. The utility of BAT in weed pollen allergy was mentioned in patients with mugwort immunotherapy [123] and mugwort pollen-related peach allergy [124]. The usefulness of BAT for bupleurum-containing Japanese herbal medicine-induced lung injury was recently published. To our knowledge, there are no other reports of BAT with HMPs in Europe [125].

6. Conclusions

To optimize the management of patients with respiratory allergies to Asteraceae weed pollen, general physicians, ENT specialists, and pulmonologists need to be updated on the diagnostic methods allergists use in clinical practice and their usefulness and limitations. A modern molecular allergology approach relying on utilizing allergen molecules as in vitro tools that complements the traditional approach based on SPT and in vitro allergen extract testing [126] may assess IgE sensitization to specific weed pollen allergens and cross-reactive allergen components in HMPs, including Asteraceae plant defensins [6,25,28,29] with good thermal and pH stability [127]. Allergists also need to become more knowledgeable about herbal therapies so that they can educate patients about the potential risks of HMPs. It is relevant to know that HMPs containing Asteraceae herbs (flowering aerial parts) preparations are usually available for oral administration in solid or liquid forms. Herbal infusions are the most frequently used liquid products. They are either loose or obtained from single-use infusion bags, considering that Asteraceae pollen grains are smaller than the pore size of woven nylon and non-woven (cellulosic, polylactic acid, nylon hybrid) infusion papers. Enemas with herbal liquid preparation are even more risky due to application to a large area of colonic mucosa [76,128,129]. Allergists must inform patients allergic to weed anemophilous pollen, such as from mugwort or ragweed, about the allergic risks of flowers/aerial parts of entomophilous Compositae plants used as HMPs consumed without or with HBPs, which may contribute to additional risks.

Author Contributions: All authors have contributed to the manuscript. All authors have read and agreed to the published version of the manuscript.

Funding: This article received no external funding.

Acknowledgments: Publication of this paper was supported by the University of Medicine and Pharmacy Carol Davila, through the institutional program Publish not Perish.

Conflicts of Interest: The authors declare no conflicts of interest.

References

1. Dramburg, S.; Hilger, C.; Santos, A.F.; de Las Vecillas, L.; Aalberse, R.C.; Acevedo, N.; Aglas, L.; Altmann, F.; Arruda, K.L.; Asero, R.; et al. EAACI Molecular Allergology User's Guide 2.0. *Pediatr. Allergy Immunol.* **2023**, *34*, e13854. [CrossRef] [PubMed]
2. D'Amato, G.; Cecchi, L.; Bonini, S.; Nunes, C.; Annesi-Maesano, I.; Behrendt, H.; Liccardi, G.; Popov, T.; van Cauwenberge, P. Allergenic pollen and pollen allergy in Europe. *Allergy* **2007**, *62*, 976–990. [CrossRef] [PubMed]
3. Lake, I.R.; Jones, N.R.; Agnew, M.; Goodess, C.M.; Giorgi, F.; Hamaoui-Laguel, L.; Semenov, M.A.; Solmon, F.; Storkey, J.; Vautard, R.; et al. Climate Change and Future Pollen Allergy in Europe. *Environ. Health Perspect.* **2017**, *125*, 385–391. [CrossRef] [PubMed]
4. Schaffner, U.; Steinbach, S.; Sun, Y.; Skjøth, C.A.; de Weger, L.A.; Lommen, S.T.; Augustinus, B.A.; Bonini, M.; Karrer, G.; Šikoparija, B.; et al. Biological Weed Control to Relieve Millions from Ambrosia Allergies in Europe. *Nat. Commun.* **2020**, *11*, 1745. [CrossRef]
5. Popescu, F.D.; Vieru, M. The presence of aeroallergens in food products: A potential risk for the patient with allergic rhinitis. *Rom. J. Rhinol.* **2018**, *8*, 11. [CrossRef]
6. Popescu, F.D. Cross-reactivity between aeroallergens and food allergens. *World J. Methodol.* **2015**, *5*, 31–50. [CrossRef]
7. Chivato, T.; Juan, F.; Montoro, A.; Laguna, R. Anaphylaxis induced by ingestion of a pollen compound. *J. Investig. Allergol. Clin. Immunol.* **1996**, *6*, 208–209. [PubMed]
8. Fuiano, N.; Incorvaia, C.; Riario-Sforza, G.G.; Casino, G. Anaphylaxis to honey in pollinosis to mugwort: A case report. *Eur. Ann. Allergy Clin. Immunol.* **2006**, *38*, 364–365. [PubMed]
9. iNaturalist. Available online: www.inaturalist.org (accessed on 12 August 2024).
10. National Center for Biotechnology Information. Taxonomy. Available online: www.ncbi.nlm.nih.gov/taxonomy (accessed on 12 August 2024).
11. Gadermaier, G.; Hauser, M.; Ferreira, F. Allergens of weed pollen: An overview on recombinant and natural molecules. *Methods* **2014**, *66*, 55–66. [CrossRef]
12. WHO/IUIS Allergen Nomenclature Sub-Committee. Allergen Nomenclature. Database: Allergen Nomenclature. Available online: www.allergen.org/index.php (accessed on 14 August 2024).
13. Fukuoka, A.; Matsushita, K.; Morikawa, T.; Adachi, T.; Yasuda, K.; Kiyonari, H.; Fujieda, S.; Yoshimoto, T. Human cystatin SN is an endogenous protease inhibitor that prevents allergic rhinitis. *J. Allergy Clin. Immunol.* **2019**, *143*, 1153–1162.e12. [CrossRef]
14. Oteros, J.; Bartusel, E.; Alessandrini, F.; Núñez, A.; Moreno, D.A.; Behrendt, H.; Schmidt-Weber, C.; Traidl-Hoffmann, C.; Buters, J. Artemisia pollen is the main vector for airborne endotoxin. *J. Allergy Clin. Immunol.* **2019**, *143*, 369–377.e5. [CrossRef] [PubMed]
15. Werfel, T.; Asero, R.; Ballmer-Weber, B.K.; Beyer, K.; Enrique, E.; Knulst, A.C.; Mari, A.; Muraro, A.; Ollert, M.; Poulsen, L.K.; et al. Position paper of the EAACI: Food allergy due to immunological cross-reactions with common inhalant allergens. *Allergy* **2015**, *70*, 1079–1090. [CrossRef] [PubMed]
16. Skypala, I.J.; Asero, R.; Barber, D.; Cecchi, L.; Diaz Perales, A.; Hoffmann-Sommergruber, K.; Pastorello, E.A.; Swoboda, I.; Bartra, J.; Ebo, D.G.; et al. Non-specific lipid-transfer proteins: Allergen structure and function, cross-reactivity, sensitization, and epidemiology. *Clin. Transl. Allergy* **2021**, *11*, e12010. [CrossRef] [PubMed]
17. Qu, L.; Zou, W.; Wang, Y.; Wang, M. European regulation model for herbal medicine: The assessment of the EU monograph and the safety and efficacy evaluation in marketing authorization or registration in Member States. *Phytomedicine* **2018**, *42*, 219–225. [CrossRef]
18. Senna, G.; Passalacqua, G.; Crivellaro, M.; Bonadonna, P.; Gani, F.; Dorizzi, R.; Dama, A.; Canonica, G.W.; Lombardi, C. Unconventional medicine: A risk of undertreatment of allergic patients. *Allergy* **1999**, *54*, 1117–1119. [CrossRef]
19. Bielory, L. Complementary and alternative interventions in asthma, allergy, and immunology. *Ann. Allergy Asthma Immunol.* **2004**, *93* (Suppl. S1), S45–S54. [CrossRef]
20. Routledge, P.A. The European Herbal Medicines Directive: Could it have saved the lives of Romeo and Juliet? *Drug Saf.* **2008**, *31*, 416–418. [CrossRef]
21. Misaka, S.; Ono, Y.; Taudte, R.V.; Hoier, E.; Ogata, H.; Ono, T.; König, J.; Watanabe, H.; Fromm, M.F.; Shimomura, K. Exposure of fexofenadine, but not pseudoephedrine, is markedly decreased by green tea extract in healthy volunteers. *Clin. Pharmacol. Ther.* **2022**, *112*, 627–634. [CrossRef]

22. Farasati Far, B.; Behzad, G.; Khalili, H. Achillea millefolium: Mechanism of action, pharmacokinetic, clinical drug-drug interactions, and tolerability. *Heliyon* **2023**, *9*, e22841. [CrossRef]
23. Caliskaner, Z.; Kartal, O.; Gulec, M.; Ozturk, S.; Erel, F.; Sener, O.; Karaayvaz, M. Awareness of allergy patients about herbal remedies: A cross-sectional study of residents of Ankara, Turkey. *Allergol. Immunopathol.* **2010**, *38*, 78–82. [CrossRef]
24. Gilissen, L.; Huygens, S.; Goossens, A. Allergic contact dermatitis caused by topical herbal remedies: Importance of patch testing with the patients' own products. *Contact Dermat.* **2018**, *78*, 177–184. [CrossRef] [PubMed]
25. de la Torre Morín, F.; Sánchez Machín, I.; García Robaina, J.C.; Fernández-Caldas, E.; Sánchez Triviño, M. Clinical cross-reactivity between Artemisia vulgaris and Matricaria chamomilla (chamomile). *J. Investig. Allergol. Clin. Immunol.* **2001**, *11*, 118–122. [PubMed]
26. Fasano, M.B. Allergenic cross-reactivity between Echinacea and ragweed. *J. Allergy Clin. Immunol.* **2007**, *119*, S270. [CrossRef]
27. Meincke, R.; Pokladnikova, J.; Straznicka, J.; Meyboom, R.H.B.; Niedrig, D.; Russmann, S.; Jahodar, L. Allergy-like immediate reactions with herbal medicines in children: A retrospective study using data from VigiBase®. *Pediatr. Allergy Immunol.* **2017**, *28*, 668–674. [CrossRef] [PubMed]
28. Reider, N.; Sepp, N.; Fritsch, P.; Weinlich, G.; Jensen-Jarolim, E. Anaphylaxis to camomile: Clinical features and allergen cross-reactivity. *Clin. Exp. Allergy* **2000**, *30*, 1436–1443. [CrossRef] [PubMed]
29. Andres, C.; Chen, W.C.; Ollert, M.; Mempel, M.; Darsow, U.; Ring, J. Anaphylactic reaction to camomile tea. *Allergol. Int.* **2009**, *58*, 135–136. [CrossRef] [PubMed]
30. European Medicines Agency. Assessment report on Chamaemelum Nobile. Available online: www.ema.europa.eu/%20en/documents/herbal-report/final-assessment-report-chamaemelum-nobile-l-all-flos_en.pdf (accessed on 14 August 2024).
31. European Medicines Agency. Matricaria Flower. *Matricaria recutita* L., flos. Available online: www.ema.europa.eu/en/documents/herbal-summary/matricaria-flower-summary-public_en.pdf (accessed on 14 August 2024).
32. Vîjan, L.E.; Mazilu, I.C.; Enache, C.; Enache, S.; Topală, C.M. Botanical origin influence on some honey physicochemical characteristics and antioxidant properties. *Foods* **2023**, *12*, 2134. [CrossRef]
33. European Medicines Agency. Tanaceti Parthenii Herba—Herbal Medicinal Product. Available online: www.ema.europa.eu/en/medicines/herbal/tanaceti-parthenii-herba (accessed on 14 August 2024).
34. Pareek, A.; Suthar, M.; Rathore, G.S.; Bansal, V. Feverfew (*Tanacetum parthenium* L.): A systematic review. *Pharmacogn. Rev.* **2011**, *5*, 103–110. [CrossRef]
35. Nakagawa, M.; Hanada, M.; Amano, H. A case of anaphylactic reaction to chamomile tea in a patient with mugwort pollinosis. *Allergol. Int.* **2019**, *68*, 396–398. [CrossRef]
36. Compes, E.; Bartolomé, B.; Fernández-Nieto, M.; Sastre, J.; Cuesta, J. Occupational asthma from dried flowers of *Carthamus tinctorious* (safflower) and *Achillea millefolium* (yarrow). *Allergy* **2006**, *61*, 1239–1240. [CrossRef]
37. European Medicines Agency. Assessment Report on *Achillea millefolium* L., flos. Available online: www.ema.europa.eu/en/documents/herbal-report/draft-assessment-report-achillea-millefolium-l-flos_en.pdf (accessed on 14 August 2024).
38. Zhumambayeva, S.; Rozenson, R.; Tawfik, A.; Awadalla, N.J.; Zhumambayeva, R. Date of birth and hay fever risk in children and adolescents of Kazakhstan. *Int. J. Pediatr. Otorhinolaryngol.* **2014**, *78*, 214–217. [CrossRef] [PubMed]
39. European Medicines Agency. Absinthii Herba—Herbal Medicinal Product. Available online: www.ema.europa.eu/%20en/medicines/herbal/absinthii-herba (accessed on 14 August 2024).
40. Ahmadi, F.; Kariman, K.; Mousavi, M.; Rengel, Z. Echinacea: Bioactive Compounds and Agronomy. *Plants* **2024**, *13*, 1235. [CrossRef] [PubMed] [PubMed Central]
41. Mullins, R.J.; Heddle, R. Adverse reactions associated with echinacea: The Australian experience. *Ann. Allergy Asthma Immunol.* **2002**, *88*, 42–51. [CrossRef]
42. Gunawardana, N.C. Risk of anaphylaxis in complementary and alternative medicine. *Curr. Opin. Allergy Clin. Immunol.* **2017**, *17*, 332–337. [CrossRef] [PubMed]
43. Myers, S.P.; Wohlmuth, H. Echinacea-associated anaphylaxis. *Med. J. Aust.* **1998**, *168*, 583–584. [CrossRef] [PubMed]
44. European Medicines Agency. Echinaceae Purpureae Herba—Herbal Medicinal Product. Available online: www.ema.europa.eu/en/medicines/herbal/echinaceae-purpureae-herba (accessed on 14 August 2024).
45. Don't take echinacea if you're allergic to ragweed. *Consum. Rep.* **2012**, *77*, 12. [PubMed]
46. Pitsios, C.; Chliva, C.; Mikos, N.; Kompoti, E.; Nowak-Wegrzyn, A.; Kontou-Fili, K. Bee pollen sensitivity in airborne pollen allergic individuals. *Ann. Allergy Asthma Immunol.* **2006**, *97*, 703–706. [CrossRef]
47. Rottem, M.; Waisel, Y. Food allergy to concealed sunflower pollen. *Allergy* **1998**, *53*, 719–720. [CrossRef]
48. Erzsébet, D.; Kursinszki, L.; Kelemen, H.; Varga, E. Phytopharmacological review of bathurst burr (*Xanthium spinosum* L.). *Acta Pharm. Hung.* **2016**, *86*, 35–40. [CrossRef]
49. Weber, R.W. Goldenrod. *Ann. Allergy Asthma Immunol.* **2003**, *91*, A6. [CrossRef]
50. Weber, R.W. Cocklebur. *Ann. Allergy Asthma Immunol.* **2004**, *93*, A6. [CrossRef] [PubMed]
51. European Medicines Agency. Calendulae flos—Herbal Medicinal Product. Available online: www.ema.europa.eu/en/medicines/herbal/calendulae-flos (accessed on 14 August 2024).
52. Gol'dman, I.I. Anaphylactic shock after gargling with an infusion of Calendula. *Klin. Med.* **1974**, *52*, 142–143. [PubMed]
53. Popescu, F.D.; Vieru, M.; Ganea, C.S. Molecular allergy explorer test based on new state-of-the-art multiplex nano-bead technology in Asteraceae-hazelnut association. *Allergy* **2018**, *74*, 547.

54. Fernández, C.; Martín-Esteban, M.; Fiandor, A.; Pascual, C.; López Serrano, C.; Martínez Alzamora, F.; Díaz Pena, J.M.; Ojeda Casas, J.A. Analysis of cross-reactivity between sunflower pollen and other pollens of the Compositae family. *J. Allergy Clin. Immunol.* **1993**, *92*, 660–667. [CrossRef]
55. European Medicines Agency. Overview of Comments Received on 'Community Herbal Monograph on *Solidago virgaurea* L. Available online: www.ema.europa.eu/en/documents/herbal-comments/overview-comments-received-community-herbal-monograph-solidago-virgaurea-l-herba-emeahmpc2857582007_en.pdf (accessed on 14 August 2024).
56. Lee, Y.W.; Choi, S.Y.; Lee, E.K.; Sohn, J.H.; Park, J.W.; Hong, C.S. Cross-allergenicity of pollens from the Compositae family: Artemisia vulgaris, Dendranthema grandiflorum, and Taraxacum officinale. *Ann. Allergy Asthma Immunol.* **2007**, *99*, 526–533. [CrossRef]
57. European Medicines Agency. Community Herbal Monograph on Taraxacum Officinale Weber ex Wigg., radix cum herba. Available online: www.ema.europa.eu/en/documents/herbal-monograph/final-community-herbal-monograph-taraxacum-officinale-weber-ex-wigg-radix-cum-herba_en.pdf (accessed on 14 August 2024).
58. Achufusi, T.G.O.; Pellegrini, M.V.; Patel, R.K. *Milk Thistle. StatPearls [Internet]*; StatPearls Publishing: Treasure Island, FL, USA, 2024. [PubMed]
59. European Medicines Agency. Silybi Mariani Fructus—Herbal Medicinal Product. Available online: www.ema.europa.eu/%20en/medicines/herbal/silybi-mariani-fructus (accessed on 14 August 2024).
60. Bousquet, J.; Heinzerling, L.; Bachert, C.; Papadopoulos, N.G.; Bousquet, P.J.; Burney, P.G.; Canonica, G.W.; Carlsen, K.H.; Cox, L.; Haahtela, T.; et al. Practical guide to skin prick tests in allergy to aeroallergens. *Allergy* **2012**, *67*, 18–24. [CrossRef]
61. Heinzerling, L.; Mari, A.; Bergmann, K.C.; Bresciani, M.; Burbach, G.; Darsow, U.; Durham, S.; Fokkens, W.; Gjomarkaj, M.; Haahtela, T.; et al. The skin prick test—European standards. *Clin. Transl. Allergy* **2013**, *3*, 3. [CrossRef]
62. Liccardi, G.; Salzillo, A.; Spadaro, G.; Senna, G.; Canonica, W.G.; D'amato, G.; Passalacqua, G. Anaphylaxis caused by skin prick testing with aeroallergens: Case report and evaluation of the risk in Italian allergy services. *J. Allergy Clin. Immunol.* **2003**, *111*, 1410–1412. [CrossRef]
63. Lieberman, P. AAAAI Allergist Resources/Ask the Expert: Tea Allergy. 20 June 2021. Available online: www.aaaai.org/allergist-resources/ask-the-expert/answers/2021/tea-allergy (accessed on 16 August 2024).
64. Antunes, J.; Borrego, L.; Romeira, A.; Pinto, P. Skin prick tests and allergy diagnosis. *Allergol. Immunopathol.* **2009**, *37*, 155–164. [CrossRef]
65. Popescu, F.D. European standards and North American practice parameters for skin prick testing panels in allergic rhinitis and asthma. *Rom. J. Rhinol.* **2015**, *5*, 19–23. [CrossRef]
66. Heinzerling, L.; Frew, A.J.; Bindslev-Jensen, C.; Bonini, S.; Bousquet, J.; Bresciani, M.; Carlsen, K.H.; van Cauwenberge, P.; Darsow, U.; Fokkens, W.J.; et al. Standard skin prick testing and sensitization to inhalant allergens across Europe—A survey from the GA2LEN network. *Allergy* **2005**, *60*, 1287–1300. [CrossRef] [PubMed]
67. Paul-Ehrlich-Institut. Available online: www.pei.de/EN/medicinal-products/allergens/prick-test/prick-test-node.html (accessed on 20 August 2024).
68. Italian Medicines Agency. Available online: www.aifa.gov.it/documents/20142/1807239/Allegato-1_02.02.2023.pdf (accessed on 20 August 2024).
69. Stallergenes. Available online: www.stagrallergy.com/wp-content/uploads/2024/05/stagr-allergy-immunotherapy-catalog.pdf (accessed on 20 August 2024).
70. Lee, S.C.; Sim, D.W.; Lee, J.; Jeong, K.Y.; Park, K.H.; Lee, J.H.; Kim, J.D.; Park, J.W. Comparison between newly developed and commercial inhalant skin prick test reagents using in vivo and in vitro methods. *J. Korean Med. Sci.* **2018**, *33*, e101. [CrossRef]
71. Klimek, L.; Hoffmann, H.J.; Kalpaklioglu, A.F.; Demoly, P.; Agache, I.; Popov, T.A.; Muraro, A.; Schmid-Grendelmeier, P.; Bonini, S.; Bonertz, A.; et al. In-vivo diagnostic test allergens in Europe: A call to action and proposal for recovery plan—An EAACI position paper. *Allergy* **2020**, *75*, 2161–2169. [CrossRef] [PubMed]
72. Zimmer, J.; Mahler, V. Regulatory framework for development and marketing authorization of allergen products for diagnosis of rare type I and type IV allergies: The current status. *Allergol. Sel.* **2024**, *8*, 212–219. [CrossRef]
73. Florido-Lopez, J.F.; Gonzalez-Delgado, P.; Saenz de San Pedro, B.; Perez-Miranda, C.; Arias de Saavedra, J.M.; Marin-Pozo, J.F. Allergy to natural honeys and camomile tea. *Int. Arc Allergy Immunol.* **1995**, *108*, 170–174. [CrossRef] [PubMed]
74. Subiza, J.; Subiza, J.L.; Hinojosa, M.; Garcia, R.; Jerez, M.; Valdivieso, R.; Subiza, E. Anaphylactic reaction after the ingestion of chamomile tea: A study of cross-reactivity with other composite pollens. *J. Allergy Clin. Immunol.* **1989**, *84*, 353–358. [CrossRef]
75. Wahl, S.; Sator, P.G. Anaphylactic reaction to camomile tea. *Hautarzt* **2018**, *69*, 938–940. [CrossRef]
76. Jensen-Jarolim, E.; Reider, N.; Fritsch, R.; Breiteneder, H. Fatal outcome of anaphylaxis to camomile-containing enema during labor: A case study. *J. Allergy Clin. Immunol.* **1998**, *102*, 1041–1042. [CrossRef]
77. Vandenplas, O.; Pirson, F.; D'Alpaos, V.; Vander Borght, T.; Thimpont, J.; Pilette, C. Occupational asthma caused by chamomile. *Allergy* **2008**, *63*, 1090–1092. [CrossRef]
78. Okuhira, H.; Nakatani, Y.; Furukawa, F.; Kanazawa, N. Anaphylaxis to ginger induced by herbal medicine. *Allergol. Int.* **2020**, *69*, 159–160. [CrossRef]
79. Ansotegui, I.J.; Melioli, G.; Canonica, G.W.; Caraballo, L.; Villa, E.; Ebisawa, M.; Passalacqua, G.; Savi, E.; Ebo, D.; Gómez, R.M.; et al. IgE allergy diagnostics and other relevant tests in allergy: A World Allergy Organization position paper. *World Allergy Organ. J.* **2020**, *13*, 100080. [CrossRef]

80. Kappen, J.; Diamant, Z.; Agache, I.; Bonini, M.; Bousquet, J.; Canonica, G.W.; Durham, S.R.; Guibas, G.V.; Hamelmann, E.; Jutel, M.; et al. Standardization of clinical outcomes used in allergen immunotherapy in allergic asthma: An EAACI position paper. *Allergy* **2023**, *78*, 2835–2850. [CrossRef]
81. Fauquert, J.L.; Jedrzejczak-Czechowicz, M.; Rondon, C.; Calder, V.; Silva, D.; Kvenshagen, B.K.; Callebaut, I.; Allegri, P.; Santos, N.; Doan, S.; et al. Conjunctival allergen provocation test: Guidelines for daily practice. *Allergy* **2017**, *72*, 43–54. [CrossRef] [PubMed]
82. Agache, I.; Antolin-Amerigo, D.; de Blay, F.; Boccabella, C.; Caruso, C.; Chanez, P.; Couto, M.; Covar, R.; Doan, S.; Fauquert, J.L.; et al. EAACI position paper on the clinical use of the bronchial allergen challenge: Unmet needs and research priorities. *Allergy* **2022**, *77*, 1667–1684. [CrossRef] [PubMed]
83. Leti. Available online: https://leti.de/fachkreise-download-public/DE_FI_Provokationstest_LETI_02-22.pdf (accessed on 20 August 2024).
84. Klimek, L.; Hammerbacher, A.S.; Hellings, P.W.; Fokkens, W.J.; Hoffmann, H.J.; Muraro, A.; Papadopoulos, N. The influence of European legislation on the use of diagnostic test allergens for nasal allergen provocation in routine care of patients with allergic rhinitis. *Rhinology* **2015**, *53*, 260–269. [CrossRef] [PubMed]
85. Augé, J.; Vent, J.; Agache, I.; Airaksinen, L.; Campo Mozo, P.; Chaker, A.; Cingi, C.; Durham, S.; Fokkens, W.; Gevaert, P.; et al. EAACI Position paper on the standardization of nasal allergen challenges. *Allergy* **2018**, *73*, 1597–1608. [CrossRef]
86. Cho, S.H.; Nanda, A.; Keswani, A.; Adinoff, A.; Baroody, F.M.; Bernstein, J.A.; Gherasim, A.; Han, J.K.; Koepke, J.W.; Ledford, D.K.; et al. Nasal allergen challenge (NAC): Practical aspects and applications from an EU/US perspective—A Work Group Report of the AAAAI Rhinitis, Rhinosinusitis and Ocular Allergy Committee. *J. Allergy Clin. Immunol.* **2023**, *151*, 1215–1222.e4. [CrossRef]
87. Patel, P.; Holdich, T.; Fischer von Weikersthal-Drachenberg, K.J.; Huber, B. Efficacy of a short course of specific immunotherapy in patients with allergic rhinoconjunctivitis to ragweed pollen. *J. Allergy Clin. Immunol.* **2014**, *133*, 121–129.e2. [CrossRef]
88. Kosowska, A.; Zemelka-Wiącek, M.; Smolińska, S.; Wyrodek, E.; Adamczak, B.; Jutel, M. Clinical validation of grass pollen exposure chamber in patients with allergic rhinitis triggered by timothy grass. *Clin. Exp. Allergy* **2024**, *54*, 489–499. [CrossRef]
89. Pfaar, O.; Zieglmayer, P. Allergen exposure chambers: Implementation in clinical trials in allergen immunotherapy. *Clin. Transl. Allergy* **2020**, *10*, 33. [CrossRef]
90. Ellis, A.K.; Cook, V.; Keith, P.K.; Mace, S.R.; Moote, W.; O'Keefe, A.; Quirt, J.; Rosenfield, L.; Small, P.; Watson, W. Focused allergic rhinitis practice parameter for Canada. *Allergy Asthma Clin. Immunol.* **2024**, *20*, 45. [CrossRef] [PubMed]
91. Popescu, F.D.; Vieru, M. Precision medicine allergy immunoassay methods for assessing immunoglobulin E sensitization to aeroallergen molecules. *World J. Methodol.* **2018**, *8*, 17–36. [CrossRef] [PubMed]
92. Mullins, R.J. Echinacea-associated anaphylaxis. *Med. J. Aust.* **1998**, *168*, 170–171. [CrossRef] [PubMed]
93. Thermo Fisher Scientifin. Immunodiagnostics Product Catalog 2024. Available online: www.abacusdx.com/media/PU_ProductCatalogue_2024.pdf (accessed on 20 August 2024).
94. Macro Array Diagnostics. ALEX2® Allergen List. Available online: https://macroarraydx.com.ua/downloads/%20alex2_allergen_list_en.pdf (accessed on 20 August 2024).
95. Siemens Healthcare. Allergy Menu. Available online: https://marketing.webassets.siemens-healthineers.com/667ff707799b2896/6da8b9913b44/30-21-DX-999-76_IMMULITE-Allergy_Menu_FINAL.pdf (accessed on 20 August 2024).
96. Preda, M.; Popescu, F.D.; Vassilopoulou, E.; Smolinska, S. Allergenic biomarkers in the molecular diagnosis of IgE-mediated wheat allergy. *Int. J. Mol. Sci.* **2024**, *25*, 8210. [CrossRef]
97. Wang, C.; Bao, Y.; Chen, J.; Chen, X.; Cheng, L.; Guo, Y.S.; Hao, C.; Lai, H.; Li, H.; Li, J.; et al. Chinese guideline on allergen immunotherapy for allergic rhinitis: The 2022 update. *Allergy Asthma Immunol. Res.* **2022**, *14*, 604–652. [CrossRef]
98. Euroimmun. Euroline Allergy—Efficient Multiparameter Profiles. Available online: www.euroimmun.com/%20documents/Indications/Allergology/Multiplex-immunoblots/Euroline/DP_3000_I_UK_D.pdf (accessed on 14 August 2024).
99. Dramburg, S.; Grittner, U.; Potapova, E.; Travaglini, A.; Tripodi, S.; Arasi, S.; Pelosi, S.; Acar Şahin, A.; Aggelidis, X.; Barbalace, A.; et al. Heterogeneity of sensitization profiles and clinical phenotypes among patients with seasonal allergic rhinitis in Southern European countries—The @IT.2020 multicenter study. *Allergy* **2024**, *79*, 908–923. [CrossRef]
100. Buzan, M.R.; Grijincu, M.; Zbîrcea, L.E.; Haidar, L.; Tamaș, T.P.; Cotarcă, M.D.; Tănasie, G.; Weber, M.; Babaev, E.; Stolz, F.; et al. Insect Cell-Expressed Major Ragweed Allergen Amb a 1.01 Exhibits Similar Allergenic Properties to Its Natural Counterpart from Common Ragweed Pollen. *Int. J. Mol. Sci.* **2024**, *25*, 5175. [CrossRef]
101. Zbîrcea, L.E.; Buzan, M.R.; Grijincu, M.; Cotarcă, M.D.; Tamaș, T.P.; Haidar, L.; Tănasie, G.; Huțu, I.; Babaev, E.; Stolz, F.; et al. Heterogenous Induction of Blocking Antibodies against Ragweed Allergen Molecules by Allergen Extract-Based Immunotherapy Vaccines. *Vaccines* **2024**, *12*, 635. [CrossRef] [PubMed]
102. Tamaș, T.P.; Buzan, M.R.; Zbîrcea, L.E.; Cotarcă, M.D.; Grijincu, M.; Păunescu, V.; Panaitescu, C.; Chen, K.W. Ragweed Major Allergen Amb a 11 Recombinant Production and Clinical Implications. *Biomolecules* **2023**, *13*, 182. [CrossRef]
103. Pablos, I.; Eichhorn, S.; Machado, Y.; Briza, P.; Neunkirchner, A.; Jahn-Schmid, B.; Wildner, S.; Soh, W.T.; Ebner, C.; Park, J.W.; et al. Distinct Epitope Structures of Defensin-Like Proteins Linked to Proline-Rich Regions Give Rise to Differences in Their Allergenic Activity. *Allergy* **2018**, *73*, 431–441. [CrossRef]
104. Grijincu, M.; Tănasie, G.; Zbîrcea, L.E.; Buzan, M.R.; Tamaș, T.P.; Cotarcă, M.D.; Huțu, I.; Babaev, E.; Stolz, F.; Dorofeeva, Y.; et al. Non-Specific Lipid Transfer Protein Amb a 6 Is a Source-Specific Important Allergenic Molecule in Ragweed Pollen. *Int. J. Mol. Sci.* **2024**, *25*, 6513. [CrossRef]

105. Cosi, V.; Gadermaier, G. The Role of Defensins as Pollen and Food Allergens. *Curr. Allergy Asthma Rep.* **2023**, *23*, 277–285. [CrossRef] [PubMed]
106. WHO/IUIS Allergen Nomenclature Sub-Committee: Allergen Nomenclature. IUIS Database. Available online: www.allergen.org (accessed on 8 August 2024).
107. Himly, M.; Jahn-Schmid, B.; Dedic, A.; Kelemen, P.; Wopfner, N.; Altmann, F.; van Ree, R.; Briza, P.; Richter, K.; Ebner, C.; et al. Art v 1, the major allergen of mugwort pollen, is a modular glycoprotein with a defensin-like and a hydroxyproline-rich domain. *FASEB J.* **2003**, *17*, 106–108. [CrossRef] [PubMed]
108. Gao, Z.; Fu, W.Y.; Sun, Y.; Gao, B.; Wang, H.Y.; Liu, M.; Luo, F.M.; Zhou, X.; Jin, J.; Zhao, L.; et al. Artemisia pollen allergy in China: Component-resolved diagnosis reveals allergic asthma patients have significant multiple allergen sensitization. *Allergy* **2019**, *74*, 284–293. [CrossRef]
109. Asero, R.; Bellotto, E.; Ghiani, A.; Aina, R.; Villalta, D.; Citterio, S. Concomitant sensitization to ragweed and mugwort pollen: Who is who in clinical allergy? *Ann. Allergy Asthma Immunol.* **2014**, *113*, 307–313. [CrossRef]
110. Gadermaier, G.; Harrer, A.; Girbl, T.; Palazzo, P.; Himly, M.; Vogel, L.; Briza, P.; Mari, A.; Ferreira, F. Isoform identification and characterization of Art v 3, the lipid-transfer protein of mugwort pollen. *Mol. Immunol.* **2009**, *46*, 1919–1924. [CrossRef] [PubMed]
111. Popescu, F.D.; Vieru, M. Polcalcins as Pollen Panallergens in Allergic Rhinitis. *Rom. J. Rhinol.* **2016**, *6*, 19–22. [CrossRef]
112. Oberhuber, C.; Ma, Y.; Wopfner, N.; Gadermaier, G.; Dedic, A.; Niggemann, B.; Maderegger, B.; Gruber, P.; Ferreira, F.; Scheiner, O.; et al. Prevalence of IgE-Binding to Art v 1, Art v 4, and Amb a 1 in Mugwort-Allergic Patients. *Int. Arch. Allergy Immunol.* **2008**, *145*, 94–101. [CrossRef]
113. Kleine-Tebbe, J.; Ackermann-Simon, J.; Hanf, G. Molecular Allergy Diagnosis Using Pollen Marker Allergens and Pollen Panallergens: Five Patterns Seen in Multiple Test Reactions to Pollen Extracts. *Allergol. Sel.* **2021**, *5*, 180–186. [CrossRef]
114. Potapova, E.; Tripodi, S.; Panetta, V.; Dramburg, S.; Bernardini, R.; Caffarelli, C.; Casani, A.; Cervone, R.; Chini, L.; Comberiati, P.; et al. IgE to Cross-Reactive Carbohydrate Determinants (CCD) in Childhood: Prevalence, Risk Factors, Putative Origins. *Clin. Exp. Allergy* **2024**, *54*, 195–206. [CrossRef]
115. Popescu, F.D. Molecular Biomarkers for Grass Pollen Immunotherapy. *World J. Methodol.* **2014**, *4*, 26–45. [CrossRef] [PubMed]
116. Gelardi, M.; Guglielmi, A.V.; Iannuzzi, L.; Quaranta, V.N.; Quaranta, N.; Landi, M.; Correale, M.; Sonnante, A.; Rossini, M.; Mariggiò, M.A.; et al. Local Allergic Rhinitis: Entopy or Spontaneous Response? *World Allergy Organ. J.* **2016**, *9*, 39. [CrossRef]
117. Mortada, M.M.; Kurowski, M. Challenges in Local Allergic Rhinitis Diagnosis, Management, and Research: Current Concepts and Future Perspectives. *Medicina* **2023**, *59*, 929. [CrossRef]
118. Campo, P.; Canonica, G.W. Local Allergic Rhinitis. *J. Allergy Clin. Immunol. Pr.* **2024**, *12*, 1430–1433. [CrossRef]
119. Krajewska-Wotys, A.; Jarzab, J.; Gawlik, R.; Bozek, A. Local Allergic Rhinitis to Pollens Is Underdiagnosed in Young Patients. *Am. J. Rhinol. Allergy* **2016**, *30*, 198–201. [CrossRef]
120. Meng, Y.; Wang, Y.; Lou, H.; Wang, K.; Meng, N.; Zhang, L.; Wang, C. Specific Immunoglobulin E in Nasal Secretions for the Diagnosis of Local Allergic Rhinitis. *Rhinology* **2019**, *57*, 313–320. [CrossRef] [PubMed]
121. Johansson, S.G.O.; Lilja, G.; Hallberg, J.; Nopp, A. A Clinical Follow-Up of Omalizumab in Routine Treatment of Allergic Asthma Monitored by CD-sens. *Immun. Inflamm. Dis.* **2018**, *6*, 382–391. [CrossRef]
122. Ebo, D.G.; Bridts, C.H.; Mertens, C.H.; Sabato, V. Principles, Potential, and Limitations of Ex Vivo Basophil Activation by Flow Cytometry in Allergology: A Narrative Review. *J. Allergy Clin. Immunol.* **2021**, *147*, 1143–1153. [CrossRef] [PubMed]
123. Kim, S.H.; Kim, S.H.; Chung, S.J.; Kim, J.H.; Lee, S.Y.; Kim, B.K.; Lim, K.W.; Chang, Y.S. Changes in Basophil Activation During Immunotherapy with House Dust Mite and Mugwort in Patients with Allergic Rhinitis. *Asia Pac. Allergy* **2018**, *8*, e6. [CrossRef]
124. Deng, S.; Yin, J. Clinical Utility of Basophil Activation Test in Diagnosis and Predicting Severity of Mugwort Pollen-Related Peach Allergy. *World Allergy Organ J.* **2019**, *12*, 100043. [CrossRef]
125. Kawahara, T.; Yamaguchi, M.; Onitsuka, C.; Kimura, T.; Homma, T.; Sagara, H. Utility of Basophil Activation Test in a Case of Daisaikoto- and Yokukansan-induced Lung Injury. *Intern. Med.* **2021**, *60*, 1573–1576. [CrossRef] [PubMed]
126. Sharma, E.; Vitte, J. A systematic review of allergen cross-reactivity: Translating basic concepts into clinical relevance. *J. Allergy Clin. Immunol. Glob.* **2024**, *3*, 100230. [CrossRef] [PubMed] [PubMed Central]
127. Kovaleva, V.; Bukhteeva, I.; Kit, O.Y.; Nesmelova, I.V. Plant Defensins from a Structural Perspective. *Int. J. Mol. Sci.* **2020**, *21*, 5307. [CrossRef] [PubMed]
128. Jha, D.K.; Dhekne, P.; Patwardhan, A.W. Characterization and evaluation of tea bag papers. *J. Food Sci. Technol.* **2020**, *7*, 3060–3070. [CrossRef]
129. Ageitos, J.M.; Robla, S.; Valverde-Fraga, L.; Garcia-Fuentes, M.; Csaba, N. Purification of Hollow Sporopollenin Microcapsules from Sunflower and Chamomile Pollen Grains. *Polymers* **2021**, *13*, 2094. [CrossRef]

medicina MDPI

Case Report

Eosinophilic Pneumonia Triggered by *Toxocara canis* in a Patient with Primary Ciliary Dyskinesia: A Clinical Case Report

Kacper Packi [1,2,3,*], Wanda Fugiel [2], Violetta Gołąbek [2], Alicja Rudek [2] and Agnieszka Śliwińska [1]

1 Department of Nucleic Acid Biochemistry, Medical University of Lodz, 92-213 Lodz, Poland; agnieszka.sliwinska@umed.lodz.pl
2 AllerGen Center of Personalized Medicine, 97-300 Piotrkow Trybunalski, Poland; wanda.jank@gmail.com (W.F.) alicjarudek@o2.pl (A.R.)
3 Wladyslaw Bieganski Collegium Medicum, Jan Dlugosz University in Czestochowa, 42-200 Czestochowa, Poland
* Correspondence: kacperpacki1@wp.pl

Abstract: Primary ciliary dyskinesia (PCD) is a rare genetic disorder that affects the structure and function of cilia, primarily impacting the respiratory system. Kartagener syndrome, a subset of PCD, is characterized by situs inversus, bronchiectasis, and chronic sinusitis. Patients with PCD are prone to recurrent respiratory infections due to impaired ciliary function, which hinders effective mucus clearance and promotes pathogen colonization. This case report describes a 24-year-old woman with congenital Kartagener syndrome who developed eosinophilic pneumonia caused by *Toxocara canis*, a rare parasitic infection that less commonly affects the lungs. Despite initial treatment for a presumed bacterial infection, the patient's symptoms persisted. Further diagnostics revealed elevated eosinophil counts, total IgE, and the presence of *Toxocara canis* antibodies. The patient was treated with albendazole, resulting in significant symptom improvement and a reduction in inflammatory markers. This case underscores the diagnostic challenges in treating PCD patients, where atypical infections must be considered, particularly when standard treatments prove ineffective. The complexity of the patient's condition required interdisciplinary management, integrating parasitological, immunological, and respiratory expertise to ensure appropriate treatment. The case highlights the need for further research into the interactions between congenital respiratory disorders such as Kartagener syndrome and parasitic infections. It also emphasizes the importance of a comprehensive diagnostic approach in managing rare genetic diseases complicated by opportunistic infections. Early detection of parasitic infections in PCD patients is crucial to preventing severe complications, and this case reinforces the necessity of considering parasitic causes in atypical pneumonia cases.

Keywords: eosinophilic pneumonia; *Toxocara canis*; Kartagener syndrome; dyskinesia

1. Introduction

Primary ciliary dyskinesia (PCD) is a rare, genetically conditioned disease affecting 1 in 10,000 to 20,000 live births, depending on the studied population [1]. In Europe and North America, the incidence of PCD varies depending on genetic background and demographic factors. This disease is characterized by the abnormal structure and/or function of cilia, leading to a range of disorders in the body, particularly in the respiratory system (Figure 1). Kartagener syndrome, which accounts for about 50% of all PCD cases, is distinguished by a characteristic triad of symptoms: situs inversus, bronchiectasis, and chronic sinusitis [2].

Cilia, microscopic hair-like structures, line the cells of the respiratory tract and play a key role in the mechanical defense of the respiratory system. Under physiological conditions, their coordinated movement enables the efficient clearance of the airways by transporting mucus along with impurities toward the throat. Disturbances in ciliary movement or a complete lack thereof, observed in PCD, lead to mucus accumulation, significantly increasing the risk of recurrent infections and inflammation [3] (Figure 2). The impaired function of cilia in PCD has far-reaching consequences for the respiratory system. Impaired airway clearance promotes colonization by pathogens, primarily bacteria but also viruses and fungi. The accumulated mucus becomes an excellent medium for microorganisms, leading to chronic and recurrent infections [4]. Furthermore, the accumulation of impurities and cellular debris can trigger and sustain inflammation, contributing to progressive lung tissue damage. Moreover, ciliary movement disorders can affect the local immune response. Studies suggest that cilia play a role in regulating immune responses, and their dysfunction may lead to abnormalities in the body's defense reactions [5]. This, in turn, can further increase susceptibility to infections and complicate the course of the disease.

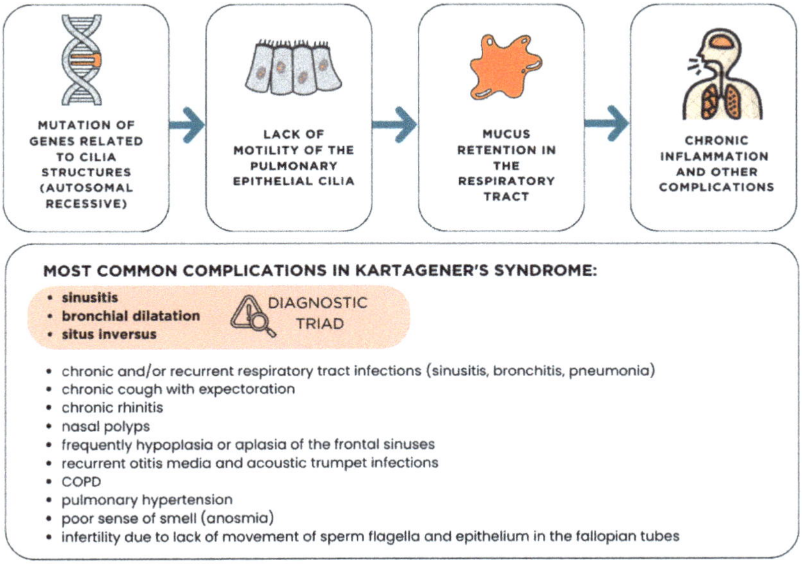

Figure 1. Etiology and complications of Kartagener's syndrome.

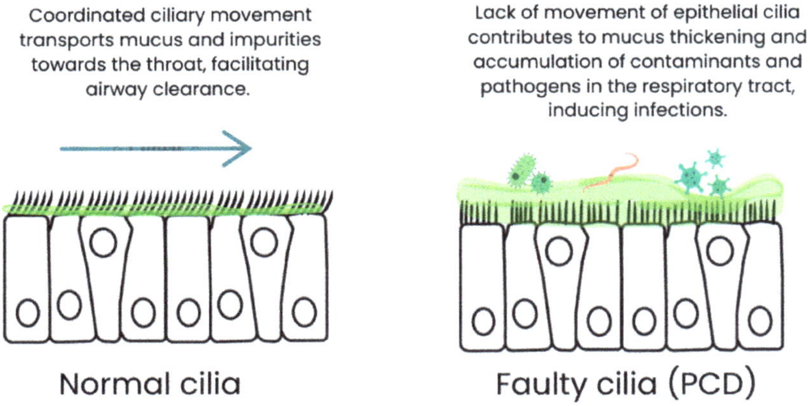

Figure 2. The role of epithelial ciliary movement in airway clearance.

In the context of PCD, infections caused by pathogens that typically rarely affect the lungs are particularly interesting. In individuals with PCD, micro- and macroorganisms such as parasites, which are normally efficiently eliminated from the respiratory tract, can more easily penetrate, accumulate, and multiply in lung tissue. The increased susceptibility to atypical lung infections in PCD patients poses an additional diagnostic and therapeutic challenge for clinicians. Overlapping symptoms and the need for differential diagnosis require advanced diagnostic techniques, as standard therapies may prove ineffective against infections unresponsive to conventional treatments [6].

One of these rare pathogens is *Toxocara canis*, a parasite commonly found in dogs that can infect humans through oral transmission, leading to visceral larva migrans. While toxocariasis most commonly affects the liver and eyes, it can also manifest in the lungs, causing eosinophilic pneumonia [7]. Documented cases of eosinophilic pneumonia due to *Toxocara canis* are rare, and statistical data on incidence remain limited. The few documented cases emphasize the complexity of diagnosing this condition, particularly in immunocompetent patients [8,9].

This publication presents a unique case of a 24-year-old woman with congenital Kartagener syndrome who was diagnosed with eosinophilic pneumonia caused by *Toxocara canis* infection. This is the first case reported in the literature of pulmonary toxocariasis in a patient with primary ciliary dyskinesia. This case not only illustrates the complexity of the health problems that PCD patients may face but also highlights the necessity of considering atypical pathogens in the differential diagnosis of lung infections in these patients.

2. Case Presentation

A 24-year-old patient with Kartagener syndrome was admitted to the hospital with symptoms of fluid in the right pleural cavity, confirmed by ultrasound examination. Her medical history included the removal of a middle lobe of the left lung, surgery for hydronephrosis of the right kidney, situs inversus (resulting in a 3-lobe left lung and a 2-lobe right lung), arterial hypertension, and two previous infections with *Toxocara canis*. A week earlier, the patient had completed a two-week hospitalization due to hypertension and chest pain. At that time, due to elevated CRP and signs of a urinary tract infection (UTI), she was treated with amoxicillin and clavulanic acid. Despite the treatment, her symptoms did not resolve, and tests showed persistent eosinophilia. The patient regularly attends specialist check-ups and occasionally requires antibiotic therapy. During the current hospitalization, three pleural punctures were performed. Due to persistent eosinophilia and elevated IgE levels, parasitological diagnostics were conducted, which confirmed *Toxocara canis* infection. Treatment with albendazole was initiated (Figure 3). This case highlights the importance of extended diagnostics in patients with Kartagener syndrome, particularly in cases of atypical infections or lack of response to standard treatment.

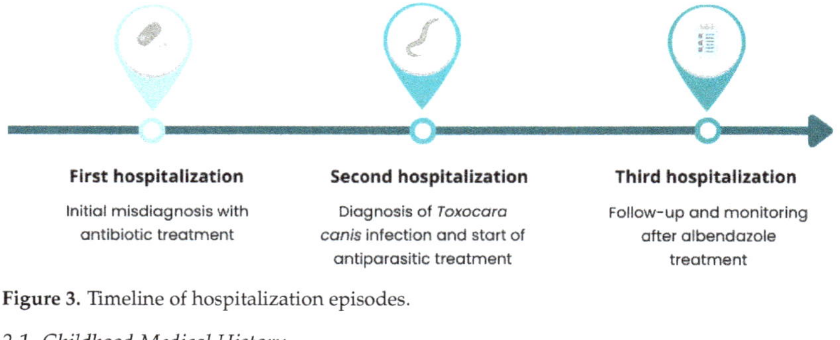

Figure 3. Timeline of hospitalization episodes.

2.1. Childhood Medical History

The patient was born at 37 weeks of gestation with a birth weight of 3400 g and an Apgar score of 9. The mother's pregnancy was complicated by gestational diabetes and a cytomegalovirus infection. Situs inversus was diagnosed on the third day of life during a hospital stay for a congenital infection. This condition also involved pulmonary inversion, with the patient having a 3-lobe left lung and a 2-lobe right lung. The infantile period was marked by recurrent respiratory infections, resulting in multiple hospitalizations. The patient was diagnosed with Kartagener syndrome at 5 months of age during hospitalization for pneumonia caused by *Pseudomonas aeruginosa*. A bronchoscopy at the time revealed immobile cilia, reversed bronchial tree arrangement, and abundant mucus secretion. In subsequent years, the girl's condition remained stable, with only mild infections occurring. Recurrent pneumonias began to appear during adolescence. At the age of 14, the patient was hospitalized due to prolonged pneumonia. At that time, an infection with *Mycoplasma pneumoniae* was diagnosed, along with coexisting parasitic infections caused by *Toxocara canis* and *Ascaris lumbricoides*. During this hospitalization, cirrhotic changes in the middle lobe of the left lung were found, which resulted in the need for a middle lobectomy that same year. Reinfection with *Toxocara canis* and *Ascaris lumbricoides* was diagnosed less than 2 years later when the patient presented with symptoms of exudative pleuritis. An ultrasound of the pleural cavity revealed the presence of 150 mL of free fluid in the left pleural cavity. Additionally, hydronephrosis of the right kidney was noted, which had been operated on when the patient was 15 years old.

2.2. *First Episode of Hospitalization—Misdiagnosis*

Further health problems reappeared at the age of 24, when recurrent respiratory infections occurred again, along with arterial hypertension. As a result, the woman presented to the hospital, where a chest X-ray and an ultrasound of the pleural cavity were performed, confirming the presence of fluid in the right pleural cavity (up to a width of 55 mm), reaching the ninth rib (Appendix B). The patient also reported a persistent cough and stabbing pain in the right side of the chest, radiating to the back and worsening with deep breaths. The maximum blood pressure readings were 180/120 mmHg. A series of laboratory tests were conducted, including a bacterial urine culture. A general urinalysis revealed the presence of numerous bacteria in the urine sediment. The CRP concentration in the serum initially measured 39.45 mg/L (immunoturbidimetric test, Integra 400 plus). Based on the diagnostic X-ray and ultrasound results, as well as the elevated CRP levels and signs of a urinary tract infection (UTI) in the urine, a decision was made to administer antibacterial treatment with amoxicillin and clavulanic acid in the form of injections, 1000 mg + 200 mg, 5 vials (1 vial per day). This decision was made without receiving the results of the bacterial culture. Despite the lack of significant improvement in the patient's condition, elevated blood parameters (including eosinophilia, 1.15 K/µL), and the absence of follow-up diagnostic tests for the presence of fluid in the pleural cavity, the patient was discharged home. The patient was instructed to continue antibiotic therapy in the form of coated amoxicillin and clavulanic acid tablets, 1000 mg (875 mg + 125 mg) once daily for the next 5 days. Additionally, probiotic support with Enterol (*Saccharomyces boulardii*) was prescribed, as well as antihypertensive medications (amlodipine 10 mg once daily, methyldopa 250 mg three times daily, indapamide 1.5 mg once daily, nebivolol 5 mg once daily).

2.3. *Second Episode of Hospitalization—Diagnosis of Toxocara canis Infection*

Due to worsening cough, shortness of breath, and a general decline in her health, the patient was readmitted to the hospital seven days after being discharged. Two anaerobic bacteriological cultures of pleural fluid were performed, and after five days of incubation, no microorganisms were grown. Ultrasound of the pleural cavity confirmed a persistent significant amount of fluid (up to 45 mm in width) in the right pleural cavity. Additionally, a non-contrast chest CT scan was performed (Figure 4), which also revealed the presence of fluid in the right pleural cavity (up to 40 mm) (Appendix B). Consolidated band-like opacities were observed in the lower lobe of the right lung, above the fluid, which was consistent with atelectasis and residual inflammatory changes. Situs inversus of the viscera and heart was also confirmed. Laboratory tests showed persistently elevated CRP levels (25.18 mg/L) and eosinophil counts (1.58 K/μL, 18%, reference value: 0.1–0.5 K/μL, 1–5%), along with a high concentration of total IgE (111.0 IU/mL, electrochemiluminescence method, Cobas). It should be noted that the eosinophil count was even higher than during the patient's first hospital stay. Due to the elevated eosinophil and total IgE levels, tests for parasitic infections were conducted. Stool parasitology did not reveal the presence of gastrointestinal parasites. An ELISA serological test (NovaTec) for *Toxocara canis* IgG antibodies was performed, and the serum showed an elevated sIgG concentration for *Toxocara canis* (16.83 NTU), indicating infection with this canine roundworm. The correlation between elevated blood parameters (*Toxocara canis* sIgG, total IgE, and eosinophils) and abnormalities observed in lung and pleural X-ray imaging led to the correct diagnosis: pleural effusion, not elsewhere classified (ICD-10 code: J90), associated with Löffler's syndrome (eosinophilic pneumonia caused by toxocariasis). The patient was treated with albendazole, an antiparasitic medication, at a dose of 400 mg/20 mL in the form of an oral suspension. During hospitalization, the patient received three doses of albendazole (once daily). She was discharged with an initial good tolerance of the treatment, with instructions to continue antiparasitic therapy for four more days (400 mg/20 mL albendazole, every morning) and to maintain her antihypertensive regimen as per the initial discharge instructions.

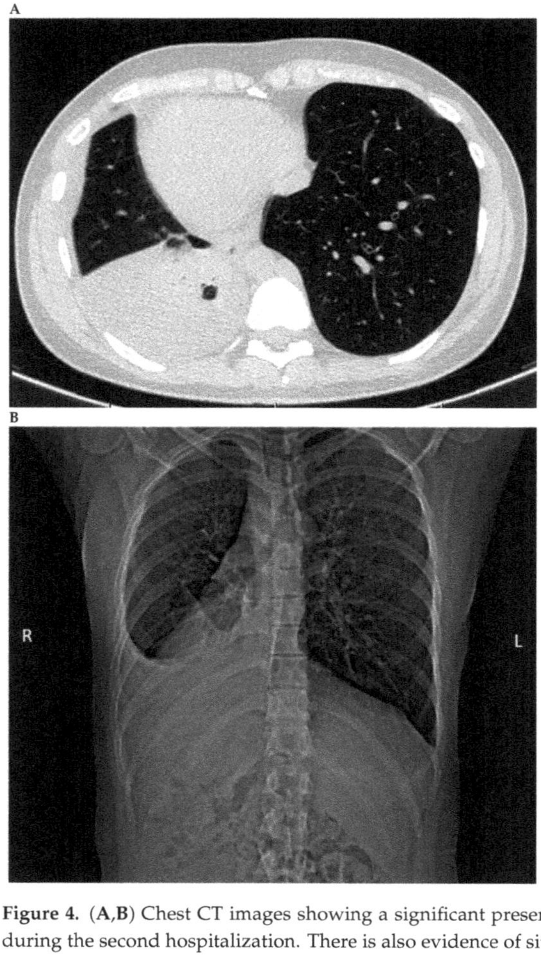

Figure 4. (**A**,**B**) Chest CT images showing a significant presence of fluid in the right lung, taken during the second hospitalization. There is also evidence of situs inversus in the patient (detailed description in Appendix B).

2.4. Third Episode of Hospitalization—Control of the Effects of Antiparasitic Treatment

Two months after the diagnosis and initiation of albendazole treatment, follow-up biochemical parameters and a chest X-ray were performed. No pleural fluid was detected (Appendix B). A decrease in eosinophil count (0.6%), CRP levels (4.63 mg/L), and *Toxocara canis* IgG antibodies (9.1 NTU) was observed (Table 1, Figure 5). All laboratory results from the three consecutive hospitalizations are summarized in Appendix A. Blood pressure readings were normal, averaging 110/75 mmHg. The patient was referred to an infectious diseases clinic for ongoing care and, in good condition, was discharged with the recommendation to continue antihypertensive medication as per the initial discharge plan. Currently, the symptoms of acute pneumonia have resolved, indicating effective antiparasitic therapy for *Toxocara canis*-induced pneumonia (Löffler's syndrome) in the patient, who also has Kartagener syndrome.

Table 1. Presentation of key laboratory parameters indicative of toxocariasis before and after appropriate therapy.

Laboratory Findings	First Hospitalization—Misdiagnosis	Second Hospitalization—*Toxocara canis* Detection	Third Hospitalization—Control of Treatment	Reference Interval
Eosinophils	1.15 (15.4)	1.58 (18.0)	0.06 (0.6)	0.1–0.5 K/μL (1–5%)
CRP	14.13	25.18	4.63	0–5 mg/L
IgE total	-	111.0	9.7	0–100 IU/mL
Toxocara canis IgG	-	16.83	9.1	>9 NTU negative 9–11 inconclusive <11 positive

increased parameter, decreased parameter.

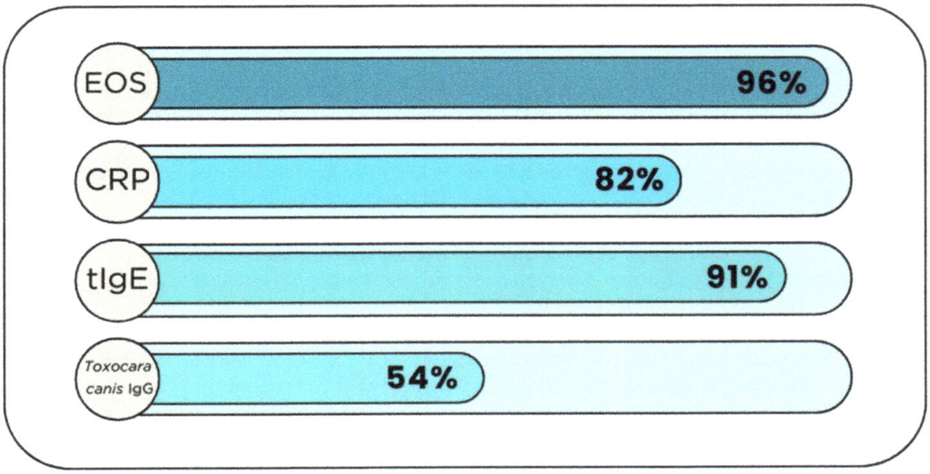

Figure 5. Percentage decrease in inflammatory and parasitic parameters after albendazole treatment (EOS—eosinophils, CRP—C-Reactive Protein, tIgE—total IgE).

3. Discussion

The clinical case of our patient demonstrates a rare combination of *Toxocara canis* infection with Kartagener syndrome, leading to eosinophilic pneumonia. This atypical clinical manifestation requires a detailed analysis of the interaction between toxocariasis pathogenesis, and the disorders related to Kartagener syndrome, in the context of current scientific and epidemiological knowledge.

Toxocariasis is a relatively common zoonotic parasitic disease. It is estimated that the seroprevalence of *Toxocara* spp. infections in Europe is 11%, while in Poland, this rate reaches 16%. Additionally, approximately 20% of Polish soils are contaminated *with Toxocara* spp. eggs [10]. Despite its prevalence, the manifestation of toxocariasis as pneumonia is rare. Typically, hepato- and splenomegaly, neurotoxocariasis, and ocular toxocariasis are observed [11]. A search of the PubMed database yielded only nine case studies (from 1994 to 2024) describing pneumonia cases caused by *Toxocara canis* (keywords: pneumonia, *Toxocara canis*, case study). This makes the described case particularly interesting from a clinical, diagnostic, and scientific perspective.

The key diagnostic parameters were:

- High antibody titer against *Toxocara canis* (1:800);
- Significant eosinophilia (18% in the peripheral blood smear);
- Elevated total IgE levels;
- Characteristic chest X-ray changes.

The primary parameter identifying *Toxocara canis* infection is the detection of sIgG antibodies. However, due to the long circulation of specific antibodies and possible cross-reactions with other nematodes, it is also recommended to assess eosinophil and total IgE levels to detect active infection. The correlation between *Toxocara canis* infection and elevated total IgE and eosinophil levels has been confirmed in many scientific studies [12,13].

The increase in eosinophil levels in alveoli and lung interstitial tissue is a common marker of the heterogeneous group of diseases known as eosinophilic pneumonias [14]. Eosinophilic pneumonia can occur as a result of autoimmune, neoplastic, or inflammatory diseases, certain medications, and parasitic infections [15]. In this case, eosinophilia (1.15–1.58 K/μL) fell within the mild (0.5 to 1.5 K/μL) to moderate (1.5–5.0 K/μL) range, which is typical for parasitic infections [16]. This increase in eosinophils, along with elevated total IgE levels, reflects the body's specific immune response to the presence of *Toxocara* larvae. These observations align with studies by Magnaval et al. [17] and Fillaux and Magnaval [18], who emphasized the importance of these parameters in diagnosing toxocariasis.

The pathogenic mechanism in this case can be classified as Löffler's syndrome, an eosinophilic pneumonia resulting from the trans-pulmonary migration of *Toxocara* larvae. This process involves the migration of larvae to lung tissue, a local inflammatory response with eosinophil infiltration, mast cell activation, the release of inflammatory mediators, and IgE antibody production leading to mast cell degranulation [19,20]. These immunological processes, as described in detail by Pinelli et al. [21], combined with the impaired ciliary function characteristic of Kartagener syndrome, led to an intensified inflammatory response in the patient's lungs. Kartagener syndrome, a rare autosomal recessive genetic disorder, played a key role in the progression of the infection. The characteristic triad of Kartagener syndrome involving situs inversus, bronchiectasis, and chronic sinusitis, created favorable conditions for parasite colonization and dissemination in the patient's lungs [22]. The dysfunction of respiratory cilia, typical of Kartagener syndrome, likely facilitated the settlement of *Toxocara canis* larvae in lung tissue, a phenomenon that is usually rare. Notably, bronchiectasis and chronic inflammation, present in Kartagener syndrome, may have created particularly conducive conditions for the development of *Toxocara* infection, leading to more severe eosinophilic pneumonia than typically observed in toxocariasis cases. This observation is consistent with the studies by Bede et al., who demonstrated increased susceptibility to infections in patients with primary ciliary dyskinesia [23]. While PCD itself does not increase susceptibility to *Toxocara canis* infection through an immunodeficiency mechanism, the impaired mucociliary clearance characteristic of PCD can exacerbate the severity of respiratory symptoms if such an infection occurs. Specifically, the reduced capacity to effectively clear mucus and pathogens from the respiratory tract in PCD patients allows parasites like *Toxocara canis* to persist longer within lung tissue, creating an environment that may intensify the local inflammatory response [24]. This prolonged presence of pathogens due to compromised airway clearance means that, although PCD patients do not face an elevated risk of acquiring *Toxocara canis*, they may experience a more severe progression of respiratory symptoms and inflammation once the infection is established.

The uniqueness of our case warrants comparison with existing literature, although documented cases of pulmonary toxocariasis in patients with primary ciliary dyskinesia (PCD) are exceptionally rare, limiting comprehensive comparative analysis. While pulmonary toxocariasis has been reported in various respiratory conditions, the combination with PCD represents a notably unusual clinical scenario [25,26]. Our observations suggest that while PCD may not increase susceptibility to Toxocara infection per se, the pre-existing impairment of mucociliary clearance can substantially amplify respiratory manifestations. This finding aligns with research by Ranasuriya et al. (2016), who documented atypical presentations of pulmonary toxocariasis in immunocompromised patients, highlighting how underlying conditions can modify disease expression [27]. Interestingly, contrary to Gonzalez-Quintela et al. [28], we observed no significant spirometric changes attributable to Toxocara infection, potentially due to the overshadowing effects of Kartagener syndrome on pulmonary function parameters.

A noteworthy aspect of our case was the elevation in hepatic enzymes (ALT, AST) following therapeutic intervention with albendazole. This observation adds to the existing literature documenting transient hepatic enzyme elevation during albendazole treatment [29]. While the precise mechanisms of albendazole-induced liver function alterations remain incompletely understood, current evidence suggests these changes are typically transient, with normalization expected post-treatment [29]. This emphasizes the importance of systematic liver function monitoring throughout the therapeutic course.

In addressing the Toxocara canis-induced eosinophilic pneumonia in our patient, albendazole was selected as the primary therapeutic agent based on its established antiparasitic efficacy. The observed clinical improvement and reduction in inflammatory markers validated this therapeutic choice. For cases presenting with severe inflammatory responses, particularly in the context of PCD where compromised airway clearance may intensify inflammation, a dual therapeutic approach incorporating both antiparasitic treatment and anti-inflammatory measures may be optimal. The potential benefit of adjunctive corticosteroid therapy in such cases, supported by the current literature [30,31], lies in its ability to modulate the inflammatory response while albendazole addresses the underlying parasitic infection. This comprehensive treatment strategy may be particularly valuable in complex cases where both infection control and inflammation management are crucial for optimal outcomes.

It is also worth noting that antibiotic therapy was initially administered, which is the most common approach to treating pneumonia. Bacteria, particularly *Streptococcus pneumoniae*, are responsible for the majority of pneumonia cases. Before the widespread use of antibiotics, *Streptococcus pneumoniae* was responsible for 95% of pneumonia cases [32]. Although bacterial causes are still the most common (24% of bacterial pneumonias in Europe), the etiology of acute pneumonia remains unidentified in about 60% of cases [33]. In this case, despite elevated eosinophil levels, which often indicate an allergic or parasitic infection, antibiotic therapy was also administered, but it did not yield the expected results (Figure 6). This situation underscores the importance of thorough differential diagnosis in cases of atypical pneumonia, especially in patients with rare genetic syndromes.

Potential long-term consequences of this case should also be considered. Kartagener syndrome itself predisposes patients to recurrent respiratory infections and may lead to permanent lung damage [34]. The superimposition of *Toxocara canis* infection may have accelerated these processes. Therefore, the patient will require special care and monitoring in the future. For patients diagnosed with PCD, preventive measures include maintaining rigorous hygiene practices, routine check-ups, relevant physiotherapy interventions, and careful monitoring for symptoms that may indicate atypical infections. Regular follow-up and immediate intervention in the case of respiratory symptoms can reduce the risk of secondary infections [35,36].

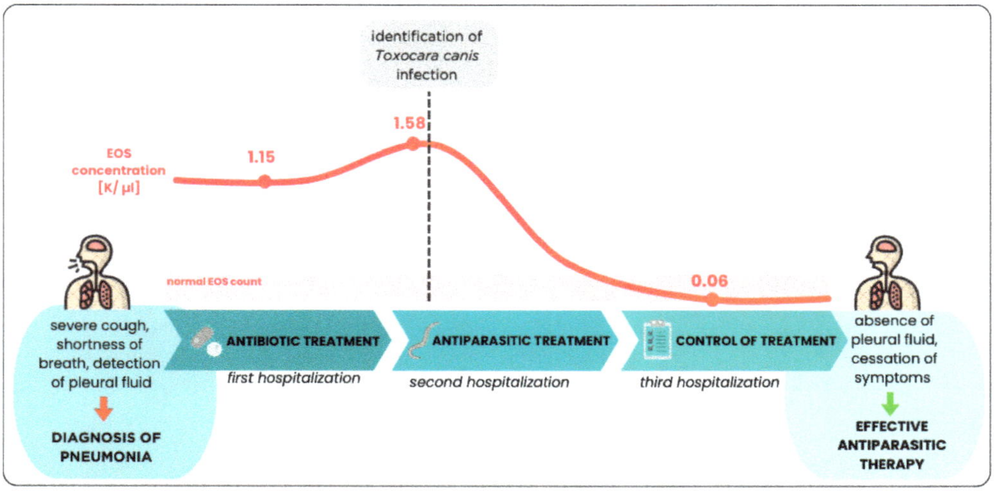

Figure 6. Effect of the treatment type on eosinophil concentration and the course of the disease.

This case also highlights the need for further research into the interactions between congenital respiratory disorders and parasitic infections. It would be particularly interesting to investigate whether patients with Kartagener syndrome are more susceptible to atypical manifestations of parasitic infections and whether these infections have long-term effects on the course of their underlying disease.

This case underscores the importance of differential diagnosis in atypical infections for patients with PCD. Key limitations include the lack of extensive data on parasitic infections within PCD populations, as most studies focus on bacterial and viral pathogens rather than parasitic agents. Additionally, the rarity of both primary ciliary dyskinesia and pulmonary toxocariasis complicates the generalizability of findings, as cases with concurrent presentation of these conditions are infrequent and underreported. The absence of large-scale studies limits our ability to draw definitive conclusions about the typical progression, optimal diagnostic approaches, and specific treatment efficacy for parasitic infections in PCD patients. Further research, including prospective studies and broader case series, is necessary to clarify the interactions between PCD and atypical infections such as toxocariasis, ultimately guiding more precise diagnostic and therapeutic strategies.

4. Conclusions

The occurrence of diseases that impair lung defense mechanisms, such as primary ciliary dyskinesia (PCD), increases the likelihood of parasitic larvae, like *Toxocara canis*, invading and proliferating in lung tissue. In cases where pneumonia-like symptoms arise in PCD patients, parasitic infection should be considered as a potential cause. Elevated eosinophil counts, total IgE levels, and specific IgG antibodies in the blood can be indicative of a *Toxocara canis* infection. Early detection of parasitic infections allows for timely treatment, significantly reducing the risk of complications that may arise from prolonged illness and pose a threat to the patient's health.

Author Contributions: Conceptualization, K.P. and W.F.; writing—original draft preparation, K.P. and W.F.; writing—review and editing, K.P., W.F., V.G., A.R. and A.Ś.; supervision, A.Ś. All authors have read and agreed to the published version of the manuscript.

Funding: This research received no external funding.

Institutional Review Board Statement: Not applicable.

Informed Consent Statement: Informed consent was obtained from subject involved in the study.

Data Availability Statement: The data supporting the findings of this study are derived from clinical observations and the medical records of the patient discussed in this case report. Due to privacy and ethical considerations, these data are not publicly available. Any additional information or details that do not compromise patient confidentiality can be provided upon reasonable request to the corresponding author, Kacper Packi, and subject to approval from the relevant ethical review board.

Conflicts of Interest: The authors declare no conflicts of interest.

Appendix A. Laboratory Test Results

Laboratory Findings	4 April 2024	10 April 2024	19 April 2024	26 April 2024	1 May 2024	24 June 2024–28 June 2024	Reference Interval
	Start of Antibiotic Therapy (First Hospital Stay)		Identification of Toxocariasis and Implementation of Appropriate Treatment (Second Hospital Stay)			Control of Treatment (Third Hospital Stay)	
Blood morphology							
Leukocytes	10.2	7.5	8.8	-	6.8	10.1	3.8–10 K/uL
Erythrocytes	5.3	5.44	5.55	-	5.4	5.09	3.7–5.1 mln/uL
Hemoglobin	15.6	15.8	16.2	-	15.6	15.0	12–16 g/dL
Haematocrit	43.5	45.3	44.9	-	44.4	43.7	37–47%
Blood platelets	225	278	264	-	258	233	140–440 K/mL
Neutrophils	-	3.70	4.70	-	-	7.33	2.5–7 K/uL
Lymphocytes	-	1.77	1.6	-	-	1.93	1–3.5 K/uL
Monocytes	-	0.83	0.87	-	-	0.76	0.2–1 K/uL
Eosinophils	-	1.15	1.58	-	-	0.06	0.1–0.5 K/uL
Basophiles	-	0.0	0.0	-	-	0.0	0–0.1 K/uL
Neutrophils	-	49.4	53.6	-	-	72.3	40–70%
Lymphocytes	-	23.7	18.2	-	-	19.1	20–45%
Monocytes	-	11.1	9.9	-	-	7.5	2–10%
Eosinophils	-	15.4	18.0	-	-	0.6	1–5%
Basophiles	-	0.4	0.3	-	-	0.5	0–2%
Biochemistry							
Toxocara canis IgG	-	-	-	16.83	-	9.1	>9 NTU—negative 9–11 inconclusive <11 positive
LDH	-	-	228	-	-	-	225–450 U/L
Total protein	-	-	7.1	-	-	-	6.4–8.3 g/dL
Total bilirubin	0.75	-	0.66	-	-	1.22	0–0.9 mg/dL
Glucose	96	-	95	-	-	93	70–99 mg/dL
GGTP	-	-	9	-	-		6–42 U/L
Urea	-	-	46.3	-	33.4	38.6	16.6–48.5 mg/dL
Sodium	136	-	140	-	141	138	136–145 mmol/L
Potassium	3.52	-	3.47	-	4.05	3.69	3.5–5.1 mmol/L
Magnesium	0.91	-	-	-	-	-	0.66–1.07 mmol/L
ALT	11	-	12	-	-	140	0–33 U/L
AST	17	-	17	-	-	86	0–32 U/L
CK-MB	-	-	-	-	-	10.2	0–25 U/L
Troponin I	<0.100	-	-	-	-	<0.100	0–0.3 ng/mL
NT-proBNP	33.44	-	21.99	-	-	-	0–125 pg/mL
Creatinine	0.87	-	1.06	-	1.13	0.98	0.5–0.9 mg/dL

eGFR	80.0		63.7	-	59.2	69.7	<90 mL/min/1.73 m^2—normal 60–89—mildly reduced 30–59 moderately reduced 15–29 severely reduced >15 renal failure
Immunochemistry							
CRP	39.45	14.13	25.18	-	5.12	4.63	0–5 mg/L
Total IgE	-	-	111.0	-	-	9.7	0–100 IU/mL
Hormones							
TSH	2.120	-	2.270	-	-	0.720	0.27–4.2 uIU/mL (non-pregnant women)
ft3	3.07	-	-	-	-	-	2.04–4.04 ng/dL (non-pregnant women)
ft4	1.28	-	-	-	-	-	0.93–1.7 ng/dL (non-pregnant women)
Arterial Blood Gas							
pH	7.44	-	7.48	-	-	7.42	7.35–7.45
pCO_2	25.4	-	34.00	-	-	32.5	35–45 mmHg
pO_2	68.6	-	62.00	-	-	60.3	80–100 mmHg
Saturation	94.7	-	93.40	-	-	91.8	90–96%
HCO_3	17.00	-	24.50	-	-	20.5	20–26 mmol/L
BE	−5.20	-	1.50	-	-	−3.00	−2.5–5.5 mmol/L
Coaguology							
D-dimers	1.56	-	-	-	-	0.41	0–0.5 ug/mL
INR	0.99	-	1.16	-	-	1.09	0.8–1.2
Prothrombin index	101	-	87	-	-	92	80–120%
Prothrombin time	10.5	-	12.2	-	-	11.3	8–12 s

increased parameter, decreased parameter.

Appendix B. Description of Diagnostic Imaging Examinations

The patient presents with situs inversus, involving pulmonary inversion, with a 3-lobe left lung, 2-lobe right lung, right-sided heart and aortic arch, liver on the left side, and spleen on the right side.

Type of Examination	First Hospitalization	Second Hospitalization	Third Hospitalization
Chest X-ray	5 April 2024: Fluid in the right pleural cavity, extending up to the ninth rib and entering the oblique fissure. Pulmonary field without focal lesions. Cardiac silhouette within normal limits.	22 April 2024: In the right pleural cavity, fluid up to 29 mm in width is present. No fluid observed in the left pleural cavity. 26 April 2024: In the right pleural cavity, fluid up to 45 mm in width is present. No fluid is observed in the left pleural cavity.	24 June 2024: No signs of fluid were observed in the right or left pleural cavity.

Abdominal ultrasound	5 April 2024: Situs inversus. The liver demonstrates normal echogenicity, is homogeneous, with no focal lesions. The gallbladder has thin walls and is free of stones. The pancreas, within the scope of the examination, is homogeneous and not enlarged. The spleen is homogeneous and not enlarged. The kidneys are of normal shape, size, and position, with no signs of nephrolithiasis. The right kidney shows an enlarged pelvicalyceal system (PCS), with calyces up to 10 mm in width and the renal pelvis up to 27 mm in width. The abdominal aorta, within the scope of the examination, shows no pathological widening of the lumen. No free fluid is observed in the peritoneal cavity. The urinary bladder is empty and cannot be assessed.	-	-
Pleural cavity ultrasound	8 April 2024: In the right pleural cavity, fluid up to 55 mm in width is present. No fluid was observed in the left pleural cavity.	-	-
Chest CT (without contrast enhancement)	-	23 April 2024: Exudative pleurisy of the right pleural cavity, associated with Löffler's syndrome (eosinophilic pneumonia in the context of toxocariasis). Situs inversus with pulmonary inversion. The heart and aortic arch are on the right side. The liver is on the left side, and the spleen is on the right. Fluid is present in the right pleural cavity, up to 40 mm in thickness. It was noted that there are atelectatic/inflammatory changes in the lower lobe of the right lung with an accompanying layer of fluid in the right pleural cavity. No enlarged lymph nodes in the mediastinum. The heart is not enlarged, there is no fluid in the pericardial sac, and the aorta is not dilated. The right kidney shows a segmentally thinned cortical layer with hypodense areas, most likely cysts. Bone structures show no pathological changes.	-

References

1. Wee, W.B.; Gatt, D.; Seidl, E.; Santyr, G.; To, T.; Dell, S.D. Estimates of primary ciliary dyskinesia prevalence: A scoping review. *ERJ Open Res.* **2024**, *10*, 00989-2023. [CrossRef]
2. Horani, A.; Ferkol, T.W. Understanding Primary Ciliary Dyskinesia and Other Ciliopathies. *J. Pediatr.* **2021**, *230*, 15–22.e1. [CrossRef]
3. Raidt, J.; Loges, N.T.; Olbrich, H.; Wallmeier, J.; Pennekamp, P.; Omran, H. Primary ciliary dyskinesia. *Presse Medicale Paris Fr. 1983* **2023**, *52*, 104171. [CrossRef]

4. Lu, D.; Yang, W.; Zhang, R.; Li, Y.; Cheng, T.; Liao, Y.; Chen, L.; Liu, H. Clinical Characteristics and Immune Responses in Children with Primary Ciliary Dyskinesia during Pneumonia Episodes: A Case–Control Study. *Children* **2023**, *10*, 1727. [CrossRef]
5. Wallmeier, J.; Nielsen, K.G.; Kuehni, C.E.; Lucas, J.S.; Leigh, M.W.; Zariwala, M.A.; Omran, H. Motile ciliopathies. *Nat. Rev. Dis. Primer* **2020**, *6*, 77. [CrossRef]
6. Mirra, V.; Werner, C.; Santamaria, F. Primary Ciliary Dyskinesia: An Update on Clinical Aspects, Genetics, Diagnosis, and Future Treatment Strategies. *Front. Pediatr.* **2017**, *5*, 135. [CrossRef]
7. Winders, W.T.; Menkin-Smith, L. Toxocara Canis. In *StatPearls*; StatPearls Publishing: Treasure Island, FL, USA, 2024. Available online: http://www.ncbi.nlm.nih.gov/books/NBK538524/ (accessed on 24 September 2024).
8. Demirci, M.Ü.M. Eosinophilic Pneumonia Due to Toxocariasis: An Adult Case Report. Available online: https://turkiyeparazitolderg.org/articles/doi/tpd.2012.61 (accessed on 29 October 2024).
9. Inoue, K.; Inoue, Y.; Arai, T.; Nawa, Y.; Kashiwa, Y. Chronic Eosinophilic Pneumonia Due to Visceral Larva Migrans. *Intern. Med.* **2002**, *41*, 478–482. [CrossRef]
10. Ma, G.; Rostami, A.; Wang, T.; Hofmann, A.; Hotez, P.J.; Gasser, R.B. Global and regional seroprevalence estimates for human toxocariasis: A call for action. *Adv. Parasitol.* **2020**, *109*, 275–290. [CrossRef]
11. Woodhall, D.M.; Fiore, A.E. Toxocariasis: A Review for Pediatricians. *J. Pediatr. Infect. Dis. Soc.* **2014**, *3*, 154–159. [CrossRef]
12. Dattoli, V.C.C.; Freire, S.M.; Mendonça, L.R.; Santos, P.C.; Meyer, R.; Alcantara-Neves, N.M. *Toxocara canis* infection is associated with eosinophilia and total IgE in blood donors from a large Brazilian centre. *Trop. Med. Int. Health* **2011**, *16*, 514–517. [CrossRef]
13. Ha, T.V.; Tang, H.K.; Ngo, B.V.; Le, T.P.; Le, D.H.; Tran, Y.M.L.; Dang, D.K.; Vo, T.T. Clinical and laboratory characteristics of Toxocara canis infection among children in Ho Chi Minh City, Vietnam. *Trans. R. Soc. Trop. Med. Hyg.* **2024**, trae057. [CrossRef]
14. Cottin, V. Eosinophilic Lung Diseases. *Immunol. Allergy Clin. N. Am.* **2023**, *43*, 289–322. [CrossRef]
15. Allen, J.; Wert, M. Eosinophilic Pneumonias. *J. Allergy Clin. Immunol. Pract.* **2018**, *6*, 1455–1461. [CrossRef]
16. Kovalszki, A.; Weller, P.F. Eosinophilia. *Prim. Care* **2016**, *43*, 607–617. [CrossRef]
17. Magnaval, J.-F.; Glickman, L.T.; Dorchies, P.; Morassin, B. Highlights of human toxocariasis. *Korean J. Parasitol.* **2001**, *39*, 1. [CrossRef]
18. Fillaux, J.; Magnaval, J.-F. Laboratory diagnosis of human toxocariasis. *Vet. Parasitol.* **2013**, *193*, 327–336. [CrossRef]
19. Kaneva, E.; Harizanov, R.; Rainova, I.; Kaftandjiev, I. Total serum Immunoglobulin E in Patients with toxocariasis and Clinically Healthy Pesrons in Bulgaria. *Acta Zool. Bulg.* **2019**, *71*, 601–609.
20. Huang, L.; Appleton, J.A. Eosinophils in Helminth Infection: Defenders and Dupes. *Trends Parasitol.* **2016**, *32*, 798–807. [CrossRef]
21. Pinelli, E.; Brandes, S.; Dormans, J.; Gremmer, E.; van Loveren, H. Infection with the roundworm Toxocara canis leads to exacerbation of experimental allergic airway inflammation. *Clin. Exp. Allergy J. Br. Soc. Allergy Clin. Immunol.* **2008**, *38*, 649–658. [CrossRef]
22. Wijers, C.D.; Chmiel, J.F.; Gaston, B.M. Bacterial infections in patients with primary ciliary dyskinesia: Comparison with cystic fibrosis. *Chron. Respir. Dis.* **2017**, *14*, 392. [CrossRef]
23. Bede, O.; Szénási, Z.; Danka, J.; Gyurkovits, K.; Nagy, D. Toxocariasis associated with chronic cough in childhood: A longitudinal study in Hungary. *J. Helminthol.* **2008**, *82*, 357–363. [CrossRef]
24. Kuek, L.E.; Lee, R.J. First contact: The role of respiratory cilia in host-pathogen interactions in the airways. *Am. J. Physiol.-Lung Cell. Mol. Physiol.* **2020**, *319*, L603. [CrossRef]
25. Aghaei, S.; Riahi, S.M.; Rostami, A.; Mohammadzadeh, I.; Javanian, M.; Tohidi, E.; Foroutan, M.; Dooki, M.E. Toxocara spp. infection and risk of childhood asthma: A systematic review and meta-analysis. *Acta Trop.* **2018**, *182*, 298–304. [CrossRef]
26. Cooper, P.J. Toxocara canis infection: An important and neglected environmental risk factor for asthma? *Clin. Exp. Allergy J. Br. Soc. Allergy Clin. Immunol.* **2008**, *38*, 551–553. [CrossRef]
27. Ranasuriya, G.; Mian, A.; Boujaoude, Z.; Tsigrelis, C. Pulmonary toxocariasis: A case report and literature review. *Infection* **2014**, *42*, 575–578. [CrossRef]
28. Gonzalez-Quintela, A.; Gude, F.; Campos, J.; Garea, M.T.; Romero, P.A.; Rey, J.; Meijide, L.M.; Fernandez-Merino, M.C.; Vidal, C. Toxocara Infection Seroprevalence and Its Relationship with Atopic Features in a General Adult Population. *Int. Arch. Allergy Immunol.* **2006**, *139*, 317–324. [CrossRef]
29. Piloiu, C.; Dumitrascu, D.L. Albendazole-Induced Liver Injury. *Am. J. Ther.* **2021**, *28*, e335–e340. [CrossRef]
30. Chen, J.; Liu, Q.; Liu, G.H.; Zheng, W.B.; Hong, S.J.; Sugiyama, H.; Zhu, X.Q.; Elsheikha, H.M. Toxocariasis: A silent threat with a progressive public health impact. *Infect. Dis. Poverty* **2018**, *7*, 59. [CrossRef]
31. Magnaval, J.-F.; Fillaux, J.; Berry, A. A Retrospective Study of the Efficacy of Albendazole and Diethylcarbamazine for the Treatment of Human Toxocariasis. *Pathogens* **2022**, *11*, 813. [CrossRef]
32. Dion, C.F.; Ashurst, J.V. Streptococcus Pneumoniae. In *StatPearls*; StatPearls Publishing: Treasure Island, FL, USA, 2024. Available online: http://www.ncbi.nlm.nih.gov/books/NBK470537/ (accessed on 24 September 2024).
33. Torres, A.; Cilloniz, C.; Niederman, M.S.; Menéndez, R.; Chalmers, J.D.; van der Poll, T. Pneumonia. *Nat. Rev. Dis. Primer* **2021**, *7*, 25. [CrossRef]
34. Gravesande, K.S.V.; Omran, H. Primary ciliary dyskinesia: Clinical presentation, diagnosis and genetics. *Ann. Med.* **2005**, *37*, 439–449. [CrossRef]

35. Schofield, L.M.; Duff, A.; Brennan, C. Airway Clearance Techniques for Primary Ciliary Dyskinesia is the Cystic Fibrosis literature portable? *Paediatr. Respir. Rev.* **2018**, *25*, 73–77. [CrossRef]
36. Paff, T.; Omran, H.; Nielsen, K.G.; Haarman, E.G. Current and Future Treatments in Primary Ciliary Dyskinesia. *Int. J. Mol. Sci.* **2021**, *22*, 9834. [CrossRef]

medicina

MDPI

Article

Long-Term Pulmonary Sequelae and Immunological Markers in Patients Recovering from Severe and Critical COVID-19 Pneumonia: A Comprehensive Follow-Up Study

Edita Strumiliene [1,*], Jurgita Urbonienė [2], Laimute Jurgauskiene [3], Ingrida Zeleckiene [4], Rytis Bliudzius [4], Laura Malinauskiene [5], Birutė Zablockiene [1], Arturas Samuilis [4] and Ligita Jancoriene [1,*]

1 Clinic of Infectious Diseases and Dermatovenerology, Faculty of Medicine, Institute of Clinical Medicine, Vilnius University, 01513 Vilnius, Lithuania; birute.zablockiene@santa.lt
2 Centre of Infectious Diseases, Vilnius University Hospital Santaros klinikos, 08661 Vilnius, Lithuania; jurgita.urboniene@santa.lt
3 Clinic of Cardiac and Vascular Diseases, Faculty of Medicine, Institute of Clinical Medicine, Vilnius University, 01513 Vilnius, Lithuania; laimute.jurgauskiene@santa.lt
4 Department of Radiology, Nuclear Medicine and Medical Physics, Faculty of Medicine, Institute of Biomedical Sciences, Vilnius University, 01513 Vilnius, Lithuania; ingrida.zeleckiene@santa.lt (I.Z.); rytis.bliudzius@santa.lt (R.B.); arturas.samuilis@santa.lt (A.S.)
5 Clinic of Chest Diseases, Immunology and Allergology, Faculty of Medicine, Institute of Clinical Medicine, Vilnius University, 01513 Vilnius, Lithuania; laura.malinauskiene@santa.lt
* Correspondence: edita.strumiliene@santa.lt (E.S.); ligita.jancoriene@santa.lt (L.J.)

Abstract: *Background and Objectives*: Severe and critical COVID-19 pneumonia can lead to long-term complications, especially affecting pulmonary function and immune health. However, the extent and progression of these complications over time are not well understood. This study aimed to assess lung function, radiological changes, and some immune parameters in survivors of severe and critical COVID-19 up to 12 months after hospital discharge. *Materials and Methods*: This prospective observational cohort study followed 85 adult patients who were hospitalized with severe or critical COVID-19 pneumonia at a tertiary care hospital in Vilnius, Lithuania, for 12 months post-discharge. Pulmonary function tests (PFTs), including forced vital capacity (FVC), forced expiratory volume in 1 s (FEV1), and diffusion capacity for carbon monoxide (DLCO), were conducted at 3, 6, and 12 months. High-resolution chest computed tomography (CT) scans assessed residual inflammatory and profibrotic/fibrotic abnormalities. Lymphocyte subpopulations were evaluated via flow cytometry during follow-up visits to monitor immune status. *Results*: The median age of the cohort was 59 years (IQR: 51–64). Fifty-three (62.4%) patients had critical COVID-19 disease. Pulmonary function improved significantly over time, with increases in FVC, FEV1, VC, TLC, and DLCO. Residual volume (RV) did not change significantly over time, suggesting that some aspects of lung function, such as air trapping, remained stable and may require attention in follow-up care. The percentage of patients with restrictive spirometry patterns decreased from 24.71% at 3 months to 14.8% at 12 months ($p < 0.05$). Residual inflammatory changes on CT were present in 77.63% at 6 months, decreasing to 69.62% at 12 months ($p < 0.001$). Profibrotic changes remained prevalent, affecting 82.89% of patients at 6 months and 73.08% at 12 months. Lymphocyte counts declined significantly from 3 to 12 months (2077 cells/µL vs. 1845 cells/µL, $p = 0.034$), with notable reductions in CD3+ ($p = 0.040$), CD8+ ($p = 0.007$), and activated CD3HLA-DR+ cells ($p < 0.001$). This study found that higher CD4+ T cell counts were associated with worse lung function, particularly reduced total lung capacity (TLC), while higher CD8+ T cell levels were linked to improved pulmonary outcomes, such as increased forced vital capacity (FVC) and vital capacity (VC). Multivariable regression analyses revealed that increased levels of CD4+/CD28+/CD192+ T cells were associated with worsening lung function, while higher CD8+/CD28+/CD192+ T cell counts were linked to better pulmonary outcomes, indicating that immune dysregulation plays a critical role in long-term respiratory recovery. *Conclusions*: Survivors of severe and critical COVID-19 pneumonia continue to experience significant long-term impairments in lung function and immune system health. Regular monitoring of pulmonary function, radiological changes, and immune parameters is essential for guiding personalized post-COVID-19 care and improving long-term outcomes. Further research is needed to explore the mechanisms behind these complications and to develop targeted interventions for long COVID-19.

Keywords: COVID-19; long COVID; pulmonary function; lymphocytes; CCR2; chest CT

1. Background

The global COVID-19 pandemic, caused by the SARS-CoV-2 virus, has led to significant morbidity and mortality since its emergence in late 2019. While most individuals experience mild to moderate symptoms, a subset of patients develops severe or critical illness, often resulting in acute respiratory distress syndrome (ARDS). This severe form of COVID-19 frequently necessitates high-flow oxygenation or mechanical ventilation in intensive care settings [1,2]. The underlying pathophysiology of severe COVID-19 involves extensive pulmonary inflammation and damage, which may lead to enduring respiratory complications even after the resolution of the acute infection [1–3].

Survivors of severe and critical COVID-19 pneumonia are at heightened risk for chronic pulmonary sequelae, including interstitial lung damage with pulmonary fibrosis and persistent pulmonary function abnormalities. Studies have documented that post-acute sequela of SARS-CoV-2 infection (PASC), commonly referred to as long COVID or post-COVID, often include sustained respiratory symptoms such as dyspnoea, cough, decreased exercise capacity, and changes in chest CT [1,4]. Long-term impacts on lung function and structure, measured by pulmonary function tests (PFTs) and radiological imaging and ongoing pathophysiological mechanisms degerming long COVID symptoms, remain an essential area of ongoing research.

Beyond pulmonary complications, severe COVID-19 also exerts profound effects on the immune system. Dysregulated immune responses, including lymphopenia and altered T-cell function, have been commonly observed in critically ill patients [5]. Lymphocytes, especially T cells, play a vital role in viral clearance and the regulation of the immune response. However, in severe COVID-19, these cells often become dysfunctional, contributing to the prolonged inflammation and immune dysregulation seen in long COVID-19 [5].

One immune marker of particular interest is the C-C chemokine receptor 2 (CCR2 or CD192, cluster of differentiation 192), a receptor expressed on various immune cells, including T cells. CCR2 is crucial for regulating cell activation and migration during infection. Studies have suggested that CCR2-dependent signaling may play a role in the development of lung fibrosis, with inhibition of this pathway shown to reduce fibrotic changes in experimental models [6,7]. Understanding the role of CCR2 in the context of post-COVID-19 immune dysregulation may provide new insights into potential therapeutic targets.

Long-term studies have highlighted that patients with severe initial COVID-19 are at higher risk for persistent abnormalities, including pulmonary fibrosis and immune dysfunction. However, independent biomarkers that could predict these outcomes are still not fully understood [3]. This study seeks to explore the longitudinal changes in lung function, radiological findings, and immunological markers over a 12-month period in patients recovering from severe or critical COVID-19 pneumonia. By identifying key predictors of poor long-term outcomes, we aim to contribute to the development of personalized post-COVID management strategies.

2. Study Rationale and Objectives

This study aims to provide a detailed evaluation of pulmonary and immunological outcomes in patients who survived severe or critical COVID-19 pneumonia. By conducting follow-up assessments at 3, 6, and 12 months post-discharge, we seek to

- Characterise the progression of lung function recovery or deterioration using pulmonary function tests (PFTs);

- Analyse the persistence and resolution of radiological abnormalities through chest CT scans;
- Investigate the longitudinal changes in immunological markers, including lymphocyte subpopulations, and their association with lung function and radiological findings;
- Identify potential predictors of long-term pulmonary impairment and immune dysregulation to inform clinical management and rehabilitation strategies for COVID-19 survivors.

3. Materials and Methods

3.1. Patients

All adult patients with a real-time reverse transcriptase polymerase chain reaction (RT-PCR) test–confirmed SARS-CoV-2 infection and severe or critical COVID-19 pneumonia, treated at Vilnius University Hospital "Santaros klinikos", a tertiary hospital, from October 2021 to October 2022, were offered to participate in this prospective follow-up study at the time of discharge if they met the following inclusion criteria:

- Radiologically confirmed lung injury via chest X-ray and/or CT scan at the onset of the disease;
- Willingness and ability to complete pulmonary function tests and to undergo chest CT and blood testing at the follow-up visits;
- No chronic lung disease prior to the infection (to avoid radiological and functional overdiagnosis);
- Ability to understand and sign the informed consent to participate in this study.

Patients with mild or moderate COVID-19, according to the WHO classification, were not included in this study, as they did not have severe lung injury and were at a lower risk for residual lung damage and long COVID-19 respiratory symptoms. Known immunosuppressive conditions were also considered as an exclusion criterion.

The follow-up visits were organized at the Respiratory Outpatient Department at 3, 6, and 12 months after discharge. Eighty-five consecutive eligible patients were included.

The patients included in this study were categorised into the following groups according to WHO criteria [6]:

- Severe disease: characterised by radiological evidence of bilateral pneumonia with lung injury > 50% and any of the following: respiratory rate $\geq$ 30 breaths/min; oxygen saturation $\leq$ 93% at rest; oxygen therapy $\leq$ 10 L/min; no need for treatment in the Intensive Care Unit (ICU);
- Critical disease: characterised by respiratory failure requiring high-flow oxygen therapy or intubation, shock, or other organ failure necessitating ICU care.

3.2. Data Collection

Medical records of the participants were reviewed from the hospital database, and demographic data and chest radiological data at the time of hospitalization (acute disease) were analysed.

Patients were evaluated at three visits: 3, 6, and 12 months after discharge from the hospital. During these visits, lung function tests and blood samples were collected and analysed. Chest CT scans were performed at 6 and 12-month visits. If pathological findings were not observed during a test, that test was not repeated in subsequent visits.

This study was approved by the Vilnius Regional Biomedical Ethics Committee (Protocol number: 2020/6-1233-718; 2020-06-22) and conducted in accordance with the ethical standards specified in the Declaration of Helsinki. All patients provided informed written consent to participate in this study.

3.2.1. Pulmonary Function Testing

The pulmonary function tests were performed using Vmax Encore (Viasys® Healthcare, Conshohocken, PA, USA). The following parameters were measured: forced vital capacity (FVC), forced expiratory volume in the first second of exhalation (FEV1), FVC/FEV1 ratio, total lung capacity (TLC), vital capacity (VC), residual volume (RV), and diffusion capacity of the lung for carbon monoxide (DLCO), measured using the single-breath test. The DLCO was corrected for haemoglobin levels. All parameters were expressed as percentages of the predicted normal value; the lower limits of normal (LLN) were taken into account.

3.2.2. Chest CT Protocols and Image Analysis

At the time of admission, all patients with suspected COVID-19 pneumonia underwent posterior–anterior and lateral chest X-rays or chest CT examinations according to the decision of the attending physician. The CT scans were performed during follow-up visits. For the portion of our cohort who did not undergo a CT scan at the initial stage of the disease, posterior–anterior and lateral chest X-rays were used to assess the extent of the disease.

All chest CT scans were performed using two helical CT scanners: (1) a 64-row GE Discovery CT750 HD (General Electric Healthcare, Waukesha, WI, USA). A low-dose lung CT protocol was used. All CT images were acquired at the end of inhalation. Acquisition parameters were set as follows: tube voltage 100 kV, automatic tube current modulation, SmartmA/AutomA, Large Body FOV, detector coverage 40 mm, slice thickness 3.75 mm, pitch 1.375, and gantry rotation time 0.4 s. All images were then reconstructed with a slice thickness of 1.25 mm using lung and standard algorithms. Adaptive Statistical Iterative Reconstruction (ASiR) with 30% mA reduction was used to reduce the X-ray dose. (2) BrainLab Airo mobile CT (Manufacturer Mobius Imaging, LLC., Shirley, MA, USA) was also used for chest CT. Acquisition parameters were set as follows: tube voltage 120 kV, tube current 50 mA, rotation time 1.92 s, Large Body FOV, detector coverage 40 mm, slice thickness 1.25 mm, and pitch 1.415. All images were reconstructed using lung and standard algorithms.

Image analysis was performed by two independent radiologists. For studies where a discordance of scoring was found, further review was performed by a third radiologist until a consensus was reached.

CT features such as ground-glass opacities (GGOs), consolidation, parenchymal bands, architectural distortion, air bronchograms, and bronchiectasis, as well as their distribution were noted. The findings were classified into two groups: inflammatory changes (including GGO and consolidation) and fibrotic/reticular changes (including parenchymal bands, architectural distortion, and bronchiectasis). The involvement of each lung lobe was quantified using a method previously employed in other studies evaluating pulmonary fibrosis caused by SARS [7,8]. Each of the five lung lobes was assigned a score of 0–5 points for inflammatory and fibrotic/reticular changes. Points were assigned as follows: 0 for a lobe without perceptible changes, 1 for lesions involving up to 5% of a lobe, 2 for lesions involving 6–25% of a lobe, 3 for lesions involving 26–50% of a lobe, 4 for lesions involving 51–75% of a lobe, and 5 for lesions involving more than 75% of a lobe [2,3]. In the analysis of images taken during the acute COVID-19 period, the scores for each lobe were summed, with a maximum total score of 25, and one score was attributed to the extent of lesions, irrespective of the type of CT features. In contrast, during follow-up, two separate scores were attributed to inflammatory and fibrotic changes, and a total radiological score was determined.

3.2.3. Blood Samples

For lymphocyte population analysis, peripheral blood samples were stained with monoclonal antibodies targeting surface markers CD3, CD4, CD8, CD19, HLA-DR, CD28 (BD Biosciences, Franklin Lakes, NJ, USA), and CD192 (BioLegend, San Diego, CA, USA). After incubating in the dark at room temperature, red blood cells were lysed using FACS lysing solution and washed with phosphate-buffered saline. Following fixation, these labelled cells were acquired on a FACSCalibur flow cytometer (BD Biosciences, Franklin Lakes, NJ, USA) using CellQestPro analysis software (Version 5.2.1) after proper instrument settings, calibration, and compensation. Analysis regions were gated using a CD45/CD14 antibody combination, and an isotype control $\gamma1/\gamma2a$ was used for negative marker settings. Absolute numbers of lymphocyte subsets were calculated using the absolute lymphocyte counts obtained from the haematology analyser and adjusted to specific subset percentages.

3.2.4. Statistical Analysis

Statistical analysis was performed using IBM SPSS version 20.0. GraphPad Prism was used to create graphics. The Shapiro–Wilk test was used to test the normality of data; the data did not exhibit a normal distribution. Continuous and categorical variables are presented as median (interquartile range (IQR)) or mean (±standard deviation (SD)) and as numbers (percentages), respectively. The Mann–Whitney U test and the Wilcoxon Signed-Rank test for paired samples were used to compare continuous variables, while the χ^2 test or Fisher's exact test was used to compare categorical variables. A multivariable linear regression model was created to determine the association between pulmonary function parameters and immunological markers. The model included pulmonary function parameter or CT change severity score as the dependent variable and age, gender, lymphocyte count, and lymphocyte subpopulation count as predictors. A multivariable binary logistic regression model was applied to determine the association between a restrictive spirometry pattern and immunological markers. The model included the presence of a restrictive spirometry pattern as the dependent variable, and age, gender, COVID-19 severity, lymphocyte count, and lymphocyte subpopulation count as predictors. The backward conditional method was used for multivariable binary logistic regression. A two-sided p-value of <0.05 was considered significant.

4. Results

A total of 85 patients were included in the analysis, comprising 40 (47.1%) women and 45 (52.9%) men. The median age was 59 years (IQR 51–64). Among these patients, 53 (62.4%) had recovered from critically severe COVID-19, and 35 (37.6%) had recovered from severe COVID-19.

4.1. Pulmonary Function Tests

Pulmonary function test results at 3, 6, and 12 months post-discharge are provided in Table 1. The pulmonary function test results showed significant improvement in lung function over time. Forced vital capacity (FVC), forced expiratory volume in one second (FEV1), and vital capacity (VC) all improved between 3, 6, and 12 months post-discharge ($p < 0.05$). The FEV1/FVC ratio remained largely unchanged and was within the range of normality in the majority of the cases.

Table 1. Pulmonary function test results at 3, 6, and 12 months post-discharge, presented as median % of the predicted value (IQR).

Parameter	Month 3	Month 6	Month 12	p1	p2	p3
FVC	95 (85–106)	99.5 (89–111.75)	101 (88.5–112.5)	<0.001	<0.001	0.123
FEV1	96 (85.5–106)	99.5 (90.3–108.75)	103.00 (88.5–110.5)	0.005	0.002	0.032
FEV1/FVC	83 (80.5–86)	83 (78–85)	82 (79–85.5)	0.007	0.181	0.214
TLC	88 (76.5–100)	90 (81–104)	90 (80.5–102)	0.086	0.333	0.223
VC	96 (84–110)	102 (92–112.75)	103 (90.5–113)	<0.001	0.001	0.431
RV	76 (56.5–104.50)	79.5 (55.25–108.25)	75 (56.5–95.5)	0.664	0.593	0.127
DLCO	76 (64–84.5)	77 (68–86.75)	79 (71.5–84.5)	0.127	0.054	0.658

Wilcoxon Signed-Rank Test for paired samples was used for calculations; FVC—forced vital capacity, FEV1 forced expiratory capacity at the first second of exhalation, TLC—total lung capacity, VC—vital capacity, RV—residual volume, DLCO—diffusion capacity of the lung for carbon monoxide; p1—comparison of month 3 vs. month 6 test results; p2—comparison of month 3 vs. month 12 test results; p3—comparison of month 6 vs. month 12 test results.

At 3 months, 24.71% of patients showed restrictive patterns in spirometry, with the rate statistically significantly decreasing to 20.24% at 6 months and 14.8% at 12 months (Figure 1).

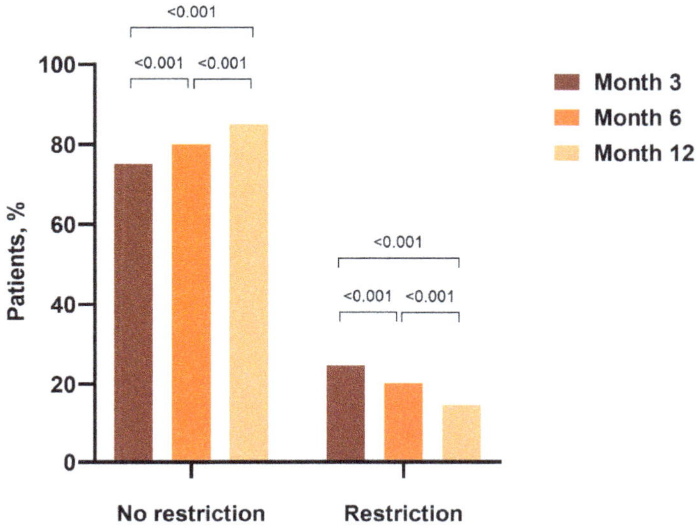

Figure 1. Rates of patients with and without restriction at 3, 6, and 12 months post-discharge.

4.2. Radiological Findings

A total of 76 out of 85 patients returned for the 6-month CT evaluation, and 79 returned for the 12-month radiological evaluation. Fibrotic/reticular changes were assessed in 78 of these patients. A total of 77.63% of patients still had residual inflammatory changes on CT at 6 months after the discharge. The lower lobes of the lungs were predominantly affected: the right lower lobe (RLL) in 73.68% of patients and the left lower lobe (LLL) in 69.74%. Additionally, inflammatory changes were observed in the right upper lobe (RUL) in 64.47% of patients, the left upper lobe (LUL) in 64.47%, and the right middle lobe (RML) in 53.95%. The total CT inflammatory change severity score was 8 (IQR 1–14).

A total of 69.62% of patients had residual inflammatory changes on CT at 12 months post-COVID-19. The RLL was affected in 64.56% of patients, the RML in 48.10%, the RUL in 53.16%, the LLL in 60.76%, and the LUL in 54.43%. The total CT inflammatory change severity score at 12 months was 6 (IQR 0–12), which was statistically significantly lower compared to the 6-month CT inflammatory change severity score ($p < 0.001$).

A total of 82.89% of patients had fibrotic/reticular changes on CT at 6 months post-discharge. The lower lobes of the lungs were mainly affected: RLL in 75% of patients and LLL in 69.74%. The RUL was affected in 64.47% of patients, the LUL in 69.74%, and the RML in 53.95%. The total CT fibrotic/reticular change severity score was 6 (IQR 2–11).

A total of 73.08% of patients had fibrotic/reticular changes on CT at 12 months post-COVID-19. The RLL was affected in 66.67% of patients, the RML in 51.28%, the RUL in 51.28%, the LLL in 61.54%, and the LUL in 56.41%. The total CT fibrotic/reticular change severity score at 12 months was 4.5 (IQR 0–10), which was statistically significantly lower compared to the 6-month CT inflammatory change severity score ($p < 0.001$).

The representative radiological changes over time are shown in Figure 2.

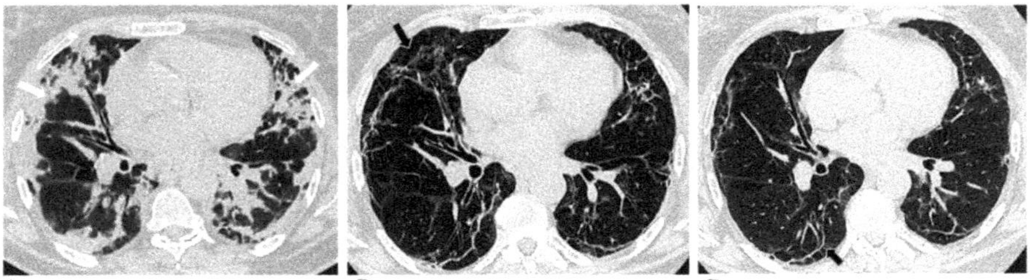

Figure 2. Evolution of chest CT features post-COVID-19 pneumonia. (**A**) Chest CT at initial presentation: bilateral multifocal organizing consolidation zones predominantly in the subpleural parts of the lung parenchyma (white arrows). (**B**) Six-month follow-up chest CT: in place of previously seen consolidation zones, we can see septal thickening and parenchymal bands with subtle ground glass opacities (black arrows). (**C**) Twelve-month follow-up chest CT: we can see almost complete resorption of ground glass opacities, with persistent subpleural curvilinear parenchymal bands (black arrows).

CT inflammatory change severity scores indicated that lobe lesions at 6 and 12 months were mostly mild, reaching 1–2 severity points, except for the RLL, where lesions were moderate, involving more than 25% of the lobe in 46.05% of patients at 6 months and in 21.52% of patients at 12 months. These scores statistically significantly decreased at 12 months compared to 6 months for the RUL, RML, RLL, and LLL. CT fibrotic/reticular change severity scores were mild and decreased at 12 months compared to 6 months for the RUL, RLL, LUL, and LLL (Table 2).

Table 2. Computed tomography severity scores in patients at 6 and 12 months post-COVID-19 by lung lobe, mean ± SD.

Lung Lobe	Inflammatory Changes			Fibrotic/Reticular Changes		
	Month 6	Month 12	*p*	Month 6	Month 12	*p*
Right upper lobe	1.59 ± 1.60	1.32 ± 1.54	0.004	1.26 ± 1.22	1.01 ± 1.21	0.004
Right middle lobe	1.38 ± 1.58	1.14 ± 1.47	0.005	1.00 ± 1.18	0.90 ± 1.14	0.157
Right lower lobe	2.17 ± 1.68	1.78 ± 1.64	<0.001	1.76 ± 1.43	1.58 ± 1.45	0.012
Left upper lobe	1.42 ± 1.46	1.30 ± 1.48	0.132	1.14 ± 1.02	0.94 ± 1.01	0.005
Left lower lobe	1.96 ± 1.79	1.56 ± 1.62	<0.001	1.63 ± 1.53	1.45 ± 1.50	0.016

Wilcoxon Signed-Rank Test for paired samples was used for calculations.

4.3. Immunological Markers

White blood cell (WBC), lymphocyte, and lymphocyte subpopulation counts were performed for 84 patients at 3 months, 65 patients at 6 months, and 59 patients at 12 months. CD4+/28+/192+ counts were conducted for 81 patients at 3 months, 59 patients at 6 months, and 55 patients at 12 months, while CD8+/28+/192+ counts were performed for 81 patients at 3 months, 60 patients at 6 months, and 55 patients at 12 months. WBC, lymphocyte, and lymphocyte subpopulation counts at 3, 6, and 12 months are shown in Table 3.

The WBC count did not change significantly between months 3, 6, and 12 post-discharge.

However, a statistically significant decrease in lymphocyte count, CD3+ cells, and CD8+ cells was observed at month 12 compared to month 3 post-COVID-19.

Additionally, CD3HLA-DR+ cells decreased significantly in month 12 compared to both month 3 and month 6. (Table 3, Figure 3).

Table 3. White blood cell, lymphocyte count, and lymphocyte subpopulation count in patients at 3, 6, and 12 months post-discharge, expressed as absolute number 10^9/L, percentage (IQR).

Parameter	Month 3	Month 6	Month 12	p1	p2	p3
WBC	**6100**	**6000**	**6000**	**0.871**	**0.613**	**0.527**
Lymphocytes	2077 36.5 (29.25–43.75)	2107 34 (27–41.5)	1845 33 (26–40.25)	0.264	0.034	0.598
CD19+	180.15 8.5 (6–11)	193.92 9 (7–12)	174.42 9 (6–12.3)	0.392	0.291	0.267
CD4+	778.95 38 (31.25–44)	862.84 40 (33–44.5)	729.28 40 (35–46)	0.909	0.284	0.413
CD8+	665.20 31 (23.25–40.75)	653.17 30 (21–38.5)	618.64 29 (22–39)	0.487	0.007	0.174
CD3+	1465.93 70 (65–76.5)	1555.2 72 (64.5–75)	1361.6 72 (66–78)	0.774	0.040	0.163
NK	344.76 16 (11–24.5)	397.60 16 (11–23.75)	300.72 14 (10–22)	0.466	0.108	0.460
CD3HLA-DR+	403.62 20.5 (14–26.75)	367.54 17 (12–22.5)	265.27 15 (10–22)	0.070	<0.001	0.003
CD4+/28+/192+	625.24 27.7 (22–35.1)	745.18 28.9 (23.5–38)	550.37 27.98 (22.5–35.12)	0.927	0.103	0.195
CD8+/28+/192+	276.64 13.2 (9.55–17.75)	297.62 13.55 (10.38–16.97)	280.29 13.70 (9.90–17.3)	0.775	0.353	0.433

Wilcoxon Signed-Rank Test for paired samples was used for calculations; p1—comparison of month 3 vs. month 6 test results; p2—comparison of month 3 vs. month 12 test results; p3—comparison of month 6 vs. month 12 test results.

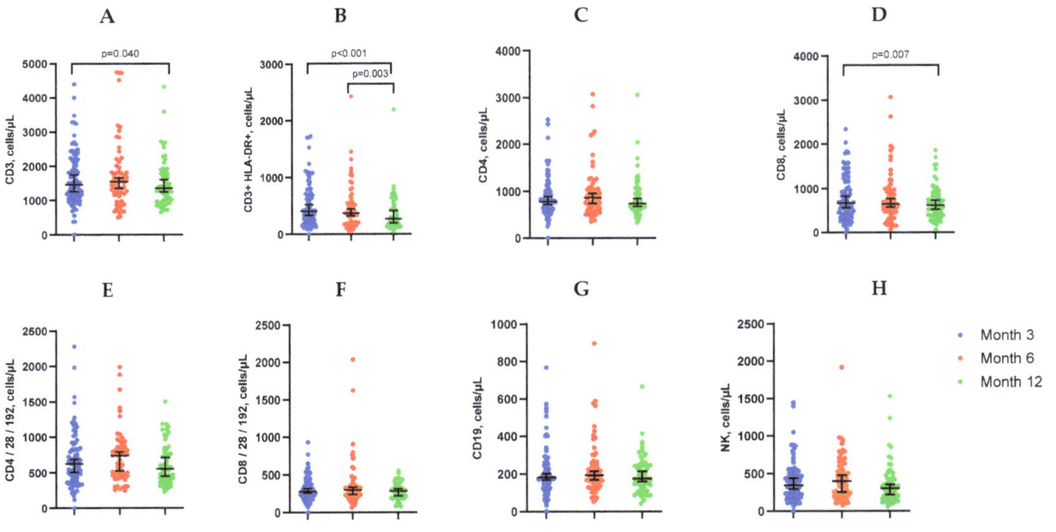

Figure 3. Concentrations of lymphocyte subpopulations CD3+ (**A**), CD3+HLA-DR+ (**B**), CD4+ (**C**), CD8+ (**D**), CD4/28/192+ (**E**), CD8/28/192+ (**F**), CD19+ (**G**) and NK (**H**) in patients at 3, 6, and 12 months post-discharge.

4.4. Association of Pulmonary Function Tests, Radiological Findings, and Immunological Markers

Patients with a restrictive spirometry pattern had higher scores for CT inflammatory and fibrotic/reticular changes at acute COVID-19 and at 6 and 12 months post-discharge compared to those without a restrictive spirometry pattern, although the differences were not statistically significant. However, patients with a restrictive spirometry pattern at 3 and 6 months had higher CT inflammatory and fibrotic/reticular change severity scores at 12 months compared to those without restriction in spirometry (Table 4).

Table 4. Computed tomography severity scores in patients at 3, 6, and 12 months post-COVID-19, grouped by restrictive spirometry pattern, median (IQR).

CT Severity Score	Restriction	No Restriction	*p*
Month 3			
Total score during acute COVID-19	17 (12–21)	15 (8.5–19)	0.140
Month 6			
Inflammatory changes at 6 months	10.5 (3.25–18.75)	7 (0.25–13)	0.129
Fibrotic/reticular changes at 6 months	9.5 (4–12.5)	5 (1.25–11)	0.090
Month 12			
Inflammatory changes at 12 months	10 (1–15)	4 (0–11)	0.211
Fibrotic/reticular changes at 12 months	11 (3–13)	4 (0–10)	0.203

Mann–Witney U Test was used for calculations; CT—computed tomography.

At 6 months, patients with a restrictive spirometry pattern had a higher CD19+ cell count compared to those without restriction (259.90 cells/µL vs. 171.12 cells/µL, $p = 0.025$). Similarly, at 12 months, patients with a restrictive spirometry pattern had a higher CD19+ cell count compared to those without restriction (279.12 cells/µL vs. 173.74 cells/µL, $p = 0.042$).

Multivariable regression was applied to evaluate the association between pulmonary function tests and the levels of immune cell subsets.

At 3 months, higher levels of CD8+/28+/192+ were associated with a slight decline in pulmonary function, as measured via the FEV1/FVC ratio: for each increase of 1×10^9/L in CD8+/28+/192+, the FEV1/FVC ratio decreased by 0.01. Increased levels of CD4+/28+/192+ were associated with lung function worsening, specifically reduced TLC at 6 months and decreased FVC, FEV1, and VC at 12 months, while increased CD8+/28+/192+ levels were associated with improved lung function (increased FVC, FEV1, and VC at 12 months). Additionally, higher levels of CD3HLA-DR+ were negatively associated with FEV1 and VC at 12 months, suggesting a decline in lung capacity (Table 5). Female gender was associated with a lower DLCO at 3, 6, and 12 months. Analysis revealed that the severity score of inflammatory changes and reticular/fibrotic changes on CT were associated with older age at 12 months (Table 5).

A decreased lymphocyte count (0.99 (95% CI 0.98–1.00, $p = 0.017$), increased CD19+ cell count (1.02 (95% CI 1.00–1.03), and increased CD4+ cell count (OR 1.01 (95% CI 1.00–1.02) were associated with a restrictive spirometry pattern at 12 months.

Patients with residual inflammatory changes on CT had a lower count of CD3HLA-DR+ cells compared to those without inflammatory changes at both 6 and 12 months. At 6 months, the count of CD3HLA-DR+ cells was 367.54 vs. 606.06, $p = 0.048$, and the percentage was 17% vs. 24%, $p = 0.014$. At 12 months, CD3HLA-DR+ cell count was 261.14 vs. 539.15, $p = 0.021$, and the percentage was 14% vs. 19.5%, $p = 0.024$.

Table 5. Association of pulmonary function tests, radiological findings, and immunological markers in patients at 3, 6, and 12 months post-COVID-19.

Parameter	Predictors	β (95% CI)	*p*
Month 3			
FEV1/FVC	CD8/28/192	−0.01 (−0.02–−0.001)	0.035
DLCO	Lymphocytes	0.06 (0.02–0.11)	0.008
	NK	−0.06 (−0.10–−0.01)	0.021
	Female gender	−8.46 (−15.33–−1.59)	0.016
Month 6			
TLC	CD4/28/192	−0.02 (−0.05–−0.004)	0.020
DLCO	Age	−0.67 (−1.14–−0.19)	0.007
	Female gender	−10.23 (−18.86–−1.61)	0.021
Month 12			
FVC	CD4/28/192	−0.07 (−0.10–−0.04)	0.001
	CD8/28/192	0.10 (0.04–0.16)	0.002
FEV1	CD3HLA-DR+	−0.04 (−0.08–−0.004)	0.031
	CD4/28/192	−0.06 (−0.09–−0.03)	0.001
	CD8/28/192	0.08 (0.01–0.15)	0.023
TLC	CD8/28/192	0.08 (0.02–0.14)	0.015
VC	CD3HLA-DR+	−0.04 (−0.07–−0.004)	0.028
	CD4/28/192	−0.06 (−0.09–−0.04)	<0.001
	CD8/28/192	0.1 (0.04–0.16)	0.002
RV	CD8	0.20 (0.03–0.36)	0.024
DLCO	Female gender	−10.16 (−18.45–−1.87)	0.017
Inflammatory changes	Age	0.22 (0.01–0.43)	0.038
Fibrotic/reticular changes	Age	0.18 (0.01–0.35)	0.044

Multivariable linear regression was used for calculations, and only statistically significant associations are included in the table. FVC—forced vital capacity, FEV1—forced expiratory capacity at the first second of exhalation, TLC—total lung capacity, VC—vital capacity, RV—residual volume, DLCO—diffusion capacity of the lung for carbon monoxide.

5. Discussion

This study offers a comprehensive evaluation of the long-term pulmonary and immunological outcomes in patients who survived severe or critical COVID-19 pneumonia, with follow-up assessments over a 12-month period. Our findings reveal that survivors often experience persistent pulmonary sequelae, including impairments in pulmonary function, particularly with the diffusion capacity of the lung for carbon monoxide (DLCO). Although there were gradual improvements in forced vital capacity (FVC), forced expiratory volume in one second (FEV1), residual volume (RV), and vital capacity (VC), complete lung function recovery remained elusive, underscoring the need for extended monitoring and rehabilitation.

Our data showed that female gender was associated with lower DLCO at 3, 6, and 12 months. Additionally, the analysis revealed that higher severity scores for inflammatory and reticular/fibrotic changes on CT at 12 months were linked to older age. These findings are consistent with existing literature, which identifies female gender and older age as risk factors for the development of long COVID [9,10].

The persistence of pulmonary abnormalities observed in our cohort aligns with previous studies on the post-COVID-19 respiratory sequelae [11–13]. For instance, Sonnweber et al. (2023) reported long-lasting pulmonary impairments, particularly in diffusion capacity, which persisted beyond 6 months after the discharge [11]. Similarly, Bocchino et al. (2022) demonstrated that 12 months post-COVID-19, many patients continued to exhibit fibrotic changes in their lung tissue, although without significant progression [12]. In contrast, Carvalho et al. (2024) [14] noted a decline in the prevalence of severe pulmonary impairments over a two-year period.

However, our data indicate a higher prevalence of residual changes at 12 months compared to some reports, although without evidence of progressive deterioration during this period [14]. The stable yet persistent fibrotic changes observed in the lower lung lobes suggest long-term structural damage, which is consistent with other findings in the literature [11–14].

Our study also demonstrated that the severity of the disease is associated with the intensity of radiological abnormalities in the lungs. Critical COVID-19 survivors showed more persistent radiological abnormalities during follow-up with higher scores of any abnormalities, including profibrotic/fibrotic changes, over time compared to those with non-severe disease. These findings are consistent with data published in a systematic review and meta-analysis by M. Babar et al. [15], showing that radiological lung changes like bronchiectasis, reticulation, and other fibrotic-like changes are highly associated with the severity of COVID-19.

Our study highlights significant long-term immunological impacts of severe COVID-19. There were significant decreases in total lymphocyte counts, including CD3+, CD8+, and CD3HLA-DR+ cells, over the 12-month follow-up period. CD4+ T cells remained relatively stable, whereas CD8+ T cells and CD3HLA-DR+ cells showed notable reductions.

This study indicates that elevated levels of CD4+ T cells, particularly the CD4+/28+/192+ subset, correlate with poorer lung function outcomes post-COVID-19. These cells are markers of immune activation and exhaustion. Increased CD4+ T cell counts are associated with reduced TLC and decreased FVC and FEV1. The persistence of high CD4+ T cell counts suggests ongoing inflammation or delayed lung tissue repair, which could contribute to structural lung changes and the exacerbation of respiratory impairment.

Conversely, CD8+ T cells appear beneficial for lung function recovery. Elevated CD8+/28+/192+ counts were positively associated with improved pulmonary parameters, such as FVC, FEV1, and VC. This suggests a potentially protective role of CD8+ T cells in mitigating fibrosis or inflammatory damage. CD8+ T cells likely contribute to a balanced immune response, aiding in the resolution of inflammation without inducing excessive fibrosis or structural changes in lung tissues.

These changes reflect ongoing immune dysregulation over 12 months and are consistent with other studies reporting prolonged alterations in lymphocyte subsets and immune activation post-COVID-19 [9].

Persistent symptoms and immune dysregulation after COVID-19 have been investigated by other authors. Carfì et al. (2020) documented persistent symptoms in patients after acute COVID-19, noting long-term immune alterations similar to our findings. Their study highlighted that lymphopenia and altered T-cell function were common among survivors [1]. Huang et al. (2021) reported that 6-month follow-ups showed sustained immune dysregulation with reductions in lymphocyte counts, similar to those observed in our cohort [2]. Chen et al. (2020) also found that severe COVID-19 is associated with significant immune dysregulation, with decreased CD3+ and CD8+ T cells, which aligns with our results of ongoing lymphocyte reduction [16].

Long-term immune alterations were investigated by Mathew et al. (2020) [17]. They identified distinct immunotypes in COVID-19 patients, with severe cases showing prolonged immune activation and altered T-cell profiles. This is consistent with our findings of reduced CD3+, CD8+, and CD3HLA-DR+ cells over the follow-up period. Davitt et al.

(2022) highlighted prolonged immune dysregulation in survivors, noting associations between lymphopenia, altered T-cell function, and ongoing inflammatory responses [5].

Sharif-Zak et al. (2022) and Ranjbar et al. (2022) explored the role of immune markers like CCR2 in COVID-19 severity and recovery, showing that dysregulated immune responses can contribute to prolonged pulmonary issues [18,19]. Our findings support this by demonstrating that specific immunological markers (e.g., CD4+/28+/192+) are associated with long-term pulmonary impairment. Milger et al. (2017) and Ranjbar et al. (2022) discussed the role of regulatory T cells in lung fibrosis, which corresponds to our observation of stable fibrotic changes and their correlation with immune dysregulation over time [19,20].

Our study's findings align closely with existing literature, reinforcing the understanding that severe COVID-19 leads to significant and persistent immune dysregulation. The observed reductions in lymphocyte counts, particularly CD3+, CD8+, and CD3HLA-DR+ cells, are consistent with other studies that highlight prolonged immune activation and altered T-cell profiles in COVID-19 survivors. The association between elevated CD4+/28+/192+ cell counts and impaired parameters of pulmonary function suggests that chronic immune dysregulation may directly impact pulmonary recovery, corroborating the need for integrated immunological and pulmonary monitoring and possible therapeutic targeting in post-COVID-19 care [15–17]. The higher counts of CD4+/28+/192+ cells were associated with impaired TLC, suggesting chronic inflammation or delayed tissue repair may directly impact lung recovery, with the possibility of lifetime residual sequela [5,18,19].

6. Clinical and Public Health Implications

The high prevalence of both pulmonary and immunological sequelae in survivors of severe COVID-19 pneumonia underscores the need for comprehensive, multidisciplinary follow-up care. Although the severity of radiological abnormalities decreases over time, many patients experience persistent lung fibrosis even after 12 months, highlighting the long-term impact of severe COVID-19 on lung structure. Immune recovery is slow in patients recovering from severe and critical COVID-19, with significant declines in key immune markers persisting even at 12 months. This underscores the need for continuous monitoring of immune function in these patients. Integrating regular lung function assessments, radiological evaluations, and immunological profiling into post-discharge care plans is essential for optimising recovery. Tailored rehabilitation strategies, including physical therapy, pulmonary rehabilitation, and potentially immunomodulatory treatments, should be considered to enhance recovery and improve quality of life [19,21]. Additionally, identifying predictors of poor long-term outcomes, such as CT severity scores and specific immunological markers, can inform personalized management approaches and early interventions for high-risk patients.

7. Limitations

This study has several limitations that should be acknowledged. The relatively small sample size and single-centre design may limit the generalisability of our findings. Additionally, the observational nature of this study precludes causal inferences. Additionally, the lack of a control group of patients who experienced mild or moderate COVID-19 makes it difficult to determine if the observed long-term effects are specific to severe and critical cases. Lastly, while we assessed several immunological markers, other relevant factors, such as genetic predispositions, comorbidities, and environmental influences, were not controlled for, which may confound the interpretation of our results. Future research should address these limitations by incorporating larger, diverse cohorts and longitudinal study designs to better elucidate the long-term immunological effects of severe COVID-19.

8. Future Directions

Longitudinal studies extending beyond 12 months are needed to fully understand the trajectory and duration of pulmonary and immunological sequelae in COVID-19 survivors. Future studies should explore interventions such as pulmonary rehabilitation and immune-modulating treatments to mitigate chronic complications. Investigating the mechanisms of immune dysregulation, particularly changes in the T-cell subset, could uncover therapeutic targets for preventing pulmonary fibrosis. Identifying biomarkers and genetic risk factors may help predict which patients are at higher risk for long-term complications. Finally, comparative studies with other respiratory conditions and analysis of factors like vaccination status, age, and gender could provide further insights into personalized post-COVID-19 care.

9. Conclusions

Our study demonstrates that the majority of survivors of severe and critical COVID-19 experience persistent pulmonary impairments and immune dysregulation even after 12 months. While lung function improves over time, many patients continue to show residual fibrotic changes and reduced diffusion capacity. Additionally, significant reductions in CD3+, CD8+, and CD3HLA-DR+ cells were observed, indicating ongoing immune dysregulation.

This study supports a model where CD4+ T cells exacerbate pulmonary sequelae, possibly through sustained activation that impairs healing, while CD8+ T cells facilitate a resolution of inflammatory damage, leading to better functional outcomes. Elevated CD4+/28+/192+ T cells, a marker of immune dysregulation, align with more severe restrictive spirometry patterns, while higher CD8+ T cells correlate with improved lung function.

This contrast underscores the importance of CD8+ T cells in recovery and highlights CD4+ T cells' potential role in chronic lung injury following severe COVID-19.

These findings highlight the importance of integrated post-COVID-19 care, combining pulmonary function monitoring and immunological assessments to identify patients at risk of long-term complications. Further research is needed to explore therapeutic strategies aimed at restoring immune balance and mitigating chronic lung damage, improving recovery and quality of life for these patients.

Author Contributions: Conceptualization, E.S., B.Z. and L.J. (Ligita Jancoriene); Methodology, E.S., J.U., L.J. (Laimute Jurgauskiene), I.Z., R.B., L.M., A.S. and L.J. (Ligita Jancoriene); Formal analysis, J.U. and A.S.; Investigation, E.S., L.J. (Laimute Jurgauskiene), I.Z. and R.B.; Resources, B.Z. and L.J. (Ligita Jancoriene); Data curation, E.S., J.U., I.Z., R.B., L.M. and A.S.; Writing—original draft, E.S., J.U., L.J. (Laimute Jurgauskiene), I.Z. and L.M.; Writing—review and editing, J.U., L.M., B.Z. and L.J. (Ligita Jancoriene); Visualization, J.U.; Supervision, A.S. and L.J. (Ligita Jancoriene); Project administration, E.S. and L.J. (Ligita Jancoriene). All authors have read and agreed to the published version of the manuscript.

Funding: This research received no external funding.

Institutional Review Board Statement: This study was approved by the Vilnius Regional Biomedical Ethics Committee (Protocol number: 2020/6-1233-718; 2020-06-22) and conducted in accordance with the ethical standards specified in the Declaration of Helsinki.

Informed Consent Statement: All patients provided informed written consent to participate in this study.

Data Availability Statement: The original contributions presented in the study are included in the article, further inquiries can be directed to the corresponding authors.

Conflicts of Interest: The authors declare no conflict of interest.

References

1. Carfi, A.; Bernabei, R.; Landi, F. Persistent Symptoms in Patients After Acute COVID-19. *JAMA* **2020**, *324*, 603–605. [CrossRef] [PubMed]
2. Huang, C.; Huang, L.; Wang, Y.; Li, X.; Ren, L.; Gu, X.; Kang, L.; Guo, L.; Liu, M.; Zhou, X.; et al. 6-month consequences of COVID-19 in patients discharged from hospital: A cohort study. *Lancet* **2021**, *397*, 220–232. [CrossRef] [PubMed]

3. McGroder, C.F.; Zhang, D.; Choudhury, M.A.; Salvatore, M.M.; D'Souza, B.M.; Hoffman, E.A.; Wei, Y.; Baldwin, M.R.; Garcia, C.K. Pulmonary fibrosis 4 months after COVID-19 is associated with severity of illness and blood leucocyte telomere length. *Thorax* **2021**, *76*, 1242–1245. [CrossRef] [PubMed]
4. Solomon, J.J.; Heyman, B.; Ko, J.P.; Condos, R.; Lynch, D.A. CT of Post-Acute Lung Complications of COVID-19. *Radiology* **2021**, *301*, E383–E395. [CrossRef] [PubMed]
5. Davitt, E.; Davitt, C.; Mazer, M.B.; Areti, S.S.; Hotchkiss, R.S.; Remy, K.E. COVID-19 disease and immune dysregulation. *Best Pract. Res. Clin. Haematol.* **2022**, *35*, 101401. [CrossRef] [PubMed]
6. WHO. Clinical Management of Severe Acute Respiratory Infection (SARI) When COVID-19 Disease Is Suspected: Interim Guidance. Available online: https://iris.who.int/handle/10665/331446 (accessed on 13 March 2020).
7. Chung, M.; Bernheim, A.; Mei, X.; Zhang, N.; Huang, M.; Zeng, X.; Cui, J.; Xu, W.; Yang, Y.; Fayad, Z.A.; et al. CT Imaging Features of 2019 Novel Coronavirus (2019-nCoV). *Radiology* **2020**, *295*, 202–207. [CrossRef] [PubMed]
8. Antonio, G.E.; Wong, K.T.; Hui, D.S.; Wu, A.; Lee, N.; Yuen, E.H.; Leung, C.B.; Rainer, T.H.; Cameron, P.; Chung, S.S.; et al. Thin-section CT in patients with severe acute respiratory syndrome following hospital discharge: Preliminary experience. *Radiology* **2003**, *228*, 810–815. [CrossRef] [PubMed]
9. Yong, S.J. Long COVID or post-COVID-19 syndrome: Putative pathophysiology, risk factors, and treatments. *Infect. Dis.* **2021**, *53*, 737–754. [CrossRef] [PubMed]
10. Rayner, D.G.; Wang, E.; Su, C.; Patel, O.D.; Aleluya, S.; Giglia, A.; Zhu, E.; Siddique, M. Risk factors for long COVID in children and adolescents: A systematic review and meta-analysis. *World J. Pediatr.* **2024**, *20*, 133–142. [CrossRef] [PubMed]
11. Sonnweber, T.; Birgit, S.; Weiss, G.; Loffler-Ragg, J. Pulmonary recovery after COVID-19—A review. *Expert Rev. Respir. Med.* **2023**, *17*, 447–457. [CrossRef] [PubMed]
12. Bocchino, M.; Lieto, R.; Romano, F.; Sica, G.; Bocchini, G.; Muto, E.; Capitelli, L.; Sequino, D.; Valente, T.; Fiorentino, G.; et al. Chest CT-based Assessment of 1-year Outcomes after Moderate COVID-19 Pneumonia. *Radiology* **2022**, *305*, 479–485. [CrossRef] [PubMed]
13. Tarraso, J.; Safont, B.; Carbonell-Asins, J.A.; Fernandez-Fabrellas, E.; Sancho-Chust, J.N.; Naval, E.; Amat, B.; Herrera, S.; Ros, J.A.; Soler-Cataluna, J.J.; et al. Lung function and radiological findings 1 year after COVID-19: A prospective follow-up. *Respir. Res.* **2022**, *23*, 242. [CrossRef] [PubMed]
14. Ribeiro Carvalho, C.R.; Lamas, C.A.; Visani de Luna, L.A.; Chate, R.C.; Salge, J.M.; Yamada Sawamura, M.V.; Toufen, C.; Garcia, M.L.; Scudeller, P.G.; Nomura, C.H.; et al. Post-COVID-19 respiratory sequelae two years after hospitalization: An ambidirectional study. *Lancet Reg. Health Am.* **2024**, *33*, 100733. [CrossRef] [PubMed]
15. Babar, M.; Jamil, H.; Mehta, N.; Moutwakil, A.; Duong, T.Q. Short- and Long-Term Chest-CT Findings after Recovery from COVID-19: A Systematic Review and Meta-Analysis. *Diagnostics* **2024**, *14*, 621. [CrossRef] [PubMed]
16. Chen, G.; Wu, D.; Guo, W.; Cao, Y.; Huang, D.; Wang, H.; Wang, T.; Zhang, X.; Chen, H.; Yu, H.; et al. Clinical and immunological features of severe and moderate coronavirus disease 2019. *J. Clin. Investig.* **2020**, *130*, 2620–2629. [CrossRef] [PubMed]
17. Mathew, D.; Giles, J.R.; Baxter, A.E.; Oldridge, D.A.; Greenplate, A.R.; Wu, J.E.; Alanio, C.; Kuri-Cervantes, L.; Pampena, M.B.; D'Andrea, K.; et al. Deep immune profiling of COVID-19 patients reveals distinct immunotypes with therapeutic implications. *Science* **2020**, *369*, eabc8511. [CrossRef] [PubMed]
18. Sharif-Zak, M.; Abbasi-Jorjandi, M.; Asadikaram, G.; Ghoreshi, Z.A.; Rezazadeh-Jabalbarzi, M.; Afsharipur, A.; Rashidinejad, H.; Khajepour, F.; Jafarzadeh, A.; Arefinia, N.; et al. CCR2 and DPP9 expression in the peripheral blood of COVID-19 patients: Influences of the disease severity and gender. *Immunobiology* **2022**, *227*, 152184. [CrossRef] [PubMed]
19. Ranjbar, M.R.A.; Baghernejadan, Z.; Ghorbani, A.; Khorramdelazad, H. Role of CCL2/CCR2 axis in the pathogenesis of COVID-19 and possible Treatments: All options on the Table. *Int. Immunopharmacol.* **2022**, *113 (Pt A)*, 109325. [CrossRef]
20. Milger, K.; Yu, Y.; Brudy, E.; Irmler, M.; Skapenko, A.; Mayinger, M.; Lehmann, M.; Beckers, J.; Reichenberger, F.; Behr, J.; et al. Pulmonary CCR2(+)CD4(+) T cells are immune regulatory and attenuate lung fibrosis development. *Thorax* **2017**, *72*, 1007–1020. [CrossRef] [PubMed]
21. Gloeckl, R.; Leitl, D.; Schneeberger, T.; Jarosch, I.; Koczulla, A.R. Rehabilitative interventions in patients with persistent post COVID-19 symptoms—A review of recent advances and future perspectives. *Eur. Arch. Psychiatry Clin. Neurosci.* **2023**, *274*, 1819–1828. [CrossRef] [PubMed]

medicina

MDPI

Review

Potential Use of GLP-1 and GIP/GLP-1 Receptor Agonists for Respiratory Disorders: Where Are We at?

Miodrag Janić [1,2,3,*], Sabina Škrgat [2,4], Matevž Harlander [2,4], Mojca Lunder [1,2], Andrej Janež [1,2], Anca Pantea Stoian [5], Mohamed El-Tanani [6], Viviana Maggio [3] and Manfredi Rizzo [3,6]

1 Department of Endocrinology, Diabetes and Metabolic Diseases, University Medical Centre Ljubljana, 1000 Ljubljana, Slovenia; mojca.lunder@kclj.si (M.L.); andrej.janez@kclj.si (A.J.)
2 Faculty of Medicine, University of Ljubljana, 1000 Ljubljana, Slovenia; sabina.skrgat@kclj.si (S.Š.); matevz.harlander@kclj.si (M.H.)
3 School of Medicine, PROMISE Department of Health Promotion Sciences Maternal and Infantile Care, Internal Medicine and Medical Specialties, University of Palermo, 90133 Palermo, Italy; viviana.maggio01@unipa.it (V.M.); manfredi.rizzo@unipa.it (M.R.)
4 Department of Pulmonary Diseases and Allergy, University Medical Centre Ljubljana, 1000 Ljubljana, Slovenia
5 Department of Diabetes, Nutrition and Metabolic Diseases, Carol Davila University of Medicine and Pharmacy, 050474 Bucharest, Romania; anca.stoian@umfcd.ro
6 College of Pharmacy, Ras Al Khaimah Medical and Health Sciences University, Ras Al Khaimah P.O. Box 11172, United Arab Emirates; eltanani@rakmhsu.ac.ae
* Correspondence: miodrag.janic@kclj.si

Abstract: Chronic respiratory disorders are the third leading cause of mortality globally. Consequently, there is a continuous pursuit of effective therapies beyond those currently available. The therapeutic potential of the glucagon-like peptide-1 (GLP-1) and the glucose-dependent insulinotropic polypeptide/GLP-1 (GIP/GLP-1) receptor agonists extends beyond the regulation of glycemia, including glucometabolic, cardiovascular, and renal effects, rendering them viable candidates, due to their mechanisms of action, for the possible treatment of respiratory disorders. This manuscript aims to provide a comprehensive evaluation of the evidence on potential direct (cellular) and indirect (metabolic) actions of GLP-1 and GIP/GLP-1 receptor agonists within the pulmonary systems. In addition, it examines their efficacy in addressing prevalent respiratory disorders, specifically chronic obstructive pulmonary disease (COPD), asthma, pneumonia, obstructive sleep apnea, pulmonary hypertension, lung cancer, and lung transplantation. Finally, the manuscript seeks to identify potential avenues for further focused research in this field.

Keywords: respiratory disorders; GLP-1 receptor agonists; GIP/GLP-1 receptor agonists; asthma; COPD

1. Introduction

Glucagon-like peptide-1 (GLP-1) and glucose-dependent insulinotropic polypeptide/GLP-1 (GIP/GLP-1) receptor agonists are well-established in various clinical settings, including glucose control in type 2 diabetes and weight loss in people with and without diabetes [1,2]. Furthermore, clinical trials have established that GLP-1 receptor agonists, including liraglutide, dulaglutide, and semaglutide, are effective in reducing major adverse cardiovascular events (MACE) in people with type 2 diabetes [3–5]. The currently available GLP-1 receptor agonists are derived either from the exendin-4 molecule (exenatide) or from the human GLP-1 scaffold (liraglutide, dulaglutide, and semaglutide). Exenatide exists in short- and long-acting formulations, whereas all human GLP-1 analogs are formulated as long-acting agents. Tirzepatide represents the only available GIP/GLP-1 receptor agonist, and it is derived primarily from the human GIP hormone, which exists as a long-acting formulation [6]. Regardless of diabetes status, semaglutide contributes to a reduction in

MACE and improves heart failure outcomes in those with mildly reduced and preserved ejection fractions, as well as effectively mitigating adverse renal events [3,4,7]. Beyond the effects validated in clinical trials, the GLP-1 and GIP/GLP-1 receptor agonists exhibit additional advantageous pleiotropic effects. The ability of these medications to reach supraphysiological concentrations relative to native GLP-1 and GIP, and their impact on receptors distributed throughout the body, has attracted increased attention. GLP-1 receptors are found in the endocrine and possibly exocrine pancreas, heart, adipose tissue, brain, lung, kidney, blood vessels, gastrointestinal tract, adrenal glands, spleen, eyes, and possibly bone. GIP receptors are present in the endocrine pancreas, heart, adipose tissue, brain, lung, kidney, bone, gastrointestinal tract, adrenal glands, and eyes [8].

Type 2 diabetes is a devastating disease that is increasing in prevalence. It has been associated with chronic obstructive pulmonary disease (COPD), asthma, and obstructive sleep apnea, while it is also accepted as an independent risk factor for pulmonary fibrosis [9]. The associations between diabetes and pulmonary diseases are complex, probably mediated by hyperglycemia, low-grade chronic inflammation, oxidative stress, hyperinsulinemia, endothelial dysfunction, autonomic neuropathy, and impaired mobility of the pulmonary muscles. Furthermore, chronic respiratory disorders represent a global health problem, as they are the third leading cause of death worldwide [10]. As diabetes and pulmonary diseases interconnect, it seems logical to search for a common denominator in their management. The GLP-1 and GIP/GLP-1 receptor agonists present one of the possibilities in this regard. Associations have been investigated in two meta-analyses. In the first meta-analysis of seven large randomized controlled trials that included 55,922 people with type 2 diabetes, 27,942 people were treated with the GLP-1 receptor agonist. The incidence of 12 types of respiratory diseases was evaluated, although their incidence was overall very low, the lowest for interstitial lung disease (0.02% in the GLP-1 receptor agonist group and 0.04% in the control group) and the highest for pneumonia (2.05% in the GLP-1 receptor agonist group and 2.31% in the placebo group). The study showed that, although not at statistical significance, there was a trend for a lower incidence of bronchitis, pneumonia, upper respiratory lung infection, lung squamous cell carcinoma, acute respiratory failure, asthma, chronic obstructive lung disease (COPD), pulmonary fibrosis, and lung oedema. The incidence of interstitial lung disease was higher in the group treated with the GLP-1 receptor agonist, while the effect was neutral for lung adenocarcinoma and obstructive sleep apnea. This study has a weakness with respect to the small incidence of respiratory disease [11]. However, as there is an increased incidence of pneumonia, asthma, and COPD in diabetes [12], this study reaffirms the beneficial effect of GLP-1 receptor agonists in reducing the number of these diseases. The second meta-analysis in 77,485 people from 28 randomized clinical trials showed that in people with type 2 diabetes, overweight, and obesity, treatment with GLP-1 receptor agonists was associated with a significant reduction of 14% in the relative risk, while separate medications, semaglutide, liraglutide, and dulaglutide, were associated with a reduction in the relative risk of 18%, 14%, and 18% for overall respiratory disease. These results were independent of the duration of treatment, the type of control, and the indication for GLP-1 receptor agonist treatment [13]. Therefore, the purpose of this manuscript is to review current evidence for possible actions of GLP-1 and GIP/GLP-1 receptor agonists in the lungs, as well as data on their efficacy in most common respiratory disorders, and to establish whether there is room for further dedicated research in this field. An extensive examination of the current body of literature within the relevant field was conducted utilizing accessible bibliographic databases.

2. Probable Mechanisms of the Beneficial Effects of GLP-1 and GIP/GLP-1 Receptor Agonists in the Lung

Both GLP-1 and GIP receptors can be found in the lung. These receptors are located within multiple lung structures (alveoli pneumocytes, ciliated and club cells, smooth muscle cells of the septa, and the airways and vascular smooth muscles as well as immune cells) and their expression levels appear to be the highest in the lung compared to other organs outside the pancreas [8,14]. Furthermore, the concentration of GLP-1 in the bronchoalveolar fluid is higher than in the serum, thus signaling its important function in the lungs [15]. The evidence on the distribution and effects of GIP receptors in the lungs is limited, and further research is necessary to elucidate their role in the pulmonary immune response [16]. The summary of probable direct and indirect effects mediated by the GLP-1 and GIP/GLP-1 receptor agonists in the lungs is presented in Figure 1.

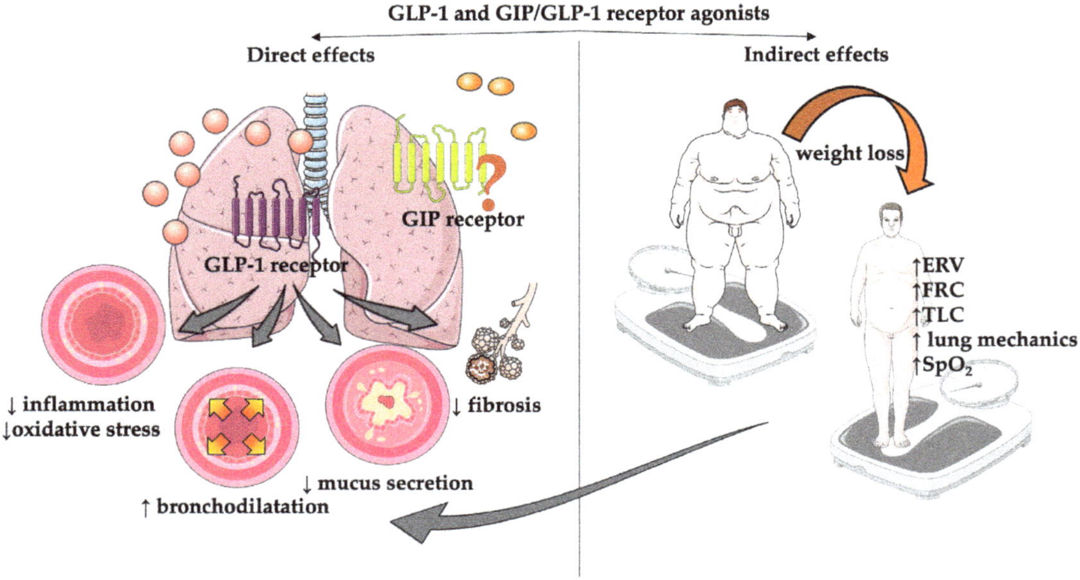

Figure 1. Summary of the direct and indirect effects of glucagon-like peptide-1 (GLP-1) and glucose-dependent insulinotropic polypeptide/GLP-1 (GIP/GLP-1) receptor agonists in lungs. The red question mark indicates that the effects mediated by GIP receptors in the lungs have not yet been fully understood, despite the confirmed presence of these receptors in the lungs. The grey arrow indicates that the indirect effects associated with weight loss also positively affect the direct effects achieved by the GLP-1 and GIP/GLP-1 receptor agonists in the lungs. ERV, expiratory residual volume; FRC, functional respiratory capacity; TLC, total lung capacity; SpO_2, blood oxygenation.

2.1. Direct Effects

The direct effects of GLP-1 receptor agonists and probably GIP/GLP-1 receptor agonists in the lungs are mediated primarily through the GLP-1 receptors, namely anti-inflammatory and antioxidant, bronchodilator, mucus-producing, and antifibrotic mechanisms (Figure 1). GLP-1 receptor agonists can modulate immune responses by influencing the signaling of immune cells and changing the signaling environment from pro-inflammatory to anti-inflammatory. This is coupled with a reduced oxidative stress, and these effects are beyond the glucose-lowering effects of these drugs.

Many immune cells, including macrophages, monocytes, eosinophils, and lymphocytes, express GLP-1 receptors. By binding to them, GLP-1 receptor agonists act in different ways. Intracellular signaling is mediated by adenylate cyclase (AC), which, through two subsequent cascades, further transmits the signal. The first cascade involves cyclic adenosine monophosphate (cAMP)-calcium that results in stimulation of the energy-sensing AMP-activated protein kinase (AMPK). Second, it involves the stimulation of protein kinase A (PKA). These both lead to reduced expression of the nuclear factor kappa B (NF-κB) and increased expression of signal transducer and activator of transcription 1 (STAT1) [17]. This is also achieved directly through the GLP-1 receptor-mediated activation of the extracellular signal-regulated kinase 1/2 (ERK1/2) pathway. Consequently, activation of these cascades leads to a reduction of the pro-inflammatory cytokine release, including tumor necrosis factor alpha (TNF-α), interleukin 6 (IL-6), IL-1β, Il-17, IL-2, and interferon γ (INF-γ), the so called non-T helper cells 2 (Th2)-mediated cytokine profile (Figure 2), and reduction in adhesion molecule release including vascular cell adhesion protein 1 (VCAM-1), intercellular adhesion molecule 1 (ICAM-1), and E-selectin. Furthermore, chemokine release is also reduced, including the C-X-C motif chemokine ligand 10 (CXCL10) and the monocyte chemoattractant protein-1 (MCP-1). Expression of IL-1β is additionally suppressed through GLP-1 receptor mediated inhibition of the protein kinase C (PKC) cascade. On the other hand, the production of anti-inflammatory cytokines, such as IL-10, increases in addition to mannose receptor-1 (MRC-1) and the release of arginine-1 (Arg-1), prostaglandin E2 (PGE2), and cyclooxygenase 2 (COX2) [18–20]. Collectively, these mechanisms lead to attenuation of inflammation.

Airway smooth muscle cells also express GLP-1 receptors. Signal transduction is mediated through the increase in adenosine-triphosphate-binding cassette transporter A1 (ABCA1) and decrease in IL-6, IL-8, TNF-α, as well as granulocyte and macrophage colony-stimulating factor (GM-CSF). The net effect is reduced proliferation and migration of smooth muscle cells in the airways, as well as their reduced secretion of inflammatory mediators [20].

GLP-1 receptor agonists also inhibit the formation of asymmetric dimethylarginine (ADMA) by modulating the advanced glycation end products (AGE) and their interaction with receptor for the AGE (RAGE), also through the PKA and blunting of NF-κB, thus suppressing the expression of the arginine methyltransferase-1 protein and inhibiting the production of reactive oxygen species. Administration of GLP-1 receptor agonists may also further inhibit dysregulated autophagy and inflammation induced by reactive oxygen species. Even more, endothelial nitric oxide (eNOS) synthesis, which is inhibited by ADMA, is thus augmented because of NF-κB and ADMA suppression [17,19]. Alternative immunomodulatory mechanisms of GLP-1 receptor agonists may encompass the modification of T cell functionality by diminishing the expression of CD28 and CD86, alongside the reduction of tissue factor (TF) and plasminogen activator inhibitor (PAI-1) production [16]. The antioxidative effects of GLP-1 receptor agonists can also be facilitated by the attenuation of lipid peroxidation, suppression of mitochondrial autophagic signaling pathways, and reduction in alpha-synuclein synthesis, which collectively lead to the inhibition of apoptosis and normalization of mitochondrial dynamic imbalance. Furthermore, the induction and upregulation of antioxidant enzymes, specifically superoxide dismutase and glutathione peroxidase, coupled with the downregulation of nicotinamide adenine dinucleotide phosphate (NADPH) oxidase and malondialdehyde levels, may represent a mechanism through which GLP-1 receptor agonists exert their antioxidative effects [20].

It is important to acknowledge that the mechanisms associated with GLP-1 receptor agonists, together with supplementary protein synthesis pathways within the smooth muscle cells of the airways, endothelial cells, and immune cells, may contribute to an imbalance in protease-antiprotease equilibrium. This occurs in addition to the indirect mechanisms that promote the synthesis of α1 antitrypsin in the liver. These processes result in the inhibition of the destruction of the alveolar septa and the development of emphysema [20].

Several studies indicate that GLP-1 receptor agonists may possess bronchodilator effects that can be facilitated through transduction pathways analogous to anti-inflammatory mechanisms. The activation of the cAMP/PKA, cAMP/guanine nucleotide exchange factor (GEF), and phosphatidylinositol-3 kinase (PI3)/PKC pathways by the GLP-1 receptor agonist in smooth muscle cells of the airways collectively facilitates the relaxation of these cells. Within the airway epithelium, specifically in goblet and airway epithelial cells, the agonism of GLP-1 receptors results in reduced expression of IL-33 and thymic stromal lymphopoietin (TSLP), which subsequently suppress group 2 innate lymphoid cells (ILC2), Th2 cells, and eosinophils from releasing IL-4, IL-5, and IL-13, the so-called Th2-mediated cytokine profile. This cascade culminates in decreased mucus secretion and increased surfactant production, complemented by thyroid transcription factor 1 (TTF-1) signaling pathway [10,17,21].

There is evidence suggesting that GLP-1 receptor agonists may possess antifibrotic properties, making them potential candidates for attenuating the progression of pulmonary fibrosis. In this context, IL-1β is recognized for its role in mediating extracellular matrix formation directly or through transforming growth factor β1 (TGF-β1). The latter, primarily derived from alveolar macrophages, is responsible for the differentiation of fibroblasts into myofibroblasts and the induction of fibrosis-related gene expression. Consequently, suppression of IL-1β via GLP-1 receptor mediation, particularly through the pathway involving PKC-mediated inhibition of the nucleotide-binding domain, leucine-rich-containing family, pyrin-domain-containing-3 (NLRP3) inflammasome, can further contribute to reducing the formation of a profibrotic environment. The antifibrotic effects are further facilitated by the altered interaction between the glycolytic pathway driven by 6-phosphofructo-2-kinase/fructose-2,6-biphosphatase 3 (PFKFB3) and the NLRP3 inflammasome, along with the subsequent inhibition of lactate-mediated histone lactylation [22].

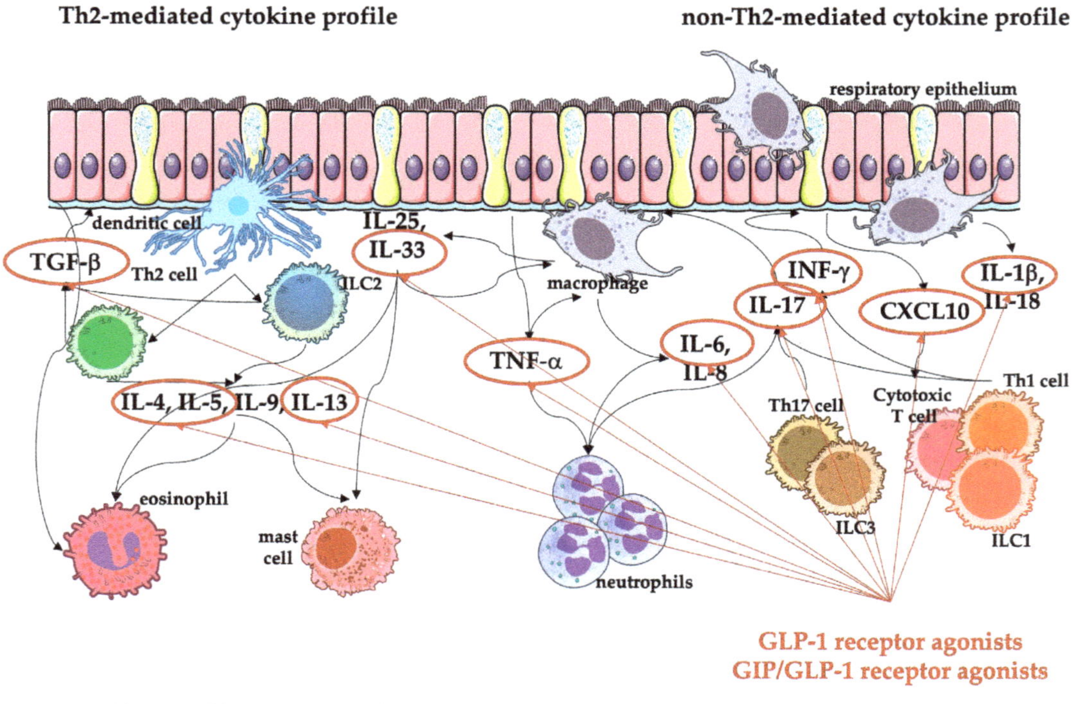

Figure 2. Main cytokine profiles attenuated by glucagon-like peptide-1 (GLP-1) and glucose-dependent insulinotropic polypeptide/GLP-1 (GIP/GLP-1) receptor agonists. The T helper cells 2 (Th2)-mediated cytokine profile is characteristic mainly for asthma and to a lesser degree for chronic obstructive pulmonary disease (COPD), while the non-Th2 mediated cytokine profile can be found in obesity-related asthma and COPD [23,24]. The red arrows show the cytokines that are affected by the GLP-1 and GIP/GLP-1 receptor agonists. TGF, transforming growth factor; IL, interleukin; TNF, tumor necrosis factor; INF, interferon; CXCL, C-X-C motif chemokine ligand; Th cell, T helper cell; ILC, innate lymphoid cell.

2.2. Indirect Effects

The indirect effects of the use of GLP-1 and GIP/GLP-1 receptor agonists on the lung are probably mediated by weight loss and improved lung mechanics. Data from weight loss studies suggest an impact on lung function. The benefits of weight loss in overweight/obese individuals are reflected in increased expiratory residual volume (ERV), functional respiratory capacity (FRC), total lung capacity (TLC), gas exchange, and consequent increase in blood oxygenation in addition to improvement in respiratory muscle strength and dyspnea [25]. Furthermore, weight loss is associated with a substantial decrease in adipose tissue generated pro-inflammatory mediators, probably enhancing the direct anti-inflammatory and antioxidant effects of these drugs [19].

Semaglutide at a dose of 2.4 mg is currently the most effective GLP-1 receptor agonist for weight reduction. In a meta-analysis involving 3087 obese individuals without diabetes, it resulted in an average weight loss difference of −12.3 kg (−12.1%) compared to a placebo for an average duration of 77 weeks. Side effects were mostly gastrointestinal in the semaglutide treated groups, but showed only mild to moderate severity and did not require discontinuation of treatment [26]. There exists biological plausibility for an association between GLP-1 receptor agonists and the development of medullary thyroid carcinomas in rodent models, as well as the formation of nonlethal thyroid C-cell tumors. Such findings were similar in two-year carcinogenicity studies involving semaglutide administered to rats and mice [27]. However, recent systematic reviews of the available evidence have indicated that there are no significant associations between semaglutide administration and thyroid cancer risk, with a reported incidence of less than 1% among patients treated with semaglutide. Furthermore, thyroid cancer has been shown to exhibit an association with overweight and obesity, implying that the population targeted for treatment with these drugs may have an increased predisposition to thyroid cancer development [28].

A pooled analysis of tirzepatide, currently the only GIP/GLP-1 receptor agonist, in 4036 participants regardless of diabetes status, for a treatment duration of 12 to 72 weeks, showed a significant weight loss of mean difference of −7.7 kg (−8.1%), −11.6 kg (−11.9%), and −11.8 kg (−12.4%) compared to placebo for doses of 5, 10, and 15 mg, respectively. Adverse events were more common in the tirzepatide-treated groups, presenting as nausea, vomiting, and diarrhea [29]. In the SURMOUNT-1 trial, 2539 people with overweight (body mass index (BMI) $\geq$ 27 kg/m^2 and one obesity related complication) and obesity BMI $\geq$ 30 kg/m^2 were treated with tirzepatide 5, 10, or 15 mg or placebo for 72 weeks. The mean percentage of weight reduction at 72 weeks ranged from −15.0%, −19.5%, and −20.9% for tirzepatide 5, 10, and 15 mg compared to −3.1% in the placebo group. Overall, 85% of the participants achieved more than 5% weight loss with a dose of 5 mg, while 57% of the participants achieved more than 20% weight loss at 15 mg. The adverse events that led to discontinuation of therapy were 4.3%, 7.1%, and 6.2% for 5, 10, and 15 mg of tirzepatide, respectively, and 2.6% in the placebo-treated group [30]. Data indicate a substantial impact on weight reduction, suggesting a promising ancillary role for GLP-1 and GIP/GLP-1 receptor agonists, which could contribute to an indirect improvement in lung function.

3. GLP-1 and GIP/GLP-1 Receptor Agonists and Common Pulmonary Diseases

3.1. Chronic Obstructive Pulmonary Disease

Chronic obstructive pulmonary disease (COPD) is characterized by airway obstruction that is poorly reversible. Chronic inflammation appears to be the primary cause. There may be obstruction of small airways leading to chronic obstructive bronchitis and destruction of the alveolar walls, known as emphysema, resulting in air trapping, dyspnea, and diminished physical capacity. It is strongly associated with smoking and air pollution. Smoking cessation is the only intervention known to reverse the progression of the disease. According to the World Health Organization (WHO), COPD ranks seventh in the leading cause of poor health and third in the leading cause of mortality globally [31]. COPD can be accompanied by diabetes, and patients with both conditions are more likely to experience severe exacerbations and death compared to COPD patients without diabetes [20]. As this is the case, there is a need for additional treatment that would lessen the burden of each disease on the others.

Potential common strategy could be based on the use of GLP-1 and GIP/GLP-1 receptor agonists. Data on the effects of GLP-1 receptor agonists have been published in patients with COPD, while no data on GIP/GLP-1 receptor agonists have been found. In one study, 1642 patients with type 2 diabetes and COPD from the US health system participated in a retrospective, observational, health record-based study. The active comparator was implemented, with a new user design, with users of the GLP-1 receptor agonist defined as the reference group. Fewer unadjusted COPD exacerbations were recorded in GLP-1 receptor users compared to significantly higher adjusted exacerbation rates with dipeptidyl peptidase 4 (DPP-4) inhibitor users and sulfonylurea users. Users of the GLP-1 receptor agonists were also less likely to experience severe exacerbations. No statistically significant differences were recorded between users of the GLP-1 receptor agonist and users of the sodium-glucose cotransporter 2 (SGLT-2) inhibitor [32]. These results were not stratified according to BMI, as this could also lead to fewer exacerbations and the possible impact due to weight loss was not considered. Furthermore, the impact of COPD overlap syndrome was not considered [33]. However, this gives a signal of a favorable effect of GLP-1 receptor agonist therapy in the COPD population, as was also previously shown in a similar study in the UK, where a 30% reduction per 100 person years of severe exacerbations was recorded in GLP-1 receptor agonist users compared to sulfonylurea users, as well as a 37% reduction per 100 person years of moderate exacerbations. There was a similar finding for the users of SGLT-2 inhibitor, but only for severe exacerbations [34]. Furthermore, among 8060 Taiwanese people with type 2 diabetes and COPD, users of the GLP-1 receptor agonist with a median follow-up duration of 2.51 years, the risk of pulmonary complication was significantly lower than in non-users. Users of the GLP-1 receptor agonists were significantly less likely to need non-invasive positive pressure ventilation, invasive mechanical ventilation, and to have bacterial pneumonia than nonusers. This observation was documented among non-obese individuals, while no notable reduction in either outcome was observed for obese individuals; this may suggest that these findings are not attributable to weight reduction. Additionally, a significantly lower risk of mortality and cardiovascular events was recorded in the users group. A longer duration of GLP-1 receptor agonist use was also associated with a lower risk of invasive mechanical ventilation, bacterial pneumonia, mortality, and cardiovascular events [35]. Only one prospective study evaluated the impact of liraglutide versus placebo in 30 people with obesity and COPD at different times on lung function tests, 6 min walk test, and responses to a questionnaire on the clinical impact of COPD (COPD assessment test—CAT score). After 40 weeks of follow-up, body weight loss was significant in users of liraglutide, forced vital capacity increased significantly, as did carbon monoxide diffusion capacity, while the CAT score improved. Other lung parameters did not reach statistical significance compared to the placebo group, but this opens the way for the preferred treatment with GLP-1 receptor agonists in this clinical setting [36].

Peripheral blood mononuclear cells (PBMC) isolated from COPD patients showed defective signaling of the GLP-1 receptor compared to subjects without COPD. The GLP-1 receptor dysfunction was characterized by decreased INF-γ expression that led to the defective T-cell functioning. When PBMC were incubated in liraglutide, the GLP-1 receptor signaling was upregulated, followed by increased INF-γ production and downregulated programmed cell death protein 1 expression on T-cells [37]. Furthermore, in female C57BL/6 mice with induced metabolic syndrome and emphysema, treatment with the GLP-1 receptor agonist has been shown to reduce the area of emphysema, as well as to increase the number of CD31+ endothelial cells, probably through reduced inflammation and positive effects on lipid and glucose metabolism. The authors propose the creation of the GLP-1-based drug focused on epithelial regeneration, as endothelial progenitor cells have been shown to be a pathogenetic and disease marker in this setting [38]. This is also in accordance with indirect mechanisms that promote the GLP-1 receptor agonists-mediated synthesis of α1 antitrypsin in the liver, as mentioned earlier [20]. Balk-Møller et al. showed improvement in lung function in COPD mice treated with the GLP-1 receptor agonist. They recorded less inflammation, but not less emphysema, compared to the study described above. Furthermore, mice treated with the GLP-1 receptor agonist had higher expression of atrial natriuretic peptide and decreased endothelin-1 expression, leading to a more bronchodilator environment [39]. Additionally, in mice, exendin-4 reinstated forkhead box protein A2 (FOXA2) expression lessened mucin production in airway cells affected by COPD and decreased both mucin and *P. aeruginosa* load in the lungs of mice, showing potential protective effect in COPD [40]. Similar findings for lixisenatide have been shown in 16 human bronchial epithelial cells (16HBE), where it reduced lipopolysaccharide-induced expression of mucin and inflammation by regulation of nuclear factor erythroid 2 related factor 2 (Nrf2) [41]. These mechanisms, shown in non-clinical environments, seem to translate into the clinical setting, as data from human trials show the positive impact of GLP-1 receptor agonists on favorable outcomes in patients with COPD.

3.2. Asthma

Asthma is a condition that involves persistent inflammation and variable structural changes in the large and small airways. It presents with a variety of symptoms, including wheezing, difficulty breathing, chest tightness, and coughing, which can change in severity and over time. The course of the disease can vary, and, in some patients, it can quickly lead to reduced lung function. Often associated with allergic diathesis, it tends to occur less frequently in association with allergies in adults. It is often accompanied by multiorgan allergies and non-allergic health problems such as obesity, gastroesophageal reflux disease, and mental health disorders. Affecting more than 4% of the world's population, it is among the most common chronic diseases [42]. Asthma is currently treated with inhalator glucocorticoids, long-acting beta agonists, leukotriene receptor antagonists, and long-acting antimuscarinic agents advancing to biologic therapies, particularly for the high-T2 (characterized by the subpopulation of CD4+ T cells—Th2 cells secreting the IL-4, IL-5, IL-13) resistant asthma phenotype. However, treatment gaps remain, as, despite therapy, some patients still have insufficiently controlled asthma. When asthma is associated with obesity and insulin resistance, the low T2 phenotype is more prevalent and is often resistant to targeted therapy [43,44]. This treatment gap, particularly in people with obesity and insulin resistance, could be at least partially overcome with GLP-1 and GIP/GLP-1 receptor agonists, as this clinical setting calls for weight loss (indirect anti-inflammatory action) and a potential direct anti-inflammatory action of these medications to reduce asthma exacerbations, possibly through some of the described mechanisms.

Khan et al. report, in 7 adherent patients with type 2 diabetes and asthma treated with liraglutide for 52 weeks, an improvement in glucometabolic parameters, as well as asthma symptoms and exacerbations, since no subject adherent to liraglutide had a significant deterioration of asthma. This was not related to changes in dose or the addition of other asthma control drugs. Two patients in that cohort dropped out due to drug-related side effects, with one of them experiencing a non-fatal severe exacerbation [45]. Foer et al. followed this with the publication of research that compared the rates of asthma exacerbations and symptoms in people with type 2 diabetes using a GLP-1 receptor agonist with those using other antidiabetic drugs (SGLT-2 inhibitors, DPP-4 inhibitors, sulfonylureas, or basal insulin) to intensify the treatment of diabetes. The study was retrospective, using a new user-based health record with an active comparator, calculating propensity scores for the use of GLP-1 receptor agonists and the use of non-GLP-1 receptor agonists. They report, after adjusting for propensity scores and other covariates, that 6 months after initiation, asthma exacerbations were lower in people who started using the GLP-1 receptor agonist compared to all other drug users; the same trend was reported for asthma symptoms. The findings remained consistent even after adjustment for variations in BMI and glucose control, indicating that these associations do not depend solely on weight or glucose management. These effects were even more pronounced in patients with moderate and severe asthma. This study suggested that GLP-1 receptor agonists could be a novel solution to manage asthma-associated metabolic dysfunction [46]. Critics of this study suggest that a comparison with metformin, previously shown to improve asthma outcomes, would be necessary to further reveal the efficacy of GLP-1 receptor agonist treatment in this setting, as well as some statistical/methodical issues [47]. However, this study encouraged further research in this field. In 2024, the investigation of new antidiabetic therapies and metformin was reported on asthma exacerbations in people with asthma and type 2 diabetes. Kimura et al. report that in the Japanese national administrative database, among 137,173 new oral antidiabetic drugs users with history of asthma, people treated with GLP-1 receptor agonists had a hazard ratio of 1.14 (95% CI: 1.01–1.28) for exacerbations requiring systemic glucocorticoid therapy compared to metformin [48]. In a recent meta-analysis of 39 randomized controlled trials involving people with obesity and/or type 2 diabetes, a trend towards a reduction in the risk of asthma was recorded in users of GLP-1 receptor agonists compared to non-users. This was significant only with light molecular weight GLP-1 receptor agonists (efpeglenatide, exenatide, liraglutide, semaglutide) [49]. The most recent study used data from the UK Clinical Practice Research Datalink Aurum (2004–2020) that included new metformin users with type 2 diabetes. The findings indicate that metformin was associated with a 32% reduction in asthma attacks as reported by the patients and a 24% reduction determined by the inverse probability weighting methodologies. These results remained unaffected by variations in HbA1c, BMI, blood eosinophil counts, or severity of asthma. Furthermore, the adjunctive use of GLP-1 receptor agonists contributed to an additional 40% reduction in the relative rates of asthma attacks. Both metformin and GLP-1 receptor agonists were effective in reducing asthma attacks, independently of glucose and weight management [50].

However, the association between GLP-1 and GIP/GLP-1 receptor agonists and asthma is not unambiguous. Among 159,705 patients in 19 randomized controlled trials, data from 218 asthma patients indicated that SGLT-2 inhibitors were associated with a markedly reduced risk of asthma, with an odds ratio of 0.59 (95% CI: 0.38–0.93). In contrast, GLP-1 receptor agonists and DPP-4 inhibitors did not demonstrate a significant impact on asthma risk [51]. Recently, data from the US Food and Drug Administration (FDA) adverse event reporting system (FAERS) revealed that in the real world, particularly exenatide, liraglutide, and semaglutide were associated with increased rates of asthma and asthma-like events (for the latter two, the association was significant). Furthermore, incidents and deaths related to asthma were reported, and exenatide was responsible for the highest share of deaths. The cause of the finding could be due to multiple factors. It may be due to the spontaneous nature of the FAERS reporting mechanism, which operates without medical review, allowing for potential misclassification of cases or the appearance of reporting bias. Furthermore, the approximate incidence of adverse events was derived from signal strength rather than exact figures. From a mechanistic perspective, the increased incidence of respiratory-related adverse events associated with exenatide can be attributed to its derivation from nonhuman GLP-1, with which it shares only 50% structural homology, potentially leading to increased immunogenicity. Furthermore, the patient populations prescribed various GLP-1 receptor agonists differ, possibly influencing the risk of asthma-related adverse events (considering factors such as age, comorbidities, preexisting respiratory conditions, smoking status, genetic predisposition). On the contrary, there were fewer respiratory and asthma-like events with tirzepatide, a dual agonist of the GIP and GLP-1 receptors. This observation may reflect an additional or synergistic anti-inflammatory effect attributed to GIP receptor agonism alongside GLP-1 receptor agonism. The authors also admit that the findings may be mainly statistical rather than causal. However, these findings require careful and cautious interpretation. It is important to remember that FAERS data can provide valuable information on the respiratory safety profile of GLP-1 receptor agonists [52].

From a mechanistic point of view, GLP-1 receptor agonists were shown to reduce airway inflammation through the NF-κB PKA-dependent inflammation pathway. They also decrease the release of IL-33 through which inflammatory Th2 are reduced and IL-5 and 13 are released, leading to a reduced number of eosinophils and reduced goblet metaplasia and mucus production (Figure 2) [53]. This is supported by research conducted on purified human neutrophils and eosinophils from healthy people and asthmatics. The expression of GLP-1 receptors in eosinophils in asthma patients was significantly lower than in healthy people's eosinophils, while the number of GLP-1 receptors in neutrophils was the same in both populations. A lipopolysaccharide challenge was carried out and significantly less surface activation markers of eosinophils were present in eosinophils treated with the GLP-1 receptor agonist, and their production of IL-4, 8, and 13, but not IL-5, decreased. This leads to the conclusion that there could be a direct effect of GLP-1 receptor agonists on eosinophils implicated in asthma exacerbation [54]. Furthermore, in obese asthma mice, the GLP-1 receptor agonist liraglutide was shown to reduce airway hyperresponsiveness and eosinophilic airway inflammation, which were associated with significant weight loss. In bronchoalveolar lavage, there was a reduction in IL-4, 5, and 33. In peribronchial tissue, a reduction in inflammation was also detected through the receptor protein 3 nucleotide oligomerization domain (NLPR3) inflammasome and IL-1β (Figure 2) [55]. Although the investigation using human isolated LPS-stimulated eosinophils did not demonstrate a reduction in IL-5, the obese asthma mouse model exhibited a decrease in IL-5 levels in bronchoalveolar lavage. The observed discrepancies are probably attributable to the different models used in their evaluation, suggesting that eosinophils are not the sole source of IL-5 production. Furthermore, the obese asthma model indicates that treatment with GLP-1 receptor agonists results in a cumulative attenuation of IL-5 production from all sources.

Similar findings have been reported for tirzepatide, showing a significant reduction in body weight, as well as glucose control and a reduction in leptin levels in the obese polygenic mouse model compared to semaglutide, GIP agonist alone, or vehicle. This was accompanied by reduction of Th2 inflammation and activation of ILC2 in tirzepatide treated mice lung compared to vehicle. There was also a reduction in IL-5, 13, and the number of Th2 cells in the lungs compared to semaglutide treatment, but with respect to IL-33, semaglutide was more powerful as its release is mediated particularly through the agonism of the GLP-1 receptor in which tirzepatide has less affinity. These findings support the fact that tirzepatide reduces allergic inflammation in the aeroallergen-induced model of asthma in obese mice [56]. In summary, GLP-1 (and possibly GIP/GLP-1) receptor agonists could improve asthma outcomes through weight reduction, decreased airway inflammation and mucus secretion, decreased type 2 inflammation signaling, reduction in IL-4, 5, 13, and 33 secretion, reduced mast cell activity, as well as increases in surfactant production and smooth muscle relaxation [57].

3.3. *Pneumonia*

Pneumonia represents a common respiratory disease that affects the alveoli and distal bronchial structures of the lungs. It is contracted primarily within the community (community-acquired) or within hospital settings (hospital-acquired), where it may also be associated with mechanical ventilation. Aspiration pneumonia accounts for 5% to 15% of community-acquired pneumonia cases, although its prevalence in hospital settings remains undetermined. The people most frequently affected are children under the age of 5 and adults over the age of 70 years, and these demographic groups also exhibit the highest mortality rates. In 2019, more than 2.5 million people were estimated to have succumbed to lower respiratory tract infections, half of these fatalities occurring in people aged 70 years or older. The etiology of pneumonia can be categorized as bacterial or viral. *Streptococcus pneumoniae* is the main causative microorganism for community-acquired pneumonia, whereas *Staphylococcus aureus* predominantly accounts for hospital-acquired cases [58,59]. The most prevalent viral pathogens responsible for pneumonia are human rhinovirus and influenza virus; recently, severe acute respiratory syndrome coronavirus 2 (SARS-CoV-2) has emerged as a significant etiological factor [58]. Individuals with diabetes exhibit an increased susceptibility to infections compared to those without diabetes, regardless of comorbid conditions and other confounding factors. People with diabetes face a two to four-fold increased risk of hospitalization due to infections, along with a 1.5-fold elevated risk of infection in outpatient settings. This pattern was particularly apparent during the COVID-19 pandemic. Diabetes is associated with more severe infection outcomes, as demonstrated by a two-fold increase in the mortality rate from COVID-19 [60].

In research carried out by Brunetti et al., they examined data from nearly 30,000 individuals, of which 705 were admitted to hospitals for community-acquired pneumonia during an average follow-up period of 1.7 years. Their findings revealed that users of SGLT-2 inhibitors faced a markedly reduced risk of hospitalization for community-acquired pneumonia compared to those using DPP-4 inhibitors. When beneficiaries were evaluated against GLP-1 receptor agonist users, no variations in risk were identified [61].

A network meta-analysis comprising 31 studies with nearly 3.7 million participants diagnosed with type 2 diabetes indicated that the incidence of adverse outcomes related to COVID-19 was the least frequent among those given SGLT-2 inhibitors, exhibiting a probability of 6% prior to their diagnosis of COVID-19. Furthermore, the use of GLP-1 receptor agonists and metformin was associated with a reduction in adverse COVID-19 outcomes compared to other antidiabetic medications, with GLP-1 receptor agonists showing a probability of 25% and metformin a probability of 28% [62]. A comprehensive meta-analysis conducted by Song et al. demonstrated that GLP-1 receptor agonists, along with SGLT-2 inhibitors and metformin, had a favorable impact on COVID-19 outcomes. The study revealed that GLP-1 receptor agonists were correlated with a 27% reduction in mortality, a 16% decrease in the risk of severe disease, and a 14% decrease in the probability of hospitalization for COVID-19 compared to insulin. The influence of various glucose-lowering medications on COVID-19 outcomes may have been moderated by their utilization in hospital settings versus nonhospital environments, their administration among elderly versus younger populations, and by geographical variations [63]. It is interesting to observe that during COVID-19, there was a notable increase in IL-6 levels, along with a marked increase in GLP-1 and procalcitonin levels at the time of admission and within 5 to 6 days after hospitalization in patients who succumbed to the disease, compared to those who survived. This phenomenon was discernible in both individuals with diabetes and without diabetes. However, the intensity of the pro-inflammatory/GLP-1 response was modulated by the presence of type 2 diabetes. Furthermore, hypoxemia specifically attenuated the GLP-1 response in people with type 2 diabetes who experienced bilateral lung damage. The authors observed that the increase in GLP-1 and procalcitonin levels indicated a bacterial infection, but the efficacy of GLP-1 receptor agonists in this particular context was not evaluated [64].

Direct application of tirzepatide in patients with COVID-19 has not yet been researched. However, potential mechanisms for reducing complications have been proposed. Tirzepatide can potentially decrease inflammation in COVID-19 cases, and its effects on weight reduction and the reduction of body fat can mitigate the severity of COVID-19. Furthermore, tirzepatide, similar to GLP-1 receptor agonists, is believed to alleviate COVID-19-induced alterations in the intestinal microbiota, thus decreasing intestinal inflammation and systemic complications in people with type 2 diabetes or obesity. Furthermore, through GIP agonism, it may inhibit the expression of IL-1β, IL-6, MCP-1, chemokines, and TNF-α [65].

A study that investigated the impact of GLP-1 receptor agonists on infectious (influenza) and non-infectious (bleomycin-induced) lung inflammation in wild-type and GLP-1 receptor knockout mice revealed that in the absence of the GLP-1 receptor, bleomycin-induced lung injury was less severe, while activation of the GLP-1 receptor was correlated with increased pulmonary inflammation mediated through the sympathetic nervous system. Administration of liraglutide led to a reduction in pathogen load in influenza-infected mice and increased survival rates [66].

In murine models of pneumonia-induced sepsis, liraglutide has been shown to significantly reduce levels of pro-inflammatory cytokines, such as TNF-α and IL-6, in the pulmonary system compared to septic control cohorts. Additionally, liraglutide significantly promoted the expression and secretion of pulmonary surfactant proteins, along with the secretion of phospholipids. These effects culminated in higher survival rates and attenuated pulmonary inflammation and damage within this specific model. GLP-1 receptor agonists have been observed to strengthen host defense mechanisms and facilitate alveolar respiratory function in the presence of acute lung injury [67].

Not unimportant, in the perioperative period, the use of GLP-1 and GIP/GLP-1 receptor agonists may be associated with an increased risk of regurgitation and aspiration of gastric contents into the lungs during induction of general anesthesia due to delayed emptying and retention of gastric contents. This is a rare but serious complication with an incidence of 1 in 3000 to 4000 elective procedures [68]. Pneumonitis, aspiration pneumonia, and other lung injuries are associated with increased morbidity and are the most common cause of anesthesia-related mortality. The greatest risk factor for them is the presence of food or fluid in the stomach immediately before the procedure [68,69]. Recommendations for the perioperative management of patients have not previously considered special measures for patients treated with GLP-1 and GIP/GLP-1 receptor agonists. However, there have been increasing reports of clinical cases of regurgitation and/or aspiration of gastric contents during induction of general anesthesia and extubation. The retention of solids and liquids in the stomach has been described during endoscopic procedures, and there are also increasing reports of gastric content retention detected by perioperative gastric ultrasound [70].

Together, it seems that treatment with GLP-1 and GIP/GLP-1 receptor agonists per se could have a protective role in respiratory infections or at least in favorable outcomes. However, on the other hand, treatment with GLP-1 and GIP/GLP-1 receptor agonists is also associated with an increased risk of gastric content retention and aspiration or regurgitation in the perioperative period. While considering the benefits of GLP-1 and GIP/GLP-1 receptor agonist therapy, caution is needed in clinical scenarios for discontinuation of drugs before procedures, as people with type 2 diabetes risk worsening diabetes control. A compromise should be accepted to bring about the greatest benefit with the least acceptable cost.

3.4. Obstructive Sleep Apnea

Obstructive sleep apnea is marked by episodes of apnea and hypopnea during sleep, leading to hypoxemia, hypercapnia, and frequent awakening. These effects result in significant drowsiness during the day. The condition affects an estimated 900 million people worldwide. It is also a risk factor for cardiovascular disease. Randomized control trials have not shown that continuous positive airway pressure (CPAP) therapy reduces the rate of cardiovascular events or mortality in this population. High body fat or adiposity is well known to be associated with obstructive sleep apnea and its related problems, and the advantages of weight loss have been recognized for a long time [71,72]. Furthermore, there also appears to be a link between the severity of obstructive sleep apnea and the reduced native GLP-1 response, which further deteriorates glucose metabolism, causes weight gain, and increases the risk of developing type 2 diabetes. Therefore, the GLP-1 and GIP/GLP-1 receptor agonists in this clinical setting have value in their weight reduction potential and glucose metabolism normalization as well as cardiovascular risk reduction and could even progress to first-line therapy for obstructive sleep apnea [73].

Liraglutide was evaluated in the SCALE sleep apnea randomized trial in non-diabetic patients. Patients with obesity and moderate-to-severe sleep apnea defined by the apnea-hypopnea index (AHI) $\geq$ 15 events per hour but unwilling to use or incapable of using CPAP therapy were randomized to receive either liraglutide 3.0 mg daily or placebo in addition to diet and exercise. After 32 weeks, the reduction in AHI was significant in the group treated with liraglutide, that is, for −12.2 events per hour compared to −6.1 events per hour in the control group, in addition to significant weight loss. Post hoc analysis revealed a significant association between weight loss and all end points of obstructive sleep apnea. Cardiometabolic parameters also improved in the group treated with liraglutide. The safety profile of liraglutide was acceptable [74]. A two-center randomized controlled study with liraglutide was conducted in people with type 2 diabetes and obstructive sleep apnea requiring CPAP. After a 3 month intervention period, in people receiving liraglutide on top of CPAP therapy, after significant weight loss, AHI significantly decreased from 31.0 ± 7.3 to 26.1 ± 7.1 events per hour, while and mean systolic blood pressure were all significantly reduced compared with the control group. The minimum oxygen saturation significantly increased from $80.3 \pm 5.8\%$ to $83.4 \pm 5.8\%$ in the liraglutide treated group compared to unsignificant changes in the placebo-controlled group only treated with CPAP. Cardiometabolic parameters also improved significantly. This was achieved without an unreasonable number of side effects [75]. An ongoing open-label prospective study is evaluating the effect of liraglutide (1.8 mg once a day) alone, liraglutide 1.8 mg daily with CPAP, CPAP alone, or without treatment in people with obstructive sleep apnea, obesity, and type 2 diabetes. This study is designed to examine the impact of weight loss-induced reductions in AHI, as well as secondary cardiometabolic parameters. It will be the first study to compare GLP-1 receptor agonist therapy and CPAP efficiency head-to-head [76].

In a recently published randomized controlled trial, SURMOUNT-OSA, tirzepatide was evaluated at maximum tolerated doses of 10 and 15 mg a week compared to placebo for its efficacy in reducing AHI in adults with obesity and moderate to severe obstructive sleep apnea. SURMOUNT-OSA was composed of two trials. The first trial enrolled participants who did not use CPAP therapy, while the second trial enrolled CPAP users at baseline. At inclusion in the study, the mean AHI of the participants in the first trial was 51.5 events per hour, while in the second trial it was 49.5 events per hour. After 52 weeks, tirzepatide significantly reduced the primary endpoint in both trials, reducing AHI by a mean of -25.3 in the first (-5.3 for placebo) and -29.3 (-5.5 for placebo) events per hour in the second trial. This was accompanied by significant body weight, hypoxic burden, high-sensitivity C-reactive protein (hsCRP), and reduction in systolic blood pressure, as well as improved sleep-related patient-reported outcomes. The safety profile of tirzepatide was in line with previous trials. The authors conclude that this result is clinically relevant, as a 50% reduction in AHI was proposed as clinically relevant [77]. Hypoxic burden is more strongly associated with cardiovascular risk than AHI. The results of SURMOUNT-OSA could, based on the reduction of hypoxic burden, translate into a reduction in cardiovascular risk. Furthermore, this reduction could be underestimated, since tirzepatide resulted in a reduction in a wide range of cardiometabolic risk factors, probably leading to even a more extensive reduction in cardiovascular risk [78].

It has also been shown that in obstructive sleep apnea models, both in vitro and in vivo, liraglutide enhanced the Nrf2 and inhibited mitogen-activated protein kinase (MAPK)/NF-κB signaling pathways, leading to alleviation of chronic intermittent hypoxia induced injury associated with cognitive defects [79].

Although we mention only a few of the most prominent clinical trials, liraglutide and tirzepatide show consistent efficacy of GLP-1 and GIP/GLP-1 receptor agonists in obstructive sleep apnea settings. These effects seem to be primarily driven by weight loss in addition to reduction in cardiometabolic risk. Unfortunately, these studies have a limited duration, so long-term efficacy in weight control, end points of obstructive sleep apnea, and cardiovascular risk remain to be seen. Adherence to therapy with respect to the safety profile is also to be considered.

3.5. Pulmonary Hypertension

Pulmonary hypertension is an entity composed of a multifactorial group of disorders that have in common an elevated mean pulmonary artery pressure (mPAP) of >20 mmHg at rest. According to etiology, it is classified into five groups: group 1—pulmonary arterial hypertension due to vascular remodeling of the pulmonary arteries, group 2—

pulmonary hypertension associated with left-sided heart failure, group 3—pulmonary hypertension associated with lung disease, group 4—pulmonary hypertension associated with pulmonary artery obstructions, and group 5—pulmonary hypertension with unclear and/or multifactorial mechanisms. Currently, it is estimated to affect approximately 1% of the world's population [80]. Group 2 is the most common. Therefore, the most pronounced effect of GLP-1 and GIP/GLP-1 receptor agonists could be expected in people with heart failure with preserved ejection fraction who have already been shown to benefit from these drugs. In a recent meta-analysis, in patients with heart failure with mildly reduced and preserved ejection fraction, most of whom had overweight or obesity, form STEP-HFpEF, STEP-HFpEF DM, and patients with investigator-reported history of heart failure with mildly reduced and preserved ejection fraction form SELECT and FLOW trials with semaglutide 2.4 mg in the first 3 and 1.0 mg in the last trial, semaglutide reduced the combined endpoint of cardiovascular death or worsening of heart failure events combined (hazard ratio 0.69, 95% CI: 0.53–0.89) and worsening heart failure alone (hazard ratio 0.59 95% CI: 0.41–0.82) compared to placebo, while there was no significant effect on reduction of cardiovascular death alone [81]. The recently published SUMMIT trial investigated the effects of tirzepatide treatment in individuals with obesity and heart failure with a preserved ejection fraction of at least 50%. The results demonstrated a relative risk reduction of 38% in the composite outcome of death from cardiovascular causes or worsening of heart failure events in participants treated with tirzepatide compared to those who received a placebo after a median follow-up period of 104 weeks. This reduction was accompanied by improved functional results. However, tirzepatide did not lead to a reduction in cardiovascular deaths alone, in line with the effects observed with semaglutide [82]. There was no report of pulmonary hypertension in these trials. As for the other groups of pulmonary hypertension, this remains to be seen. Data are scarce, and are mainly found in non-clinical models.

In non-diabetic rats with flow-induced pulmonary hypertension (monocrotaline injection followed by aorto-caval fistula), a 3-week treatment with exendin-4 significantly reduced right ventricle mass and pulmonary artery pressure, thus improving right ventricular function and reducing overall mortality in rats. These effects were achieved through direct vasoactive and anti-inflammatory effects of exendin, as well as modulation of the pulmonary artery smooth muscle cell phenotype. These responses were also associated with the reduction of interleukin-1beta and downstream signaling molecules [83]. Similar findings have been reported for liraglutide that prevented and reversed monocrotaline-induced pulmonary hypertension, right ventricular hypertrophy, and remodeling of the pulmonary artery wall in rats. These effects were mediated by the endothelial nitric oxide synthase (eNOS)/soluble guanylate cyclase/protein kinase G and Rho kinase pathways [84]. This was further explained by showing that liraglutide significantly inhibited platelet-derived BB growth factor proliferation, migration, and motility in smooth muscle cells of the pulmonary artery. These results are mitigated by inhibiting the cellular Drp1/nicotinamide adenine dinucleotide phosphate (NADPH) oxidases (NOX) pathways and Atg-5/Atg-7/Beclin-1/LC3β-dependent autophagy pathways in pulmonary hypertension [85]. Additionally, it was shown that in hypoxia-induced pulmonary hypertension, liraglutide reduced pulmonary artery systolic pressure and right ventricular hypertrophy through the activation of eNOS by normalizing the endothelin B pathway and activation of the AMP-activated protein kinase (AMPK) pathway in mice [86].

Based on non-clinical and clinical data, in 2021, Lee proposed a hypothesis that GLP-1 receptor agonists could be potential therapeutic candidates in pulmonary hypertension patients recovering from COVID-19 by regulating the right ventricular systolic pressure and pulmonary artery remodeling [87]. This hypothesis remains to be confirmed, and no studies have been reported that tested it.

3.6. Lung Cancer

According to the WHO, lung cancer was the most commonly diagnosed cancer in 2022 (12.4% of all cancer cases worldwide) and the leading cause of cancer-related death (18.7%) [88]. There is evidence that the incidence of lung cancer increases in people with prediabetes and diabetes [89]. GLP-1 receptor agonists may have a neutral or beneficial effect on lung cancer [90–93]. In a study by Tabernacky et al., de-identified electronic health records of more than 1,000,000 people with type 2 diabetes were analyzed over a 15-year period. They showed that among patients treated with non-insulin antidiabetic drugs (with the exception of alpha-glucosidase inhibitors), GLP-1 receptor agonists had the lowest risk ratio for lung cancer (0.49, 95% CI: 0.41–0.59) compared to insulin regardless of histological type, gender, race, or smoking status; regrettably, records did not include information on the duration of use or dose of GLP-1 receptor agonists, thereby precluding a thorough analysis of the impact of these variables on the outcomes. [94]. These beneficial effects could be partly explained by the effect of liraglutide in the non-clinical setting. Liraglutide was shown to inhibit lung cancer cell proliferation, cell cycle, and migration compared to control in cell cultures, in addition to inhibiting the epithelial-mesenchymal transition process. There was also evidence that liraglutide suppressed lung cancer cell proliferation in vivo. Furthermore, liraglutide also abrogated high glucose-induced cell senescence, as well as suppressed lung aging and stress of the endoplasmic reticulum [95].

3.7. Lung Transplantation

There is no evidence on the effect of incretin-based therapy on lung transplant outcomes. GLP-1 receptor agonists can be used in weight loss strategies prior to lung transplantation [96], as it has been shown that mortality risk increases with BMI > 35 kg/m^2 and that the magnitude of pre-transplant weight loss is directly correlated with improved post-transplant survival [97]. A small retrospective study evaluated 21 patients with an average BMI of 36.34 kg/m^2 using GLP-1 receptor agonists to lose weight before lung transplant. They found that 14 (66.7%) of the patients achieved the desired weight loss in this group and lost on average 11.8% of their initial body weight. On the other hand, there was no report on post-transplant outcomes [98]. Considering the tolerability of GLP-1 receptor agonists in the clinical setting after lung transplantation, 58 lung transplant recipients were evaluated, starting GLP-1 receptor agonists (41% semaglutide, 38% dulaglutide) in the median year 2.1 after transplantation. The median duration of GLP-1 receptor agonists therapy was 1.4 years, and 31% of the patients discontinued the drug, 7% due to nausea and 5% due to vomiting. During GLP-1 receptor agonists therapy, 9% of the patients had cell rejection and 14% had lung allograft dysfunction. The median weight loss was 5 kg. They demonstrated the safety and relatively good tolerability of GLP-1 receptor agonists in this clinical circumstance, but the discontinuation was more common than in general population, most probably due to the overlap and multiplication of side effects of lung transplant medications with those of GLP-1 receptor agonists [99].

Management of post-transplant diabetes can be challenging, as immunosuppressive drugs such as glucocorticoids, calcineurin inhibitors, and mTOR (mammalian target of rapamycin) inhibitors are associated with induction of hyperglycemia or worsening of glucose control. Several clinical trials evaluated the use of GLP-1 receptor agonists in the treatment of solid organ post-transplant diabetes. The number of lung transplant patients was minor among the generally small number of patients included. There is consistency in the efficacy and safety of these drugs in the post-solid organ transplant period in both glycemia and weight management. In addition, there is evidence of no interference with immunosuppressive therapy [100,101]. Data show that use of GLP-1 receptor agonists in the post-transplant setting may be beneficial in ameliorating immunosuppression induced beta cells dysfunction as well as positively affecting the immune function in metabolic disorders through suppression of the activation of the CD4+ T lymphocyte cytokine expression [102].

4. Future Directions and Possibilities

Based on the data presented, we can establish that the use of GLP-1 and GIP/GLP-1 receptor agonists seems to be safe and beneficial in many respiratory disorders. Despite this, there is undoubtedly ground for further research on the use of GLP-1 and GIP/GLP-1 receptor agonists in the broad field of respiratory disease. Several questions remain to be answered. First, although data show that they beneficially influence metabolic and inflammatory pathways in the lung, mediating both Th2-mediated and non-Th2-mediated inflammatory profiles (Figure 2), the complete mechanism of action in the lungs has not yet been fully elucidated. Second, long-term safety with regard to adipose tissue loss and, in particular, muscle mass loss must be determined, as chronic pulmonary diseases due to continuous inflammation are known to lead to sarcopenia. Third, the optimal dose of these drugs remains to be established; as in clinical scenarios primarily of lung problems, the doses do not need to be the same as for cardiometabolic treatment. Fourth, the respiratory disease patient subpopulations that would benefit the most from the treatment of the GLP-1 and GIP/GLP-1 receptor agonists must be determined. Fifth, according to the present data, most of the studies were retrospective in nature and focused on findings without a primary focus on analyzing the effects of these drugs on lung function; the lung findings were based on secondary or additional analysis. Consequently, prospective studies are necessary to directly assess the impact of GLP-1 and GIP/GLP-1 receptor agonists on the lungs, with primary endpoints focused on lung-related outcomes. Sixth, there is a need for prospective clinical trials that evaluate their use in particular clinical settings, including uncontrolled non-Th2 asthma in obese individuals; influence on respiratory control and upper airway muscle tone, sleep architecture, and quality, and whether they have a potential synergistic effect not only with CPAP, but also with other devices used in the treatment of obstructive sleep apnea treatment; and regulation of right ventricular systolic pressure and remodeling of the pulmonary arteries in pulmonary hypertension, as well as their effects in pulmonary hypertension outside group 2, to name just a few. These future studies must be strictly designed and sufficiently powered to provide as straightforward and clear as possible information on the future use and establishment of GLP-1 and GIP/GLP-1 receptor agonists in daily pulmonary clinical practice.

5. Conclusions

GLP-1 and GIP/GLP-1 receptor agonists constitute a promising opportunity for the treatment of respiratory disorders. Due to their multifaceted beneficial properties, these agents appear to be viable candidates for the treatment of a variety of respiratory conditions in addition to the well-established lung-directed therapies. As research progresses, these agents could become more central in the treatment of respiratory diseases.

Author Contributions: Conceptualization, M.J. and S.Š.; writing—original draft preparation, M.J. and S.Š.; writing—review and editing, M.J., S.Š., M.H., M.L., A.J., A.P.S., M.E.-T., V.M. and M.R.; visualization, M.J. All authors have read and agreed to the published version of the manuscript.

Funding: This research received no external funding.

Institutional Review Board Statement: Not applicable.

Informed Consent Statement: Not applicable.

Data Availability Statement: Not applicable.

Acknowledgments: Parts of the figures were generated using Servier Medical Art, provided by Servier (https://smart.servier.com/), licensed under CC BY 4.0 (https://creativecommons.org/licenses/by/4.0/) and NIH BIOART Source (https://bioart.niaid.nih.gov/).

Conflicts of Interest: The authors declare that they have no known competing financial interests or personal relationships that could have appeared to influence the work reported in this manuscript.

References

1. Muzurovic, E.; Yumuk, V.D.; Rizzo, M. GLP-1 and dual GIP/GLP-1 receptor agonists in overweight/obese patients for atherosclerotic cardiovascular disease prevention: Where are we now? *J. Diabetes Complicat.* **2023**, *37*, 108647. [CrossRef] [PubMed]
2. Gomez-Peralta, F.; Abreu, C.; Rizzo, M. GLP-1 receptor agonists and SGLT2 inhibitors: The need to shed light on their safety risks real dimension and possible mechanisms. *J. Diabetes Complicat.* **2023**, *37*, 108553. [CrossRef] [PubMed]
3. Janez, A.; Muzurovic, E.; Bogdanski, P.; Czupryniak, L.; Fabryova, L.; Fras, Z.; Guja, C.; Haluzik, M.; Kempler, P.; Lalic, N.; et al. Modern Management of Cardiometabolic Continuum: From Overweight/Obesity to Prediabetes/Type 2 Diabetes Mellitus. Recommendations from the Eastern and Southern Europe Diabetes and Obesity Expert Group. *Diabetes Ther.* **2024**, *15*, 1865–1892. [CrossRef]
4. Rangraze, I.; Patoulias, D.; Karakasis, P.; El-Tanani, M.; Rizzo, M. Tirzepatide, a novel, dual glucose-dependent insulinotropic polypeptide/glucagon-like peptide-1 receptor agonist for the ongoing diabesity epidemic: The dawn of a new era? *Expert. Rev. Clin. Pharmacol.* **2024**, *17*, 853–856. [CrossRef]
5. Patoulias, D.; Popovic, D.S.; Stoian, A.P.; Janez, A.; Sahebkar, A.; Rizzo, M. Effect of semaglutide versus other glucagon-like peptide-1 receptor agonists on cardio-metabolic risk factors in patients with type 2 diabetes: A systematic review and meta-analysis of head-to-head, phase 3, randomized controlled trials. *J. Diabetes Complicat.* **2023**, *37*, 108529. [CrossRef]
6. Nachawi, N.; Rao, P.P.; Makin, V. The role of GLP-1 receptor agonists in managing type 2 diabetes. *Cleve Clin. J. Med.* **2022**, *89*, 457–464. [CrossRef]
7. Apperloo, E.M.; Gorriz, J.L.; Soler, M.J.; Cigarran Guldris, S.; Cruzado, J.M.; Puchades, M.J.; Lopez-Martinez, M.; Waanders, F.; Laverman, G.D.; van der Aart-van der Beek, A.; et al. Semaglutide in patients with overweight or obesity and chronic kidney disease without diabetes: A randomized double-blind placebo-controlled clinical trial. *Nat. Med.* **2024**. [CrossRef]
8. Nauck, M.A.; Quast, D.R.; Wefers, J.; Pfeiffer, A.F.H. The evolving story of incretins (GIP and GLP-1) in metabolic and cardiovascular disease: A pathophysiological update. *Diabetes Obes. Metab.* **2021**, *23* (Suppl. S3), 5–29. [CrossRef] [PubMed]
9. De Santi, F.; Zoppini, G.; Locatelli, F.; Finocchio, E.; Cappa, V.; Dauriz, M.; Verlato, G. Type 2 diabetes is associated with an increased prevalence of respiratory symptoms as compared to the general population. *BMC Pulm. Med.* **2017**, *17*, 101. [CrossRef]
10. Kantreva, K.; Katsaounou, P.; Saltiki, K.; Trakada, G.; Ntali, G.; Stratigou, T.; Tzanela, M.; Psaltopoulou, T.; Paschou, S.A. The possible effect of anti-diabetic agents GLP-1RA and SGLT-2i on the respiratory system function. *Endocrine* **2024**. [CrossRef]
11. Wei, J.P.; Yang, C.L.; Leng, W.H.; Ding, L.L.; Zhao, G.H. Use of GLP1RAs and occurrence of respiratory disorders: A meta-analysis of large randomized trials of GLP1RAs. *Clin. Respir. J.* **2021**, *15*, 847–850. [CrossRef] [PubMed]
12. Ehrlich, S.F.; Quesenberry, C.P., Jr.; Van Den Eeden, S.K.; Shan, J.; Ferrara, A. Patients diagnosed with diabetes are at increased risk for asthma, chronic obstructive pulmonary disease, pulmonary fibrosis, and pneumonia but not lung cancer. *Diabetes Care* **2010**, *33*, 55–60. [CrossRef] [PubMed]
13. Yu, M.; Wang, R.; Pei, L.; Zhang, X.; Wei, J.; Wen, Y.; Liu, H.; Ye, H.; Wang, J.; Wang, L. The relationship between the use of GLP-1 receptor agonists and the incidence of respiratory illness: A meta-analysis of randomized controlled trials. *Diabetol. Metab. Syndr.* **2023**, *15*, 164. [CrossRef]
14. Korner, M.; Stockli, M.; Waser, B.; Reubi, J.C. GLP-1 receptor expression in human tumors and human normal tissues: Potential for in vivo targeting. *J. Nucl. Med.* **2007**, *48*, 736–743. [CrossRef] [PubMed]
15. Mendivil, C.O.; Koziel, H.; Brain, J.D. Metabolic hormones, apolipoproteins, adipokines, and cytokines in the alveolar lining fluid of healthy adults: Compartmentalization and physiological correlates. *PLoS ONE* **2015**, *10*, e0123344. [CrossRef]
16. Webber, T.; Ronacher, K.; Conradie-Smit, M.; Kleynhans, L. Interplay Between the Immune and Endocrine Systems in the Lung: Implications for TB Susceptibility. *Front. Immunol.* **2022**, *13*, 829355. [CrossRef]
17. Nguyen, D.V.; Linderholm, A.; Haczku, A.; Kenyon, N. Glucagon-like peptide 1: A potential anti-inflammatory pathway in obesity-related asthma. *Pharmacol. Ther.* **2017**, *180*, 139–143. [CrossRef]
18. Lee, Y.S.; Jun, H.S. Anti-Inflammatory Effects of GLP-1-Based Therapies beyond Glucose Control. *Mediat. Inflamm.* **2016**, *2016*, 3094642. [CrossRef]
19. Alharbi, S.H. Anti-inflammatory role of glucagon-like peptide 1 receptor agonists and its clinical implications. *Ther. Adv. Endocrinol. Metab.* **2024**, *15*, 20420188231222367. [CrossRef]
20. Wang, W.; Mei, A.; Qian, H.; Li, D.; Xu, H.; Chen, J.; Yang, H.; Min, X.; Li, C.; Cheng, L.; et al. The Role of Glucagon-Like Peptide-1 Receptor Agonists in Chronic Obstructive Pulmonary Disease. *Int. J. Chron. Obs. Pulmon Dis.* **2023**, *18*, 129–137. [CrossRef]
21. Wu, A.Y.; Peebles, R.S. The GLP-1 receptor in airway inflammation in asthma: A promising novel target? *Expert. Rev. Clin. Immunol.* **2021**, *17*, 1053–1057. [CrossRef] [PubMed]
22. Liu, C.; Zhang, Q.; Zhou, H.; Jin, L.; Liu, C.; Yang, M.; Zhao, X.; Ding, W.; Xie, W.; Kong, H. GLP-1R activation attenuates the progression of pulmonary fibrosis via disrupting NLRP3 inflammasome/PFKFB3-driven glycolysis interaction and histone lactylation. *J. Transl. Med.* **2024**, *22*, 954. [CrossRef] [PubMed]
23. Barnes, P.J. Targeting cytokines to treat asthma and chronic obstructive pulmonary disease. *Nat. Rev. Immunol.* **2018**, *18*, 454–466. [CrossRef] [PubMed]
24. Liu, T.; Woodruff, P.G.; Zhou, X. Advances in non-type 2 severe asthma: From molecular insights to novel treatment strategies. *Eur. Respir. J.* **2024**, *64*, 2300826. [CrossRef] [PubMed]
25. Mafort, T.T.; Rufino, R.; Costa, C.H.; Lopes, A.J. Obesity: Systemic and pulmonary complications, biochemical abnormalities, and impairment of lung function. *Multidiscip. Respir. Med.* **2016**, *11*, 28. [CrossRef]

26. Moiz, A.; Levett, J.Y.; Filion, K.B.; Peri, K.; Reynier, P.; Eisenberg, M.J. Long-Term Efficacy and Safety of Once-Weekly Semaglutide for Weight Loss in Patients Without Diabetes: A Systematic Review and Meta-Analysis of Randomized Controlled Trials. *Am. J. Cardiol.* **2024**, *222*, 121–130. [CrossRef]
27. Espinosa De Ycaza, A.E.; Brito, J.P.; McCoy, R.G.; Shao, H.; Singh Ospina, N. Glucagon-Like Peptide-1 Receptor Agonists and Thyroid Cancer: A Narrative Review. *Thyroid* **2024**, *34*, 403–418. [CrossRef]
28. Feier, C.V.I.; Vonica, R.C.; Faur, A.M.; Streinu, D.R.; Muntean, C. Assessment of Thyroid Carcinogenic Risk and Safety Profile of GLP1-RA Semaglutide (Ozempic) Therapy for Diabetes Mellitus and Obesity: A Systematic Literature Review. *Int. J. Mol. Sci.* **2024**, *25*, 4346. [CrossRef]
29. de Mesquita, Y.L.L.; Pera Calvi, I.; Reis Marques, I.; Almeida Cruz, S.; Padrao, E.M.H.; Carvalho, P.E.P.; da Silva, C.H.A.; Cardoso, R.; Moura, F.A.; Rafalskiy, V.V. Efficacy and safety of the dual GIP and GLP-1 receptor agonist tirzepatide for weight loss: A meta-analysis of randomized controlled trials. *Int. J. Obes.* **2023**, *47*, 883–892. [CrossRef]
30. Jastreboff, A.M.; Aronne, L.J.; Ahmad, N.N.; Wharton, S.; Connery, L.; Alves, B.; Kiyosue, A.; Zhang, S.; Liu, B.; Bunck, M.C.; et al. Tirzepatide Once Weekly for the Treatment of Obesity. *N. Engl. J. Med.* **2022**, *387*, 205–216. [CrossRef]
31. Barnes, P.J.; Burney, P.G.; Silverman, E.K.; Celli, B.R.; Vestbo, J.; Wedzicha, J.A.; Wouters, E.F. Chronic obstructive pulmonary disease. *Nat. Rev. Dis. Primers* **2015**, *1*, 15076. [CrossRef] [PubMed]
32. Foer, D.; Strasser, Z.H.; Cui, J.; Cahill, K.N.; Boyce, J.A.; Murphy, S.N.; Karlson, E.W. Association of GLP-1 Receptor Agonists with Chronic Obstructive Pulmonary Disease Exacerbations among Patients with Type 2 Diabetes. *Am. J. Respir. Crit. Care Med.* **2023**, *208*, 1088–1100. [CrossRef] [PubMed]
33. Li, Q.; Chen, Y.; Jiang, H.; Xi, Y.; Wang, J.; Zhu, X.; Lai, J.; Zhang, N.; Zhao, D. A Daunting and Challenging Task to Prove the Effectiveness of Reducing Acute Exacerbation in COPD Patients with Type 2 Diabetes by GLP-1 Receptor Agonists. *Am. J. Respir. Crit. Care Med.* **2023**, *208*, 1345–1346. [CrossRef]
34. Pradhan, R.; Lu, S.; Yin, H.; Yu, O.H.Y.; Ernst, P.; Suissa, S.; Azoulay, L. Novel antihyperglycaemic drugs and prevention of chronic obstructive pulmonary disease exacerbations among patients with type 2 diabetes: Population based cohort study. *BMJ* **2022**, *379*, e071380. [CrossRef]
35. Yen, F.S.; Hsu, C.C.; Wei, J.C.; Tsai, F.J.; Huang, Y.; Yu, T.S.; Hwu, C.M. Glucagon-like peptide-1 receptor agonists may benefit cardiopulmonary outcomes in patients with COPD. *Thorax* **2024**, *79*, 1017–1023. [CrossRef]
36. Altintas Dogan, A.D.; Hilberg, O.; Hess, S.; Jensen, T.T.; Bladbjerg, E.M.; Juhl, C.B. Respiratory Effects of Treatment with a Glucagon-Like Peptide-1 Receptor Agonist in Patients Suffering from Obesity and Chronic Obstructive Pulmonary Disease. *Int. J. Chron. Obs. Pulmon Dis.* **2022**, *17*, 405–414. [CrossRef] [PubMed]
37. Huang, J.; Yi, H.; Zhao, C.; Zhang, Y.; Zhu, L.; Liu, B.; He, P.; Zhou, M. Glucagon-like peptide-1 receptor (GLP-1R) signaling ameliorates dysfunctional immunity in COPD patients. *Int. J. Chron. Obs. Pulmon Dis.* **2018**, *13*, 3191–3202. [CrossRef]
38. Skurikhin, E.G.; Pershina, O.V.; Pakhomova, A.V.; Pan, E.S.; Krupin, V.A.; Ermakova, N.N.; Vaizova, O.E.; Pozdeeva, A.S.; Zhukova, M.A.; Skurikhina, V.E.; et al. Endothelial Progenitor Cells as Pathogenetic and Diagnostic Factors, and Potential Targets for GLP-1 in Combination with Metabolic Syndrome and Chronic Obstructive Pulmonary Disease. *Int. J. Mol. Sci.* **2019**, *20*, 1105. [CrossRef]
39. Balk-Moller, E.; Windelov, J.A.; Svendsen, B.; Hunt, J.; Ghiasi, S.M.; Sorensen, C.M.; Holst, J.J.; Kissow, H. Glucagon-like Peptide 1 and Atrial Natriuretic Peptide in a Female Mouse Model of Obstructive Pulmonary Disease. *J. Endocr. Soc.* **2020**, *4*, bvz034. [CrossRef]
40. Choi, W.; Choe, S.; Lin, J.; Borchers, M.T.; Kosmider, B.; Vassallo, R.; Limper, A.H.; Lau, G.W. Exendin-4 restores airway mucus homeostasis through the GLP1R-PKA-PPARgamma-FOXA2-phosphatase signaling. *Mucosal Immunol.* **2020**, *13*, 637–651. [CrossRef]
41. Xu, L.; Chen, G.; Zhang, L.; He, A.; Li, Y. Lixisenatide ameliorated lipopolysaccharide (LPS)-induced expression of mucin and inflammation in bronchial epithelial cells. *J. Biochem. Mol. Toxicol.* **2024**, *38*, e23618. [CrossRef] [PubMed]
42. Holgate, S.T.; Wenzel, S.; Postma, D.S.; Weiss, S.T.; Renz, H.; Sly, P.D. Asthma. *Nat. Rev. Dis. Primers* **2015**, *1*, 15025. [CrossRef] [PubMed]
43. Skrgat, S.; Harlander, M.; Janic, M. Obesity and Insulin Resistance in Asthma Pathogenesis and Clinical Outcomes. *Biomedicines* **2024**, *12*, 173. [CrossRef]
44. Kaplan, A.G.; Kim, J.W. Asthma Exacerbations and Glucagon-Like Peptide-1 Receptor Agonists: A Review of the Current Evidence. *Pulm. Ther.* **2022**, *8*, 343–358. [CrossRef]
45. Khan, F.; Mat, A.; Hogan, A.E.; Kent, B.D.; Eigenheer, S.; Corrigan, M.A.; O'Shea, D.; Butler, M.W. Preliminary asthma-related outcomes following glucagon-like peptide 1 agonist therapy. *QJM* **2017**, *110*, 853–854. [CrossRef]
46. Foer, D.; Beeler, P.E.; Cui, J.; Karlson, E.W.; Bates, D.W.; Cahill, K.N. Asthma Exacerbations in Patients with Type 2 Diabetes and Asthma on Glucagon-like Peptide-1 Receptor Agonists. *Am. J. Respir. Crit. Care Med.* **2021**, *203*, 831–840. [CrossRef] [PubMed]
47. Forno, E. A Potential New Treatment Option for Asthma in the Setting of Obesity or Insulin Resistance? *Am. J. Respir. Crit. Care Med.* **2021**, *203*, 788–789. [CrossRef]
48. Kimura, Y.; Jo, T.; Inoue, N.; Suzukawa, M.; Hashimoto, Y.; Kumazawa, R.; Ishimaru, M.; Matsui, H.; Yokoyama, A.; Tanaka, G.; et al. Association of Novel Antihyperglycemic Drugs Versus Metformin With a Decrease in Asthma Exacerbations. *J. Allergy Clin. Immunol. Pract.* **2024**, *12*, 2035–2044. [CrossRef] [PubMed]

49. Zhang, M.Q.; Lin, C.; Cai, X.L.; Jiao, R.Y.; Bai, S.Z.; Li, Z.L.; Hu, S.Y.; Lyu, F.; Yang, W.J.; Ji, L.N. The Association between GLP-1 Receptor-Based Agonists and the Incidence of Asthma in Patients with Type 2 Diabetes and/or Obesity: A Meta-Analysis. *Biomed. Environ. Sci.* **2024**, *37*, 607–616. [CrossRef]
50. Lee, B.; Man, K.K.C.; Wong, E.; Tan, T.; Sheikh, A.; Bloom, C.I. Antidiabetic Medication and Asthma Attacks. *JAMA Intern. Med.* **2024**. [CrossRef]
51. Wang, A.; Tang, H.; Zhang, N.; Feng, X. Association between novel Glucose-Lowering drugs and risk of Asthma: A network Meta-Analysis of cardiorenal outcome trials. *Diabetes Res. Clin. Pract.* **2022**, *183*, 109080. [CrossRef]
52. Cazzola, M.; Matera, M.G.; Calzetta, L.; Lauro, D.; Rogliani, P. Can glucagon-like peptide-1 receptor agonists induce asthma? An analysis of the FAERS database. *J. Asthma* **2024**, *61*, 1638–1645. [CrossRef]
53. Chiarella, S.E.; Barnes, P.J. Endogenous inhibitory mechanisms in asthma. *J. Allergy Clin. Immunol. Glob.* **2023**, *2*, 100135. [CrossRef]
54. Mitchell, P.D.; Salter, B.M.; Oliveria, J.P.; El-Gammal, A.; Tworek, D.; Smith, S.G.; Sehmi, R.; Gauvreau, G.M.; Butler, M.; O'Byrne, P.M. Glucagon-like peptide-1 receptor expression on human eosinophils and its regulation of eosinophil activation. *Clin. Exp. Allergy* **2017**, *47*, 331–338. [CrossRef]
55. Hur, J.; Kang, J.Y.; Kim, Y.K.; Lee, S.Y.; Lee, H.Y. Glucagon-like peptide 1 receptor (GLP-1R) agonist relieved asthmatic airway inflammation via suppression of NLRP3 inflammasome activation in obese asthma mice model. *Pulm. Pharmacol. Ther.* **2021**, *67*, 102003. [CrossRef]
56. Toki, S.; Zhang, J.; Printz, R.L.; Newcomb, D.C.; Cahill, K.N.; Niswender, K.D.; Peebles, R.S., Jr. Dual GIPR and GLP-1R agonist tirzepatide inhibits aeroallergen-induced allergic airway inflammation in mouse model of obese asthma. *Clin. Exp. Allergy* **2023**, *53*, 216–221. [CrossRef]
57. Kanwar, M.K.; Sunku, R.; Alruwaili, F.; Mufti, M.A.; Raji, M. Beneficial Effects of Glucagon-Like Peptide-1 Receptor Agonists in Patients With Asthma: A Literature Review. *Cureus* **2022**, *14*, e30812. [CrossRef]
58. Torres, A.; Cilloniz, C.; Niederman, M.S.; Menendez, R.; Chalmers, J.D.; Wunderink, R.G.; van der Poll, T. Pneumonia. *Nat. Rev. Dis. Primers* **2021**, *7*, 25. [CrossRef]
59. Cilloniz, C.; Torres, A. Diabetes Mellitus and Pneumococcal Pneumonia. *Diagnostics* **2024**, *14*, 859. [CrossRef]
60. Holt, R.I.G.; Cockram, C.S.; Ma, R.C.W.; Luk, A.O.Y. Diabetes and infection: Review of the epidemiology, mechanisms and principles of treatment. *Diabetologia* **2024**, *67*, 1168–1180. [CrossRef]
61. Brunetti, V.C.; Reynier, P.; Azoulay, L.; Yu, O.H.Y.; Ernst, P.; Platt, R.W.; Filion, K.B. SGLT-2 inhibitors and the risk of hospitalization for community-acquired pneumonia: A population-based cohort study. *Pharmacoepidemiol. Drug Saf.* **2021**, *30*, 740–748. [CrossRef] [PubMed]
62. Zhu, Z.; Zeng, Q.; Liu, Q.; Wen, J.; Chen, G. Association of Glucose-Lowering Drugs With Outcomes in Patients With Diabetes Before Hospitalization for COVID-19: A Systematic Review and Network Meta-analysis. *JAMA Netw. Open* **2022**, *5*, e2244652. [CrossRef] [PubMed]
63. Song, Z.H.; Huang, Q.M.; Xu, S.S.; Zhou, J.B.; Zhang, C. The Effect of Antihyperglycemic Medications on COVID-19: A Meta-analysis and Systematic Review from Observational Studies. *Ther. Innov. Regul. Sci.* **2024**, *58*, 773–787. [CrossRef] [PubMed]
64. Bloch, O.; Kobi, P.; Ben Shimol, A.; Rotmensh, A.; Kagansky, D.; Zelnik-Yovel, D.; Yehudah, G.B.; Cantrell, D.; Rapoport, M.J. Severe and fatal COVID-19 is characterised by increased circulating glucagon like peptide 1 and procalcitonin modulated by type 2 diabetes. *Diabetes Metab. Res. Rev.* **2023**, *39*, e3635. [CrossRef] [PubMed]
65. Batiha, G.E.; Al-Kuraishy, H.M.; Al-Gareeb, A.I.; Ashour, N.A.; Negm, W.A. Potential role of tirzepatide towards Covid-19 infection in diabetic patients: A perspective approach. *Inflammopharmacology* **2023**, *31*, 1683–1693. [CrossRef]
66. Sato, T.; Shimizu, T.; Fujita, H.; Imai, Y.; Drucker, D.J.; Seino, Y.; Yamada, Y. GLP-1 Receptor Signaling Differentially Modifies the Outcomes of Sterile vs Viral Pulmonary Inflammation in Male Mice. *Endocrinology* **2020**, *161*, bqaa201. [CrossRef]
67. Guo, J.; Chen, X.; Wang, C.; Ruan, F.; Xiong, Y.; Wang, L.; Abdel-Razek, O.; Meng, Q.; Shahbazov, R.; Cooney, R.N.; et al. Liraglutide Alleviates Acute Lung Injury and Mortality in Pneumonia-Induced Sepsis through Regulating Surfactant Protein Expression and Secretion. *Shock* **2024**, *61*, 601–610. [CrossRef]
68. Warner, M.A.; Meyerhoff, K.L.; Warner, M.E.; Posner, K.L.; Stephens, L.; Domino, K.B. Pulmonary Aspiration of Gastric Contents: A Closed Claims Analysis. *Anesthesiology* **2021**, *135*, 284–291. [CrossRef]
69. Cook, T.M.; Woodall, N.; Frerk, C.; Fourth National Audit, P. Major complications of airway management in the UK: Results of the Fourth National Audit Project of the Royal College of Anaesthetists and the Difficult Airway Society. Part 1: Anaesthesia. *Br. J. Anaesth.* **2011**, *106*, 617–631. [CrossRef]
70. Milder, D.A.; Milder, T.Y.; Liang, S.S.; Kam, P.C.A. Glucagon-like peptide-1 receptor agonists: A narrative review of clinical pharmacology and implications for peri-operative practice. *Anaesthesia* **2024**, *79*, 735–747. [CrossRef]
71. Grunstein, R.R.; Wadden, T.A.; Chapman, J.L.; Malhotra, A.; Phillips, C.L. Giving weight to incretin-based pharmacotherapy for obesity-related sleep apnea: A revolution or a pipe dream? *Sleep* **2023**, *46*, zsad224. [CrossRef] [PubMed]
72. Le, K.D.R.; Le, K.; Foo, F. The Impact of Glucagon-like Peptide 1 Receptor Agonists on Obstructive Sleep Apnoea: A Scoping Review. *Pharmacy* **2024**, *12*, 11. [CrossRef] [PubMed]
73. Papaetis, G.S. GLP-1 receptor agonists, SGLT-2 inhibitors, and obstructive sleep apnoea: Can new allies face an old enemy? *Arch. Med. Sci. Atheroscler. Dis.* **2023**, *8*, e19–e34. [CrossRef] [PubMed]

74. Blackman, A.; Foster, G.D.; Zammit, G.; Rosenberg, R.; Aronne, L.; Wadden, T.; Claudius, B.; Jensen, C.B.; Mignot, E. Effect of liraglutide 3.0 mg in individuals with obesity and moderate or severe obstructive sleep apnea: The SCALE Sleep Apnea randomized clinical trial. *Int. J. Obes.* **2016**, *40*, 1310–1319. [CrossRef]
75. Jiang, W.; Li, W.; Cheng, J.; Li, W.; Cheng, F. Efficacy and safety of liraglutide in patients with type 2 diabetes mellitus and severe obstructive sleep apnea. *Sleep. Breath.* **2023**, *27*, 1687–1694. [CrossRef]
76. Sprung, V.S.; Kemp, G.J.; Wilding, J.P.; Adams, V.; Murphy, K.; Burgess, M.; Emegbo, S.; Thomas, M.; Needham, A.J.; Weimken, A.; et al. Randomised, cOntrolled Multicentre trial of 26 weeks subcutaneous liraglutide (a glucagon-like peptide-1 receptor Agonist), with or without contiNuous positive airway pressure (CPAP), in patients with type 2 diabetes mellitus (T2DM) and obstructive sleep apnoEa (OSA) (ROMANCE): Study protocol assessing the effects of weight loss on the apnea-hypnoea index (AHI). *BMJ Open* **2020**, *10*, e038856. [CrossRef]
77. Malhotra, A.; Grunstein, R.R.; Fietze, I.; Weaver, T.E.; Redline, S.; Azarbarzin, A.; Sands, S.A.; Schwab, R.J.; Dunn, J.P.; Chakladar, S.; et al. Tirzepatide for the Treatment of Obstructive Sleep Apnea and Obesity. *N. Engl. J. Med.* **2024**, *391*, 1193–1205. [CrossRef]
78. Beccuti, G.; Bioletto, F.; Parasiliti-Caprino, M.; Benso, A.; Ghigo, E.; Cicolin, A.; Broglio, F. Estimating Cardiovascular Benefits of Tirzepatide in Sleep Apnea and Obesity: Insight from the SURMOUNT-OSA Trials. *Curr. Obes. Rep.* **2024**, *13*, 739–742. [CrossRef]
79. Lv, R.; Zhao, Y.; Wang, X.; He, Y.; Dong, N.; Min, X.; Liu, X.; Yu, Q.; Yuan, K.; Yue, H.; et al. GLP-1 analogue liraglutide attenuates CIH-induced cognitive deficits by inhibiting oxidative stress, neuroinflammation, and apoptosis via the Nrf2/HO-1 and MAPK/NF-kappaB signaling pathways. *Int. Immunopharmacol.* **2024**, *142*, 113222. [CrossRef]
80. Mocumbi, A.; Humbert, M.; Saxena, A.; Jing, Z.-C.; Sliwa, K.; Thienemann, F.; Archer, S.L.; Stewart, S. Pulmonary hypertension. *Nat. Rev. Dis. Primers* **2024**, *10*, 1. [CrossRef]
81. Kosiborod, M.N.; Deanfield, J.; Pratley, R.; Borlaug, B.A.; Butler, J.; Davies, M.J.; Emerson, S.S.; Kahn, S.E.; Kitzman, D.W.; Lingvay, I.; et al. Semaglutide versus placebo in patients with heart failure and mildly reduced or preserved ejection fraction: A pooled analysis of the SELECT, FLOW, STEP-HFpEF, and STEP-HFpEF DM randomised trials. *Lancet* **2024**, *404*, 949–961. [CrossRef] [PubMed]
82. Packer, M.; Zile, M.R.; Kramer, C.M.; Baum, S.J.; Litwin, S.E.; Menon, V.; Ge, J.; Weerakkody, G.J.; Ou, Y.; Bunck, M.C.; et al. Tirzepatide for Heart Failure with Preserved Ejection Fraction and Obesity. *N. Engl. J. Med.* **2024**. [CrossRef] [PubMed]
83. Roan, J.N.; Hsu, C.H.; Fang, S.Y.; Tsai, H.W.; Luo, C.Y.; Huang, C.C.; Lam, C.F. Exendin-4 improves cardiovascular function and survival in flow-induced pulmonary hypertension. *J. Thorac. Cardiovasc. Surg.* **2018**, *155*, 1661–1669.e4. [CrossRef] [PubMed]
84. Lee, M.Y.; Tsai, K.B.; Hsu, J.H.; Shin, S.J.; Wu, J.R.; Yeh, J.L. Liraglutide prevents and reverses monocrotaline-induced pulmonary arterial hypertension by suppressing ET-1 and enhancing eNOS/sGC/PKG pathways. *Sci. Rep.* **2016**, *6*, 31788. [CrossRef] [PubMed]
85. Wu, Y.C.; Wang, W.T.; Lee, S.S.; Kuo, Y.R.; Wang, Y.C.; Yen, S.J.; Lee, M.Y.; Yeh, J.L. Glucagon-Like Peptide-1 Receptor Agonist Attenuates Autophagy to Ameliorate Pulmonary Arterial Hypertension through Drp1/NOX- and Atg-5/Atg-7/Beclin-1/LC3beta Pathways. *Int. J. Mol. Sci.* **2019**, *20*, 3435. [CrossRef]
86. Honda, J.; Kimura, T.; Sakai, S.; Maruyama, H.; Tajiri, K.; Murakoshi, N.; Homma, S.; Miyauchi, T.; Aonuma, K. The glucagon-like peptide-1 receptor agonist liraglutide improves hypoxia-induced pulmonary hypertension in mice partly via normalization of reduced ET(B) receptor expression. *Physiol. Res.* **2018**, *67*, S175–S184. [CrossRef]
87. Lee, J.H. Potential therapeutic effect of glucagon-like peptide-1 receptor agonists on COVID-19-induced pulmonary arterial hypertension. *Med. Hypotheses* **2022**, *158*, 110739. [CrossRef]
88. Hendriks, L.E.L.; Remon, J.; Faivre-Finn, C.; Garassino, M.C.; Heymach, J.V.; Kerr, K.M.; Tan, D.S.W.; Veronesi, G.; Reck, M. Non-small-cell lung cancer. *Nat. Rev. Dis. Primers* **2024**, *10*, 71. [CrossRef]
89. Hua, J.; Lin, H.; Wang, X.; Qian, Z.M.; Vaughn, M.G.; Tabet, M.; Wang, C.; Lin, H. Associations of glycosylated hemoglobin, pre-diabetes, and type 2 diabetes with incident lung cancer: A large prospective cohort study. *Diabetes Metab. Syndr.* **2024**, *18*, 102968. [CrossRef]
90. Sun, Y.; Liu, Y.; Dian, Y.; Zeng, F.; Deng, G.; Lei, S. Association of glucagon-like peptide-1 receptor agonists with risk of cancers-evidence from a drug target Mendelian randomization and clinical trials. *Int. J. Surg.* **2024**, *110*, 4688–4694. [CrossRef]
91. Wang, J.; Kim, C.H. Differential Risk of Cancer Associated with Glucagon-like Peptide-1 Receptor Agonists: Analysis of Real-world Databases. *Endocr. Res.* **2022**, *47*, 18–25. [CrossRef] [PubMed]
92. Rouette, J.; Yin, H.; Yu, O.H.Y.; Bouganim, N.; Platt, R.W.; Azoulay, L. Incretin-based drugs and risk of lung cancer among individuals with type 2 diabetes. *Diabet. Med.* **2020**, *37*, 868–875. [CrossRef] [PubMed]
93. Song, J.; Cali Daylan, A.E.; Chi, K.Y.; Prem Anand, D.; Chang, Y.; Chiang, C.H.; Cheng, H. Association Between GLP-1 Receptor Agonists and Incidence of Lung Cancer in Treatment-Naive Type 2 Diabetes. *J. Gen. Intern. Med.* **2024**. [CrossRef]
94. Tabernacki, T.; Wang, L.; Kaelber, D.C.; Xu, R.; Berger, N.A. Non-Insulin Antidiabetic Agents and Lung Cancer Risk in Drug-Naive Patients with Type 2 Diabetes Mellitus: A Nationwide Retrospective Cohort Study. *Cancers* **2024**, *16*, 2377. [CrossRef]
95. Pu, Z.; Yang, Y.; Qin, S.; Li, X.; Cui, C.; Chen, W. The Effect of Liraglutide on Lung Cancer and Its Potential Protective Effect on High Glucose-Induced Lung Senescence and Oxidative Damage. *Front. Biosci.* **2023**, *28*, 259. [CrossRef]
96. Callaghan, M.; Le Roux, C.; Fabre, A.; McCarthy, C. Weight loss with GLP-1 analogues in preparation for transplantation. *BMJ Case Rep.* **2024**, *17*, e256099. [CrossRef] [PubMed]

97. Leard, L.E.; Holm, A.M.; Valapour, M.; Glanville, A.R.; Attawar, S.; Aversa, M.; Campos, S.V.; Christon, L.M.; Cypel, M.; Dellgren, G.; et al. Consensus document for the selection of lung transplant candidates: An update from the International Society for Heart and Lung Transplantation. *J. Heart Lung Transplant.* **2021**, *40*, 1349–1379. [CrossRef]
98. Long, M.; Paplaczyk, K.; Tomic, R.; Venkata Subramani, M.; Arunachalam, A.; Myers, C. (1401)-Evaluating the Utility of Glucagon-Like Peptide 1 Receptor Agonists in Potential Lung Transplant Candidates Requiring Weight Loss Prior to Transplant. *J. Heart Lung Transplant.* **2024**, *43*, S642–S643. [CrossRef]
99. Walshe, C.; Anderson, M.; Diamond, J.; Witek, S. (1402)-Evaluating the Tolerability of Glucagon-Like Peptide-1 Receptor Agonists in Lung Transplant Recipients. *J. Heart Lung Transplant.* **2024**, *43*, S643. [CrossRef]
100. Sweiss, H.; Hall, R.; Zeilmann, D.; Escamilla, J.; Bhayana, S.; Patel, R.; Long, C. Single-center Evaluation of Safety & Efficacy of Glucagon-Like Peptide-1 Receptor Agonists in Solid Organ Transplantation. *Prog. Transplant.* **2022**, *32*, 357–362. [CrossRef]
101. Thangavelu, T.; Lyden, E.; Shivaswamy, V. A Retrospective Study of Glucagon-Like Peptide 1 Receptor Agonists for the Management of Diabetes After Transplantation. *Diabetes Ther.* **2020**, *11*, 987–994. [CrossRef] [PubMed]
102. Bertera, S.; Knoll, M.F.; Eicher, D.; Knoll, C.A.; Trucco, M.; Bottino, R. GLP-1 receptor agonists can reverse immunosuppression-induced beta-cell dysfunction. *CellR4* **2020**, *8*, e2943. [CrossRef]

medicina

MDPI

Article

Gender-Based Differences in COPD Patients with Type 2 Respiratory Failure—Impact on Clinical Practice

Tarkan Ozdemir [1,*], Murat Yıldız [1], Maşide Arı [1], Emrah Arı [2], Güler Eraslan Doğanay [3], Mustafa Özgür Cırık [3], Melek Doğancı [3], Çiğdem Özdilekcan [4], Derya Kızılgöz [1] and Yusuf Tuğrul Şipit [1]

1 Department of Chest Diseases, Ankara Sanatoryum Training and Research Hospital, Ankara 06290, Turkey; drmuratyildiz85@gmail.com (M.Y.); masidetuten@icloud.com (M.A.); derya.ozaydin999@gmail.com (D.K.); yusuftugrulsipit@yahoo.com (Y.T.Ş.)

2 Department of Emergency Medicine, Mamak Public Hospital, Ankara 06620, Turkey; dremrahari25@gmail.com

3 Department of Anesthesiology, Ankara Sanatoryum Training and Research Hospital, Ankara 06290, Turkey; gulerdoganay@hotmail.com.tr (G.E.D.); dr.ozgurr@hotmail.com (M.Ö.C.); melekdidik@hotmail.com (M.D.)

4 Department of Chest Diseases, Ankara Oncology Training and Research Hospital, Ankara 06200, Turkey; cigdemozdilekcan@yahoo.com.tr

* Correspondence: tarkanozdemir78@gmail.com

Abstract: *Background and Objectives:* To contribute to clinical practice by identifying gender-based differences in patients diagnosed with chronic obstructive pulmonary disease (COPD) who are monitored in the intensive care unit due to type 2 respiratory failure. *Materials and Methods:* The study was planned as a prospective, observational, and cross-sectional investigation. A total of 258 patients, 91 females and 167 males, were included in the study between 2023 and 2024. Demographic data and clinical parameters of COPD patients admitted to intensive care due to hypercapnic respiratory failure and treated with noninvasive ventilation (NIV) were compared between genders. *Results*: The number of male patients was higher than female patients, while the mean age of female patients was higher than that of males. The body mass index (BMI), morbid obesity, atrial fibrillation, renal disease, heart failure, hypertension, hypothyroidism, the Charlson Comorbidity Index (CCI), and the cardiothoracic ratio were found to be significantly higher in female patients. Emphysema and steroid use in treatment were more common in male patients. In laboratory analyses conducted at the time of admission, the average D-dimer and brain natriuretic peptide (BNP) levels were higher in female patients. The mean arterial carbon dioxide pressure ($PaCO_2$) level assessed prior to discharge was also higher in female patients. *Conclusions*: Heart failure and risk factors that may lead to heart failure are more prominent in female COPD patients with type 2 respiratory failure. Despite the lower number of female patients compared to males, the significantly higher comorbidity burden in females, as per CCI scores, suggests that medical processes may be more challenging to manage in females. We believe that these findings will contribute to clinical practice and provide clinicians with insights for patient management.

Keywords: hypercapnia; NIV; BPAP; comorbidity; sex; female

1. Introduction

Chronic obstructive pulmonary disease (COPD) ranks among the leading causes of morbidity and mortality globally [1]. COPD is the third leading cause of death in the United States (US) [2]. The prevalence and burden of COPD are expected to increase in the coming decades due to continued exposure to risk factors and an aging global population [3]. The Global Initiative for Chronic Obstructive Lung Disease (GOLD) reports an overall prevalence of COPD at 11.8% in men and 8.5% in women [4], with significantly higher prevalence in men than women [5]. However, from 2001 to 2019, COPD prevalence has been steadily rising among women [6]. Although COPD is still primarily considered a "male disease", mortality rates among men have been decreasing in some countries, such as the US and the United Kingdom, while remaining relatively unchanged among women [7,8].

Hypercapnic respiratory failure (HRF), also known as type 2 respiratory failure (T2RF), is characterized by an increase in the arterial carbon dioxide (CO_2) pressure ($PaCO_2$). CO_2 levels in arterial blood are directly proportional to CO_2 production and inversely proportional to alveolar ventilation. Increased dead space and decreased minute ventilation are common causes of hypercapnia [9]. During exacerbations, ventilation–perfusion (VA/Q) mismatches occur, potentially leading to arterial hypoxemia with or without hypercapnia [10]. Hypercapnia should always be suspected in individuals at risk of hypoventilation (e.g., sedative use, history of sleep apnea) or with increased physiological dead space and limited pulmonary reserve (e.g., COPD exacerbation) presenting with symptoms, such as dyspnea or altered mental status [9]. Acute or acute-on-chronic hypercapnia may develop during exacerbations or in response to oxygen therapy in some COPD patients [9]. Immediate admission to the intensive care unit (ICU) may be necessary for some cases. Ventilatory support during a COPD exacerbation can be provided via noninvasive (nasal or facial mask) or invasive ventilation [11]. Noninvasive ventilation (NIV) is the preferred first-line treatment for acute respiratory failure due to COPD exacerbations, with an 80–85% success rate in hypercapnic patients [12].

Many funding agencies in Europe and North America have implemented policies to encourage or mandate the consideration of sex and gender in medical research at all levels [13]. Despite significant advances in intensive care medicine, limited attention has been given to gender differences in the management and outcomes of ICU patients [14]. Although half of the global population comprises women, they account for only 35–45% of ICU patients [15]. Clinical presentations, comorbidities, and prognoses may differ by gender, potentially affecting treatment decisions [16].

A review of the literature reveals numerous studies on gender–COPD and gender–ICU topics. In these studies, multiple parameters, including demographic data, the severity of illness, comorbidities, Charlson Comorbidity Index (CCI), clinical and laboratory parameters, treatment responses, the need for mechanical ventilation, the length of hospital stay, mortality, and readmission rates, were compared among patients diagnosed with COPD or those followed in the ICU, stratified by gender, to identify similarities and differences [15–30].

However, no study has specifically compared COPD patients with T2RF treated with NIV based on gender. This study aims to identify gender-based differences in patients with HRF treated with NIV and to contribute findings to clinical practice.

2. Materials and Methods

2.1. Study Design and Inclusion and Exclusion Criteria

Our study is prospective, observational, and cross-sectional. Since the study was observational, it was planned according to routine laboratory and radiologic examinations. Patients admitted to the second-level pulmonary ICU between 30 March 2023 and 30 March 2024 for T2RF and clinically stabilized with NIV before discharge were included. The hospital where the study was conducted is located in Ankara, the second largest city and capital of Türkiye. The estimated population of Ankara in 2025 is 5,909,658. The study was conducted in a university hospital with a capacity of 500 beds, which serves as a reference hospital for the pulmonology department. The secondary-level pulmonary intensive care department consists of two separate units with 11 and 12 beds, respectively. The patients included in the study were those followed in the 11-bed unit. There are a total of 14 NIV devices, 4 high flow oxygen devices, and 2 mechanical ventilator devices in the ward. The healthcare staff in the unit is trained and experienced in NIV application. There are 16 nurses working in shifts in the ward; 1 specialist physician and 2 assistant physicians work during the day, and 1 specialist physician and 1 assistant physician work on duty. In addition, to assist the nurses, 3 patient care personnel work during the daytime and 1 patient care personnel works during the on-call hours; 91 female and 167 male patients were enrolled in the study. Inclusion criteria were as follows: patients were over 40 years of age; patients had previously been diagnosed with COPD; patients had previously received a medication report for COPD medications; patients presented with hypercapnic respiratory failure. Exclusion criteria were as follows: included patients with type 1 respiratory failure (T1RF) alone; patients without a COPD diagnosis; those requiring intubation after NIV; patients transferred to third-level ICUs; COVID-19 PCR-positive patients transferred to COVID ICUs; patients who died during hospitalization for unrelated reasons; and patients with chronic hypercapnia previously using home BPAP. The inclusion and exclusion criteria of patients in the study were shown as a flowchart (Figure 1).

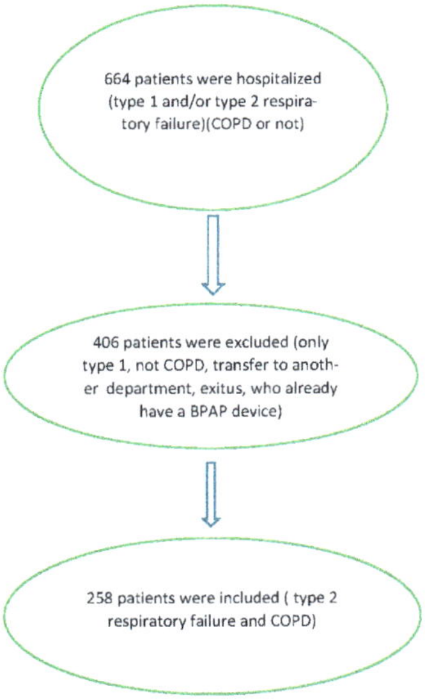

Figure 1. Flowchart of the study. COPD: chronic obstructive pulmonary disease.

2.2. Data Collection and Study Protocol

Informed consent was obtained from patients prior to data collection. Patient files and the hospital information-management system served as data sources. In addition to demographic data, comorbidities, treatments received, long-term device use reports, length of stay, and routine laboratory parameters were recorded. To make a diagnosis of emphysema, new or previous thorax computed tomography scans of the patients were analyzed together with their reports through the radiological imaging system.

2.3. Descriptions

Standardized variables, such as the body mass index, Charlson comorbidity index, and cardiothoracic ratio, were used to compare the study groups.

Body Mass Index (BMI): BMI values were calculated as the ratio of height squared to body weight (kg/m^2). The classification recommended by the World Health Organization was used: underweight below 18.5 kg/m^2 was considered underweight, normal between 18.5–24.9 kg/m^2, overweight between 25–29.9 kg/m^2, obese above 30 kg/m^2 and morbidly obese above 40 kg/m^2 [31].

The Charlson comorbidity index (CCI) is one of the most commonly used methods to assess comorbid factors and predict mortality. The CCI takes into account many underlying conditions, such as age, kidney diseases, malignancies, cerebrovascular diseases, liver diseases, and lung diseases. Scoring is based on 19 medical conditions and is calculated based on variable morbidity rates in the patient population. The severity of morbidities is graded from 1 to 4 [32].

Cardiothoracic ratio: The cardiothoracic ratio (CTR), which expresses the relationship between the transverse size of the chest and the size of the heart measured on postero-anterior chest radiography, is a commonly used parameter in the evaluation of cardiomegaly and has a cut-off value of 0.5. A value greater than 0.5 should be interpreted as an enlarged heart [33].

Classification of disease groups was made according to the ICD 10 coding system used in Türkiye [34]: C34, malignant neoplasm of the bronchus and lung; D50, iron deficiency anemia; D51, vitamin B12 deficiency anemia; D52, folate deficiency anemia; D53, other nutritional anemias; E02, subclinical iodine-deficiency hypothyroidism; E03, other hypothyroidism; E66.2, extreme obesity with alveolar hypoventilation; E10, type 1 diabetes mellitus; E11, type 2 diabetes mellitus; F03, unspecified dementia; F20, schizophrenia; F41, other anxiety disorders; F41.2, anxiety depression; F32, depressive episode; G47.3, sleep apnea; G20, Parkinson disease; G30, dementia in Alzheimer disease; I10, essential (primary) hypertension; I25.1, atherosclerotic heart disease; I48, atrial fibrillation and flutter; I50, heart failure; I69, sequelae of cerebrovascular disease; I26, pulmonary embolism; J44.1, COPD with acute exacerbation; J96.0, acute respiratory failure; J47, bronchiectasis; J09-J18, pneumonia; J43, emphysema; M40.0, postural kyphosis; M40.1, other secondary kyphosis; M40.2, other and unspecified kyphosis; M41.3, thoracogenic scoliosis; N17, acute renal failure; N18, chronic kidney disease; N19, unspecified kidney failure; Q76.3, congenital scoliosis due to congenital bony malformation.

2.4. Statistical Analysis

The data were analyzed using the Statistical Package for Social Sciences (SPSS) Windows 27.0 software (Chicago, IL, USA). The normality of data distribution was evaluated using the Kolmogorov–Smirnov test and histograms. Numerical data with a normal distribution were presented as the mean $\pm$ standard deviation, while non-normally distributed numerical data were presented as the median and minimum–maximum values (IQR 25–75%). Categorical variables were expressed as numbers (n) and percentages (%). Categorical variables were compared using the Chi-square or Fisher's Exact test, while continuous variables were compared using the Student's *t*-test or Mann–Whitney U test. The Kruskal–Wallis analysis was used to compare more than two continuous variables. A p-value < 0.05 was considered statistically significant for all tests.

2.5. Ethical Considerations

Ethical approval for the study was obtained from the Ethics Committee of Ankara Sanatorium Training and Research Hospital (Date: 22 February 2023; No: 2012-KAEK-15/2644).

3. Results

Table 1 evaluates the gender distribution, ages, comorbidities, treatments, and hospital stay durations of the patients. The study was conducted with a total of 258 patients. Of these, 91 (35.3%) were female and 167 (64.7%) were male ($p < 0.01$). The mean age of the patients was 69 ± 10 years. The mean age of female patients was 72 ± 12 years, significantly higher than that of male patients (68 ± 8 years, $p = 0.003$) (Table 1). When comorbidities were compared by gender, body mass index (BMI) ($p < 0.001$), morbid obesity ($p < 0.001$), atrial fibrillation ($p = 0.023$), renal disease ($p = 0.027$), neurological diseases ($p = 0.005$), heart failure ($p < 0.001$), hypertension ($p < 0.001$), hypothyroidism ($p = 0.024$), CCI ($p = 0.02$), and CTR ($p < 0.001$) were significantly higher in female patients than in males (Table 2). Emphysema was significantly higher in male patients than in females ($p < 0.001$) (Table 1).

No significant differences were found in the gender comparison of patients prescribed long-term bilevel positive airway pressure (BPAP) at home ($p = 0.730$) or long-term oxygen therapy (LTOT) at home ($p = 0.765$) (Table 1).

When comparing treatments (antibiotics, steroids, antidepressants, anxiolytics, nutritional support), the number of male patients receiving steroid therapy was significantly higher than female patients ($p = 0.004$) (Table 1).

There were no significant differences in hospital stay durations between genders ($p = 0.926$) (Table 1).

Table 2 evaluates the laboratory parameters of the patients. In the analysis of laboratory parameters at admission, the average D-dimer value ($p = 0.036$) and brain natriuretic peptide (BNP) value ($p = 0.04$) were significantly higher in female patients than in males (Table 2). No significant differences were found in the comparison of pH compensation-decompensation in blood gas analysis at admission by gender (Table 2).

In the hemogram analyses conducted at admission and prior to discharge, the mean hemoglobin levels were significantly higher in male patients than in females ($p < 0.001$, $p < 0.001$) (Table 2).

In the blood gas analyses performed before discharge, the mean partial carbon dioxide pressure ($PaCO_2$) ($p = 0.036$), actual bicarbonate ($aHCO_3$) ($p = 0.031$), actual base excess (aBe) ($p = 0.021$), and standard base excess (sBE) ($p = 0.035$) values were significantly higher in female patients than in males. Additionally, in the biochemistry analysis, the mean sodium levels ($p = 0.003$) were significantly higher in female patients (Table 2).

Although not shown in the table, the lymphocyte/WBC ratio at admission, lymphocyte/WBC ratio at discharge, monocyte/WBC ratio at admission, monocyte/WBC ratio at discharge, neutrophil/WBC ratio at admission, neutrophil/WBC ratio at discharge, eosinophil/WBC ratio at admission, eosinophil/WBC ratio at discharge, basophil/WBC ratio at admission, and basophil/WBC ratio at discharge showed no significant differences between males and females ($p = 0.25$, $p = 0.19$, $p = 0.34$, $p = 0.96$, $p = 0.52$, $p = 0.09$, $p = 0.75$, $p = 0.37$, $p = 0.89$, $p = 0.24$, respectively). Additionally, no significant differences were found in blood group parameters (A, B, O, AB) when compared by gender ($p = 0.92$).

Table 1. Comparison of comorbidities, treatments, and hospital stay durations by gender.

	General	Female	Male	p
n (%)	258 (100%)	91 (35.3%)	167 (64.7%)	<0.01
Age	69 ± 10	72 ± 12	68 ± 8	0.03
Kyphoscoliosis	8 (3.1%)	5 (5.5%)	3 (1.8%)	0.102
Morbid obesity	26 (10.1%)	17 (18.7%)	9 (5.4%)	<0.001

Table 1. *Cont.*

	General	Female	Male	*p*
OSAS	13 (5%)	6 (6.6%)	7 (4.2%)	0.400
Hypertension	147 (57%)	65 (71.4%)	82 (49.1%)	<0.001
Diabetes Mellitus	81 (31.4%)	32 (35.2%)	49 (29.3%)	0.336
Coronary artery disease	52 (20.2%)	20 (22.0%)	32 (19.2%)	0.591
Atrial fibrillation	39 (15.1%)	20 (22.0%)	19 (11.4%)	0.023
Kidney disease	72 (27.9%)	33 (36.2%)	39 (23.3%)	0.027
Neurological disease	7 (2.7%)	6 (6.6%)	1 (0.6%)	0.005
Depression/anxiety	44 (17.1%)	17 (18.7%)	27 (16.2%)	0.609
Bronchiectasis	19 (7.4%)	3 (3.3%)	16 (9.6%)	0.065
Pneumonia	17 (6.6%)	8 (8.8%)	9 (5.4%)	0.294
History of previous tuberculosis	12 (4.7%)	2 (2.2%)	10 (6.0%)	0.168
Pulmonary embolism	16 (6.2%)	8 (8.8%)	8 (4.8%)	0.204
Heart failure	124 (48.1%)	59 (64.8%)	65 (38.9%)	<0.001
Lung cancer	22 (8.5%)	4 (4.4%)	18 (10.8%)	0.080
Hypothyroidism	18 (7.0%)	11 (12.8%)	7 (4.7%)	0.024
Emphysema	69 (26.7%)	5 (5.5%)	64 (38.3%)	<0.001
Anemia	65 (25.2%)	27 (29.7%)	38 (22.9%)	0.233
Body mass index (Mean ± SD)	28 ± 8	31 ± 9	27 ± 7	<0.001
Charlson comorbidity index (Mean ± SD)	5 ± 2	5 ± 2	4 ± 1	0.002
Cardiothoracic ratio (Mean ± SD)	0.56 ± 0.09	0.61 ± 0.07	0.53 ± 0.09	<0.001
Length of stay (Mean ± SD)	9 ± 5	10 ± 7	9 ± 7	0.926
Systemic steroid treatment	184 (71.3%)	55 (60.4%)	129 (77.2%)	0.004
Antibiotic treatment	222 (86%)	77 (84.6%)	145(68.8%)	0.625
Anxiolytic/antidepressant treatment	38 (14.7%)	14 (15.4%)	24 (14.4%)	0.827
Nutritional support	19 (7.4%)	6 (6.6%)	13 (7.8%)	0.727
Number of patients prescribed BPAPs at home	138 (53.5%)	50 (54.9%)	88 (52.7%)	0.730
Number of patients prescribed OCs at homes	91 (35.3%)	31 (34.1%)	60 (35.9%)	0.765

OSAS: obstructive sleep apnea syndrome, BPAP: bilevel positive airway pressure, OC: oxygen concentrator.

Table 2. Analysis of laboratory parameters by gender.

	General 258 (100%)	Female 91 (35.3%)	Male 167 (64.7%)	*p*
Compensation in Hospitalization				0.761
Compensated (PH = 7.35–7.45) n (%)	187 (72.5%)	67 (73.6%)	120 (71.9%)	
Decompensated (PH < 7.35) n (%)	71 (27.5%)	24 (26.4%)	47 (28.1%)	
Admission PH	7.29 ± 0.08	7.28 ± 0.07	7.29 ± 0.08	0.686
Discharged PH	7.46 ± 0.05	7.47 ± 0.04	7.46 ± 0.05	0.402
Admission $PaCO_2$	79.1 ± 15.7	77.5 ± 15.2	79.8 ± 16.0	0.239
Discharged $PaCO_2$	50.4 ± 7.7	51.6 ± 6.1	49.8 ± 7.4	0.036
Admission $aHCO_3$	37.8 ± 7.7	37.0 ± 9.0	38.3 ± 6.9	0.160

Table 2. *Cont.*

	General 258 (100%)	Female 91 (35.3%)	Male 167 (64.7%)	p
Discharged $aHCO_3$	36.1 ± 5.3	37.0 ± 5.3	35.7 ± 5.3	0.031
Admission $aHCO_3$	31.9 ± 7.3	31.9 ± 8.0	31.9 ± 6.8	0.680
Discharged $aHCO_3$	34.5 ± 4.9	35.3 ± 4.4	34.1 ± 5.1	0.038
Admission aBe	8.5 ± 7.6	8.2 ± 8.4	8.6 ± 7.1	0.679
Discharged aBe	11.0 ± 5.3	11.7 ± 4.3	10.6 ± 5.8	0.021
Admission sBe	11.3 ± 7.9	10.4 ± 8.7	11.8 ± 7.3	0.208
Discharged sBe	12.9 ± 6.3	13 ± 5	12 ± 6	0.035
Admission CRP	77 ± 88	62 ± 76	86 ± 94	0.086
Discharged CRP	24 ± 29	20 ± 22	25 ± 32	0.792
Admission BUN	59 ± 34	66 ± 35	55 ± 33	0.006
Discharged BUN	52 ± 25	52 ± 23	52 ± 25	0.848
Admission creatinine	1.15 ± 0.59	1.16 ± 0.52	1.15 ± 0.63	0.591
Discharged creatinine	0.94 ± 0.50	0.87 ± 0.27	0.98 ± 0.59	0.136
Admission sodium	138.6 ± 4.8	139.0 ± 4.2	138.4 ± 5.1	0.500
Discharged sodium	138.6 ± 3.4	139.4 ± 3.4	138.2 ± 3.4	0.003
Admission potassium	4.58 ± 0.78	4.56 ± 0.72	4.60 ± 0.81	0.237
Discharged potassium	4.19 ± 0.63	4.14 ± 0.58	4.21 ± 0.67	0.229
Admission chloride	96.5 ± 6.7	96.3 ± 6.3	96.7 ± 7.0	0.399
Discharged chloride	96.1 ± 4.3	95.9 ± 4.7	96.1 ± 4.1	0.683
Admission magnesium	2.03 ± 0.35	2.00 ± 0.35	2.04 ± 0.36	0.636
Discharge magnesium	1.95 ± 0.24	1.91 ± 0.26	1.96 ± 0.22	0.183
Admission calcium	8.76 ± 0.76	8.67 ± 0.85	8.81 ± 0.70	0.594
Discharge calcium	8.69 ± 0.60	8.73 ± 0.61	8.67 ± 0.60	0.501
Admission albumin	3.50 ± 0.52	3.48 ± 0.50	3.51 ± 0.54	0.518
Discharge albumin	3.16 ± 0.45	3.14 ± 0.39	3.17 ± 0.48	0.465
Admission leukocyte	10.92 ± 4.39	11.01 ± 4.27	10.87 ± 4.46	0.753
Dischage leukocyte	9.08 ± 3.41	8.68 ± 2.91	9.30 ± 3.64	0.294
Admission lymphocyte	1.27 ± 1.06	1.36 ± 0.98	1.22 ± 1.10	0.127
Discharge lymphocyte	1.36 ± 1.39	1.29 ± 0.73	1.40 ± 1.65	0.680
Admission monocyte	0.611 ± 0.254	0.601 ± 0.352	0.616 ± 0.376	0.695
Discharge monocyte	0.589 ± 0.254	0.573 ± 0.234	0.598 ± 0.265	0.618
Admission neutrophil	8.81 ± 3.94	8.78 ± 3.91	8.83 ± 3.97	0.827
Discharge neutrophil	7.05 ± 2.96	6.62 ± 2.76	7.29 ± 3.05	0.119
Admission eosinophil	0.082 ± 0.185	0.073 ± 0.118	0.087 ± 0.213	0.938
Discharge eosinophil	0.123 ± 0.154	0.144 ± 0.191	0.111 ± 0.129	0.485
Admission basophil	0.037 ± 0.035	0.036 ± 0.026	0.038 ± 0.039	0.599
Discharge basophil	0.028 ± 0.022	0.029 ± 0.024	0.027 ± 0.021	0.493
Admission hemoglobin	13.2 ± 2.6	12.1 ± 2.3	13.8 ± 2.6	<0.001

Table 2. *Cont.*

	General 258 (100%)	Female 91 (35.3%)	Male 167 (64.7%)	p
Discharge hemoglobin	12.2 ± 2.6	11.4 ± 2.2	12.7 ± 2.7	<0.001
Admission platelet	244 ± 92	253 ± 94	239 ± 91	0.162
Discharge platelet	233 ± 87	229 ± 90	234 ± 85	0.456
Admission procalcitonin	0.81 ± 4.90	0.35 ± 0.99	1.07 ± 6.06	0.510
Discharge procalcitonin	0.11 ± 0.27	0.10 ± 0.24	0.11 ± 0.28	0.822
Admission D-dimer	2497 ± 4667	3535 ± 6411	1933 ± 3255	0.036
Admission troponin	347 ± 1660	249 ± 697	401 ± 2005	0.702
Admission BNP	355 ± 519	469 ± 603	294 ± 458	0.004
Admission T4	0.98 ± 0.23	0.95 ± 0.21	0.99 ± 0.24	0.381
Admission TSH	2.05 ± 9.32	3.42 ± 15	1.27 ± 2	0.640

$PaCO_2$: partial arterial carbon dioxide pressure, $aHCO_3$: actual bicarbonate, aBe: actual base excess, sBe: standard base excess, BNP: brain natriuretic peptide, TSH: thyroid-stimulating hormone.

4. Discussion

Our study is the first to compare clinical parameters by gender in COPD patients treated with NIV and other medical therapies for T2RF in the ICU and subsequently discharged. The strength of the study is that it was conducted prospectively in an intensive care unit where a team experienced in NIV application worked and specialized in this field. The number of male patients was higher than that of females. The mean age of female patients was significantly higher than that of males. BMI, morbid obesity, atrial fibrillation, renal disease, heart failure, hypertension, hypothyroidism, CCI, BNP, BUN, D-dimer, CTR assessed on the first day of hospitalization, and $PaCO_2$ measured before discharge were significantly higher in females. The presence of emphysema and the use of steroids in treatment were significantly more common in males. No significant gender differences were observed in patients prescribed long-term BPAP or oxygen therapy for home use.

A study examining the epidemiology of COPD in Türkiye using health insurance data found that 56.2% of physician-diagnosed COPD patients were male and 43.8% were female [35]. Another study on COPD exacerbations in Türkiye reported that 85% of the patients were male, while 15% were female [36]. Studies examining ICU patients have shown that the number of male patients is consistently higher [16–19,22,25,37]. In our study, consistent with the literature, the number of male patients was significantly higher than that of females.

A meta-analysis evaluating hospital admissions due to COPD exacerbations showed that the gender distribution varied widely, with mean ages ranging from 63.0 ± 14.5 to 76.3 ± 10.6 years [30]. Studies by Zetterstein et al. on ICU patients and Grabicki et al. on COPD patients found no differences in the mean age between males and females [16,25]. However, Todorov et al. reported a significantly higher mean age in female ICU patients than in males [75 (64;82) years in women vs. 68 (58;77) years in men, $p < 0.001$] [28]. In our study, the mean age of females was significantly higher than that of males. The life expectancy at birth in Türkiye is 80 years for women and 74.7 years for men, which may have influenced the results [38].

Comorbidities are common in all stages of COPD, from mild to severe [1]. A study evaluating COPD patients by gender found that the comorbidity burden, based on the CCI, was higher in women with severe and very severe COPD [26]. A study on ICU patients found fewer comorbidities in females than in males (5.4 vs. 6.4, $p = 0.002$) [26]. Among four studies examining CCI by gender, three found no significant differences [19,39,40], while one reported a higher comorbidity burden in males [25]. In our study, CCI was higher in females than in males. The higher average age in female patients compared to males is believed to impact the CCI, both directly due to age and indirectly due to the increased burden of comorbidities associated with aging.

Cardiovascular diseases are common and significant comorbidities in COPD [1]. The prevalence of systolic and diastolic heart failure in COPD patients ranges from 20% to 70% [41]. COPD is frequently associated with cardiac arrhythmias, which contribute to increased dyspnea [42]. Atrial fibrillation is common in COPD and can exacerbate dyspnea [43]. Hypertension is likely the most common comorbidity in COPD and can significantly impact disease progression [44]. Grabicki et al. found that cardiovascular diseases were more prevalent in females, while coronary artery disease was more common in males [16]. A study conducted in northern Sweden on COPD patients found a higher prevalence of cardiovascular disease in males [45]. Roche et al. found no gender differences in hypertension, ischemic heart disease, or left heart failure [21]. Todorov et al. reported no significant differences between genders in arrhythmias and heart failure [28]. In our study, heart failure, hypertension, atrial fibrillation, increased CTR (a radiological indicator of heart failure), and elevated BNP (a laboratory marker of heart failure) were significantly more common in females. No significant differences were observed between genders in coronary artery disease. It is thought that the higher prevalence of heart failure in women may be related to the frequency of hypertension and atrial fibrillation.

Patients with pulmonary etiologies and increased BMI are considered at risk for ICU admission [46]. Pulmonary causes are the most frequent reasons for hospital admission in patients with an elevated BMI [47]. A study by Kumar et al. on ICU patients found that among patients with a BMI of 30–39, 51.4% were male and 48.6% were female; for a BMI of 40–49, 41.5% were male and 58.5% were female; for a BMI $\geq$50, 41.9% were male and 58.1% were female [46]. Grabicki et al. found that females had lower BMIs than males [16]. In contrast, Roche et al. reported higher BMIs in females with COPD but no gender differences in the obesity prevalence [21]. In our study, females had significantly higher BMIs than males, and the number of morbidly obese female patients was greater than that of males. A higher age and comorbid disease burden in female patients may contribute to mobility restrictions, which, in turn, may be associated with a higher BMI.

In our study, renal failure and hypothyroidism were significantly more common in females. Matera et al. reported a higher prevalence of renal disease in males [27], and Grabicki et al. found thyroid diseases to be more common in females [16].

When we evaluated the relationship between an increased BMI, hypothyroidism, renal failure, and heart failure, all three conditions were found to be associated with heart failure and an increased heart failure risk. Heart failure often coexists with reduced renal function, and the relationship between the two conditions is bidirectional [47]. Being overweight (BMI $\geq$ 25 kg/m^2) and having obesity (BMI $\geq$ 30 kg/m^2) independently increase the risk of heart failure [48]. Hypothyroidism is also a risk factor for heart failure [49].

Other laboratory parameters significantly higher in females were D-dimer levels assessed on admission and $PaCO_2$ levels measured before discharge. Elevated D-dimer levels are known to correlate with renal failure [50]. The higher $PaCO_2$ levels before discharge in females may be due to the higher BMI and obesity prevalence, making hypercapnia more challenging to control in this group. In males, parameters significantly higher than in females included steroid use and the presence of emphysema. Males and females may exhibit phenotypically different responses to tobacco smoke exposure, with males being more prone to the emphysematous phenotype and females to the airway-dominant phenotype [51]. A review of the literature revealed no studies comparing systemic steroid use between men and women. In our study, the higher prevalence of steroid use in men could be attributed to the prioritization of diuretic therapy in women due to the higher incidence of heart failure as a comorbidity, relegating the anti-inflammatory steroid therapy to secondary importance.

The findings of this study are expected to guide future research. Furthermore, larger, multicenter studies focusing on gender-based comparisons across different age groups would contribute more significantly to clinical practice.

5. Limitations

The study was conducted at a single center. As this was an observational study, only routinely evaluated parameters were examined. Additional tests (e.g., echocardiography, spirometry) could not be performed. Due to the poor general condition of patients at the time of admission, a detailed medical history could not be obtained. Instead, anamnesis was collected from patient relatives and/or previous medical records were reviewed. The smoking history (amount, duration, age of initiation), biomass exposure, GOLD stage, alpha-1 antitrypsin levels, and frequency of exacerbations were not available. Due to the limited sample size, comparisons could not be made based on age groups. Chest radiographs used in the evaluation of CTR were performed with portable devices under intensive care conditions. The weight and height values used in the BMI calculation were either based on information obtained from patients/relatives or estimated. In cases where current data are not sufficient for the parameters used in the calculation of CCI, old records were also examined and included in the calculation.

Strength of the Study

The strength of the study is that it was conducted prospectively in an intensive care unit where a team experienced in NIV application worked and specialized in this field.

6. Conclusions

In our study examining gender-based differences in COPD patients treated with NIV for T2RF, heart failure and risk factors for heart failure were found to be more prominent in female patients. Consistent with the literature, although the number of female patients was lower than that of males, the significantly higher comorbidity burden in females based on CCI scores suggests that medical processes may be more challenging to manage in women. We believe that these findings will contribute to clinical practice and provide clinicians with valuable insights into patient management.

Author Contributions: Conceptualization, T.O., M.Y., M.A., G.E.D., M.Ö.C., and Ç.Ö.; Methodology, T.O., M.Y., M.A., and E.A.; Software, T.O.; Validation, T.O., M.Y., and M.A.; Formal analysis, T.O., M.A., and E.A.; Investigation, T.O., M.Y., E.A., G.E.D., M.Ö.C., and M.D.; Resources, T.O.; Data curation, T.O., M.Y., G.E.D., M.Ö.C., M.D., D.K., and Y.T.Ş.; Writing—original draft, T.O.; Writing—review and editing, T.O., M.Y., M.A., E.A., G.E.D., M.Ö.C., M.D., Ç.Ö., D.K., and Y.T.Ş.; Supervision, T.O.; Project administration, T.O. All authors have read and agreed to the published version of the manuscript.

Funding: This research received no external funding.

Institutional Review Board Statement: The study was conducted in accordance with the Declaration of Helsinki and approved by the Ethics Committee of Ankara Sanatorium Training and Research Hospital (date: 22 February 2023; No: 2012-KAEK-15/2644).

Informed Consent Statement: Informed consent was obtained from patients prior to data collection.

Data Availability Statement: The original contributions presented in this study are included in the article. Further inquiries can be directed to the corresponding author.

Conflicts of Interest: The authors declare no conflict of interest.

References

1. Venkatesan, P. GOLD COPD Report: 2024 Update. *Lancet Respir. Med.* **2024**, *12*, 15–16. [PubMed]
2. Hoyert, D.L.; Xu, J.Q. Deaths: Preliminary data for 2011. *Natl. Vital. Stat. Rep.* **2011**, *61*, 1–65.
3. Mathers, C.D.; Loncar, D. Projections of global mortality and burden of disease from 2002 to 2030. *PLoS Med.* **2006**, *3*, e442. [PubMed]
4. Lamprecht, B.; McBurnie, M.A.; Vollmer, W.M.; Gudmundsson, G.; Welte, T.; Nizankowska-Mogilnicka, E.; Studnicka, M.; Bateman, E.; Anto, J.M.; Burney, P.; et al. COPD in never smokers: Results from the population-based burden of obstructive lung disease study. *Chest* **2011**, *139*, 752–763. [PubMed]
5. Menezes, A.M.; Perez-Padilla, R.; Jardim, J.R.; Muiño, A.; Lopez, M.V.; Valdivia, G.; Montes de Oca, M.; Talamo, C.; Hallal, P.C.; Victora, C.G. Chronic obstructive pulmonary disease in five Latin Ameri-can cities (the PLATINO study): A prevalence study. *Lancet* **2005**, *366*, 1875–1881.
6. Marshall, D.C.; Al Omari, O.; Goodall, R.; Shalhoub, J.; Adcock, I.M.; Chung, K.F.; Salciccioli, J.D. Trends in prevalence, mortality, and disability-adjusted life years relating to chronic obstructive pulmonary disease in Europe: An observational study of the global burden of disease database, 2001–2019. *BMC Pulm. Med.* **2022**, *22*, 289.
7. Agusti, A.; Faner, R. COPD beyond smoking: New paradigm, novel opportunities. *Lancet Respir. Med.* **2018**, *6*, 324–326.
8. Lozano, R.; Naghavi, M.; Foreman, K.; Lim, S.; Shibuya, K.; Aboyans, V.; Abraham, J.; Adair, T.; Aggarwal, R.; Ahn, S.Y.; et al. Global and regional mortality from 235 causes of death for 20 age groups in 1990 and 2010: A systematic analysis for the Global Burden of Disease Study 2010. *Lancet* **2012**, *380*, 2095–2128.
9. Feller-Kopman, D.J.; Schwartzstein Richard, M. The evaluation, diagnosis, and treatment of the adult patient with acute hypercapnic respiratory failure. In *UpToDate*; Stoller, J.K., Geraldine, F., Eds.; Wolters Kluwer: Alphen aan den Rijn, The Netherlands, 2022. Available online: https://www.uptodate.com/contents/the-evaluation-diagnosis-and-treatment-of-the-adult-patient-with-acute-hypercapnic-respiratory-failure (accessed on 17 March 2025).
10. Barberà, J.A.; Roca, J.; Ferrer, A.; Félez, M.A.; Díaz, O.; Roger, N.; Rodriguez-Roisin, R. Mechanisms of worsening gas exchange during acute exacerbations of chronic obstructive pulmonary disease. *Eur. Respir. J.* **1997**, *10*, 1285–1291.
11. National Institute for Health and Care Excellence. Chronic Obstructive Pulmonary Disease in over 16s: Diagnosis and Management. 2018. Available online: https://www.nice.org.uk/guidance/NG115 (accessed on 14 March 2025).
12. Rochwerg, B.; Brochard, L.; Elliott, M.W.; Hess, D.; Hill, N.S.; Nava, S.; Navalesi, P.; Members of The Steering Committee; Antonelli, M.; Brozek, J.; et al. Official ERS/ATS clinical practice guidelines: Noninvasive ventilation for acute respiratory failure. *Eur. Respir. J.* **2017**, *50*, 1602426.
13. Mauvais-Jarvis, F.; Bairey Merz, N.; Barnes, P.J.; Brinton, R.D.; Carrero, J.J.; DeMeo, D.L.; De Vries, G.J.; Epperson, C.N.; Govindan, R.; Klein, S.L.; et al. Sex and gender: Modifiers of health, disease, and medicine. *Lancet* **2020**, *396*, 565–582. [CrossRef] [PubMed]
14. Merdji, H.; Long, M.T.; Ostermann, M.; Herridge, M.; Myatra, S.N.; De Rosa, S.; Metaxa, V.; Kotfis, K.; Robba, C.; De Jong, A.; et al. Sex and gender differences in intensive care medicine. *Intensive Care Med.* **2023**, *49*, 1155–1167.
15. Modra, L.; Higgins, A.; Vithanage, R.; Abeygunawardana, V.; Bailey, M.; Bellomo, R. Sex differences in illness severity and mortality among adult intensive care patients: A systematic review and meta-analysis. *J. Crit. Care* **2021**, *65*, 116–123.
16. Grabicki, M.; Kuźnar-Kamińska, B.; Rubinsztajn, R.; Brajer-Luftmann, B.; Kosacka, M.; Nowicka, A.; Piorunek, T.; Kostrzewska, M.; Chazan, R.; Batura-Gabryel, H. COPD Course and Comorbidities: Are There Gender Differences? *Adv. Exp. Med. Biol.* **2019**, *1113*, 43–51. [PubMed]
17. Valentin, A.; Jordan, B.; Lang, T.; Hiesmayr, M.; Metnitz, P.G. Gender-related differences in intensive care: A multiple-center cohort study of therapeutic interventions and outcome in critically ill patients. *Crit. Care Med.* **2003**, *31*, 1901–1907.
18. Reinikainen, M.; Niskanen, M.; Uusaro, A.; Ruokonen, E. Impact of gender on treatment and outcome of ICU patients. *Acta Anaesthesiol. Scand* **2005**, *49*, 984–990. [CrossRef] [PubMed]
19. Fowler, R.A.; Sabur, N.; Li, P.; Juurlink, D.N.; Pinto, R.; Hladunewich, M.A.; Adhikari, N.K.; Sibbald, W.J.; Martin, C.M. Sex-and age-based differences in the delivery and outcomes of critical care. *CMAJ* **2007**, *177*, 1513–1519. [CrossRef]
20. Mahmood, K.; Eldeirawi, K.; Wahidi, M.M. Association of gender with outcomes in critically ill patients. *Crit. Care* **2012**, *16*, R92.
21. Roche, N.; Deslée, G.; Caillaud, D.; Brinchault, G.; Court-Fortune, I.; Nesme-Meyer, P.; Surpas, P.; Escamilla, R.; Perez, T.; Chanez, P.; et al. Impact of gender on COPD expression in a real-life cohort. *Respir. Res.* **2014**, *15*, 20.

22. Kristensen, M.L.; Vestergaard, T.R.; Bülow, H.H. Gender differences in randomised, controlled trials in intensive care units. *Acta Anaesthesiol. Scand.* **2014**, *58*, 788–793.
23. Liao, K.M.; Chen, Y.C.; Cheng, K.C.; Wang, J.J.; Ho, C.H. Trends in intensive care unit admissions of COPD patients from 2003 to 2013 in Taiwan. *Int. J. Chron. Obstruct. Pulmon. Dis.* **2018**, *13*, 2007–2012.
24. Hill, A.; Ramsey, C.; Dodek, P.; Kozek, J.; Fransoo, R.; Fowler, R.; Doupe, M.; Wong, H.; Scales, D.; Garland, A. Examining mechanisms for gender differences in admission to intensive care units. *Health Serv. Res.* **2020**, *55*, 35–43. [PubMed]
25. Zettersten, E.; Jäderling, G.; Bell, M.; Larsson, E. Sex and gender aspects on intensive care. A cohort study. *J. Crit. Care* **2020**, *55*, 22–27. [PubMed]
26. Backman, B.H.; Virchow, J.C.; Lundbäck, B. COPD in women—New results presented. *Respir. Med.* **2021**, *176*, 106238.
27. Matera, M.G.; Ora, J.; Calzetta, L.; Rogliani, P.; Cazzola, M. Sex differences in COPD management. *Expert Rev. Clin. Pharmacol.* **2021**, *14*, 323–332. [PubMed]
28. Todorov, A.; Kaufmann, F.; Arslani, K.; Haider, A.; Bengs, S.; Goliasch, G.; Zellweger, N.; Tontsch, J.; Sutter, R.; Buddeberg, B.; et al. Gender differences in the provision of intensive care: A Bayesian approach. *Intensive Care Med.* **2021**, *47*, 577–587.
29. Rogliani, P.; Cavalli, F.; Ritondo, B.L.; Cazzola, M.; Calzetta, L. Sex differences in adult asthma and COPD therapy: A systematic review. *Respir. Res.* **2022**, *23*, 222.
30. Ruan, H.; Zhang, H.; Wang, J.; Zhao, H.; Han, W.; Li, J. Readmission rate for acute exacerbation of chronic obstructive pulmonary disease: A systematic review and meta-analysis. *Respir. Med.* **2023**, *206*, 107090.
31. Physical status: The use and interpretation of anthropometry. Report of a WHO Expert Committee. *World Health Organ Tech. Rep. Ser.* **1995**, *854*, 1–452.
32. Charlson, M.E.; Pompei, P.; Ales, K.L.; MacKenzie, C.R. A new method of classifying prognostic comorbidity in longitudinal studies: Development and validation. *J. Chronic Dis.* **1987**, *40*, 373–383.
33. Danzer, C.S. The Cardiothoracic Ratio. *Am. J. Med. Sci.* **1919**, *157*, 513–554. [CrossRef]
34. World Health Organization. International Statistical Classification of Diseases and Related Health Problems 10th Revision. Available online: https://iris.who.int/handle/10665/246208 (accessed on 3 March 2025).
35. Özdemir, T.; Yilmaz Demirci, N.; Kiliç, H.; Koç, O.; Kaya, A.; Öztürk, C. An epidemiologic study of physician-diagnosed chronic obstructive pulmonary disease in the Turkish population: COPDTURKEY-1. *Turk. J. Med. Sci.* **2020**, *50*, 132–140. [PubMed]
36. Ozyilmaz, E.; Kokturk, N.; Teksut, G.; Tatlicioglu, T. Unsuspected risk factors of frequent exacerbations requiring hospital admission in chronic obstructive pulmonary disease. *Int. J. Clin. Pract.* **2013**, *67*, 691–697. [PubMed]
37. Samuelsson, C.; Sjoberg, F.; Karlstrom, G.; Nolin, T.; Walther, S.M. Gender differences in outcome and use of resources do exist in Swedish intensive care, but to no advantage for women of premenopausal age. *Crit. Care* **2015**, *19*, 129.
38. Başara, B.B.; Aygün, A.; Özdemir, T.A.; Kulali, B. *Health Statistics Yearbook 2023*; Ministry of Health: Ankara, Turkey, 2023. Available online: https://sbsgm.saglik.gov.tr/TR-93567/health-statistics-yearbook.html (accessed on 3 March 2025).
39. Hollinger, A.; Gayat, E.; Feliot, E.; Paugam-Burtz, C.; Fournier, M.C.; Duranteau, J.; Lefrant, J.Y.; Leone, M.; Jaber, S.; Mebazaa, A.; et al. Gender and survival of critically ill patients: Results from the FROG-ICU study. *Ann. Intensive Care* **2019**, *9*, 43.
40. Shen, H.N.; Lu, C.L.; Yang, H.H. Women receive more trials of noninvasive ventilation for acute respiratory failure than men: A nationwide population-based study. *Crit. Care* **2011**, *15*, R174.
41. Bhatt, S.P.; Dransfield, M.T. Chronic obstructive pulmonary disease and cardiovascular disease. *Transl. Res.* **2013**, *162*, 237–251.
42. Liu, X.; Chen, Z.; Li, S.; Xu, S. Association of Chronic Obstructive Pulmonary Disease with Arrhythmia Risks: A Systematic Review and Meta-Analysis. *Front. Cardiovasc. Med.* **2021**, *8*, 732349.
43. Terzano, C.; Romani, S.; Conti, V.; Paone, G.; Oriolo, F.; Vitarelli, A. Atrial fibrillation in the acute hypercapnic exacerbations of COPD. *Eur. Rev. Med. Pharmacol. Sci.* **2014**, *18*, 2908–2917.
44. Divo, M.; Cote, C.; de Torres, J.P.; Paone, G.; Oriolo, F.; Vitarelli, A. Comorbidities and risk of mortality in patients with chronic obstructive pulmonary disease. *Am. J. Respir. Crit. Care Med.* **2012**, *186*, 155–161.
45. Sawalha, S.; Hedman, L.; Backman, H. The impact of comorbidities on mortality among men and women with COPD: Report from the OLIN COPD study. *Ther. Adv. Respir. Dis.* **2019**, *13*, 1753466619860058. [CrossRef] [PubMed]
46. Kumar, S.I.; Doo, K.; Sottilo-Brammeier, J.; Lane, C.; Liebler, J.M. Super Obesity in the Medical Intensive Care Unit. *J. Intensive Care Med.* **2020**, *35*, 478–484. [CrossRef] [PubMed]
47. Szlagor, M.; Dybiec, J.; Młynarska, E.; Rysz, J.; Franczyk, B. Chronic Kidney Disease as a Comorbidity in Heart Failure. *Int. J. Mol. Sci.* **2023**, *24*, 2988. [CrossRef]
48. Mandviwala, T.; Khalid, U.; Deswal, A. Obesity and Cardiovascular Disease: A Risk Factor or a Risk Marker? *Curr. Atheroscler. Rep.* **2016**, *18*, 21. [CrossRef]

49. Ning, N.; Gao, D.; Triggiani, V.; Iacoviello, M.; Mitchell, J.E.; Ma, R.; Zhang, Y.; Kou, H. Prognostic Role of Hypothyroidism in Heart Failure: A Meta-Analysis. *Medicine* **2015**, *94*, e1159. [CrossRef] [PubMed]
50. Robert-Ebadi, H.; Bertoletti, L.; Combescure, C.; Le Gal, G.; Bounameaux, H.; Righini, M. Effects of impaired renal function on levels and performance of D-dimer in patients with suspected pulmonary embolism. *Thromb. Haemost.* **2014**, *112*, 614–620.
51. Han, M.K.; Postma, D.; Mannino, D.M.; Giardino, N.D.; Buist, S.; Curtis, J.L.; Martinez, F.J. Gender and Chronic Obstructive Pulmonary Disease: Why It Matters. *Am. J. Respir. Crit. Care Med.* **2007**, *176*, 1179–1184. [CrossRef]

medicina

MDPI

Systematic Review

Efficacy of Long-Term Use of Azithromycin in the Management of Cystic Fibrosis in Pediatric Patients with or Without *Pseudomonas aeruginosa*: A Systematic Review and Meta-Analysis Article

Hassan Al-shehri *,† and Dana Albassam †

Department of Pediatrics, College of Medicine, Imam Mohammad Ibn Saud Islamic University (IMSIU), Riyadh 13317, Saudi Arabia; daalbassam@imamu.edu.sa

* Correspondence: haalshehri@imamu.edu.sa

† Equally contributed to the first author.

Abstract: *Background and Objectives:* In the present systematic review and meta-analysis, we aimed to discover the overall efficacy of azithromycin in children with cystic fibrosis (CF) and with or without *Pseudomonas aeruginosa* infection, specifically regarding its effect on respiratory parameters such as forced expiratory volume in 1 s (FEV1) and forced vital capacity (FVC) in addition to its effect on exacerbations and the need to use additional antibiotics. *Materials and Method:* We conducted this systematic review and meta-analysis by searching for all eligible articles on PubMed, Web of Science, and Scopus published between inception and September 2024. We used the following search strategy for our searching process: "Cystic fibrosis" AND "Azithromycin" and "Children" OR "Pediatric" OR "Infant". We conducted the meta-analysis by pooling the mean difference (MD) and comparing the continuous variables and odds ratio (OR) for dichotomous variables at 95% confidence intervals (CI), at a p-value of 0.05. *Results:* Azithromycin was observed to be associated with increased FEV1 compared with the control, showing an MD of 1.91 (95% CI: 1.09, 2.74, $p < 0.00001$) and non-significant heterogeneity. However, no significant difference was observed between azithromycin and control groups regarding FVC with MD = 0.62 (95% CI: −0.01, 1.25, $p = 0.06$). Compared with the control group, azithromycin was significantly associated with lower risk and a lower number of exacerbations, with OR = 0.48 (95% CI: 0.34, 0.67, $p < 0.0001$) and MD = −0.82 (95% CI: −1.32, −0.33, $p = 0.001$), respectively, with non-significant heterogeneity. Regarding the need for new antibiotic usage, azithromycin showed a significantly lower need, with OR = 0.35 (95% CI: 0.13, 0.94, $p = 0.04$), $I^2 = 75\%$, $p = 0.02$. No significant difference was observed between both groups regarding hospitalization rate, with OR = 0.88 (95% CI: 0.55, 1.4, $p = 0.59$). *Conclusions:* This systematic review and meta-analysis showed the efficacy of azithromycin in pediatric patients with CF, as it improved lung function by increasing FEV1, reduced exacerbations of CF, which is the most common symptom of CF that leads to mortality, and reduced the number of antibiotics that needed to be administered to patients with CF, which reduces the risk of antibiotic resistance. Therefore, the long-term use of azithromycin is recommended for pediatric patients with CF as part of their treatment regimen.

Keywords: azithromycin; cystic fibrosis; children; pulmonary function; *Pseudomonas aeruginosa*

1. Introduction

Cystic fibrosis (CF) is an autosomal recessive multisystem disorder characterized by severe symptoms in the respiratory, urogenital, and gastrointestinal systems. The cumulative symptoms significantly impair the quality of life for many individuals and necessitate several hospitalizations during the course of their illness. Research indicates that most hospitalizations result from pulmonary symptoms, thereby exacerbating the disease's burden [1,2]. It is the most prevalent cause of early mortality among autosomal recessive illnesses in the global Caucasian population [3].

CF is linked to mutations in the CF transmembrane conductance regulator (CFTR) gene situated on the long arm of chromosome 7. CFTR encodes a protein present in the epithelial cells of the lungs, sweat glands, pancreas, intestines, and liver. It is part of the Adenosine triphosphate (ATP-) binding cassette transporter family and operates as a Cyclic adenosine monophosphate (cAMP) dependent chloride channel that enables Cl^-/HCO_3^- exchange in exocrine epithelia [4]. It functions to sustain an alkaline pH and dilute fluid secretions [5]. Mutations in CFTR result in dehydrated secretions and hyperviscous mucus, leading to a multisystem disorder that significantly impacts the respiratory, gastrointestinal, and hepatobiliary systems. The fundamental flow in ion transport creates a continuous loop of compromised airway clearance, persistent endobronchial infection, and excessive inflammatory response in the lungs [6]. Chronic high-intensity inflammation causes irreversible structural damage to CF airways and deteriorates lung function, ultimately leading to respiratory failure and mortality. Numerous impaired inflammatory responses have been associated with CFTR loss, encompassing innate and adaptive immunological dysregulation, anomalies in cell membrane lipids, different transcription factor signaling deficiencies, and altered kinase and toll-like receptor responses [7]. Lung inflammation in CF is characterized by neutrophils that secrete oxidants and proteases, including elastase. Neutrophil elastase in airway secretions precedes bronchiectasis and correlates with the decline in lung function and respiratory exacerbations in CF [8].

Pulmonary exacerbation is the most prevalent acute occurrence in patients with CF [9]. Clinical trials have shown *Pseudomonas aeruginosa* as the most often implicated bacteria in acute exacerbations [10,11].

Macrolides, including azithromycin, have been extensively researched in patients with CF, both with [12] and without [13] *Pseudomonas aeruginosa* infection. This research consistently demonstrates a clinically significant decrease in the incidence of pulmonary exacerbation for up to 6 months. Macrolides have not exhibited bactericidal activity against *Pseudomonas aeruginosa* and are not deemed suitable as a singular or first-line antibiotic for eradication therapy. Macrolides exhibit anti-inflammatory properties [14] and may diminish *Pseudomonas aeruginosa* biofilm formation [15], which could partially elucidate their influence on pulmonary exacerbations. In the present systematic review and meta-analysis, we aimed to discover the overall efficacy of azithromycin in children with CF with or without *Pseudomonas aeruginosa* infection, specifically regarding its effect on respiratory parameters such as forced expiratory volume in 1 s (FEV1) and forced vital capacity (FVC), in addition to its effect on exacerbations and the need to use additional antibiotics.

2. Materials and Methods

2.1. Database Searching and Screening

By adhering to the Preferred Reporting Items for Systematic Reviews and Meta-Analyses (PRISMA, File S1) guidelines [16], we conducted this systematic review and meta-analysis by searching for all eligible articles on PubMed, Web of Science, and Scopus published between inception and September 2024. We used the following search strategy for our searching process: "Cystic fibrosis" AND "Azithromycin" and "Children" OR "Pediatric" OR "Infant".

2.2. Eligibility Criteria

We selected studies based on the following inclusion criteria: studies published without time frame limitations, randomized controlled trial (RCT) studies, and observational cohort studies comparing the use of azithromycin against a control group (those receiving no azithromycin) or a placebo in pediatric patients with CF. We excluded reviews, case reports, studies with no comparison groups, and studies analyzing drugs other than azithromycin.

2.3. Screening

For the screening process, the search results were uploaded on Rayyan [17] to facilitate title and abstract screening. The eligible articles underwent full-text screening after the previous step to examine the eligibility of the whole article. Any disagreement was resolved by consensus, and, if it persisted, it was referred to the senior author.

2.4. Data Extraction

Using Microsoft Excel spreadsheets, we conducted the process of data extraction to extract the baseline data and outcomes of interest. Regarding the baseline data, we collected data on study design, population, age, gender, sample size, follow-up, and the use of other drugs. For the outcomes, we extracted data on changes in FEV1 and FVC, exacerbations, hospitalization, and the use of antibiotics.

2.5. Quality and Risk of Bias Assessments

Utilizing the Newcastle–Ottawa Scale (NOS), which rates each study from 0 to 9 stars, quality evaluation for the observational cohort studies was carried out. With the exception of the comparability question, the answer to which can receive zero, one, or two stars, each answer can be given a star. A study is rated as low quality if it receives 0–3 stars, moderate quality if it receives 4–6 stars, and high quality if it receives 7–9 stars [18]. We also utilized the Cochrane risk-of-bias instrument (Rob-2) [19], comprising five domains with associated sets of questions. These domains include randomization, deviations from intended interventions, outcome measurement, missing outcome data, and outcome selection of the reported result. A study can only be considered to have an overall low risk of bias if each of the five domains is classified as low risk individually. If concerns are expressed in any domain, then the study is considered to have problems. Additionally, if any domain is judged to be at high risk or if multiple domains raise red flags, the study is labeled as having a high risk of bias.

2.6. Statistical Analysis

Using Review Manager Version 5.4 [20], we conducted a meta-analysis by pooling the mean difference (MD) and comparing the continuous variables and odds ratio (OR) for dichotomous variables. The random effect model was used for heterogenous variables and the fixed effect model was used for homogenous ones, with 95% confidence intervals (CI) and a p-value of 0.05. The heterogeneity was assessed using the I^2 and a p-value of 0.05.

3. Results

3.1. Search Results and Screening

The applied search strategy resulted in a total of 264 articles with 158 duplicates. After title and abstract screening, 15 articles were found to be eligible for full-text screening, and a final 7 articles were eligible to undergo systematic review and meta-analysis [13,21–26] (Figure 1).

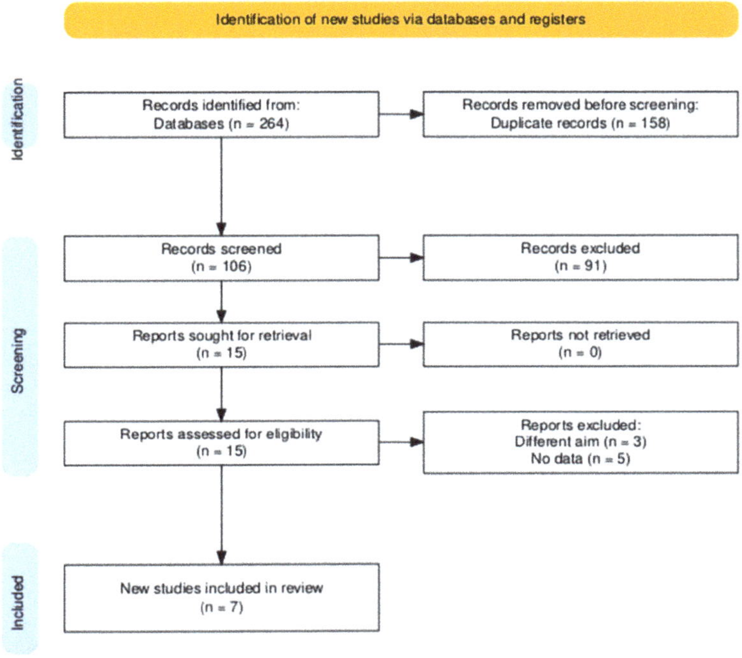

Figure 1. PRISMA flow diagram of the searching and screening processes.

3.2. Quality and Risk of Bias Assessments

According to Rob-2, the four included RCTs were found to have a low risk of bias across all domains (Figure 2). The three included cohort studies were deemed to have high quality according to the NOS (Table 1).

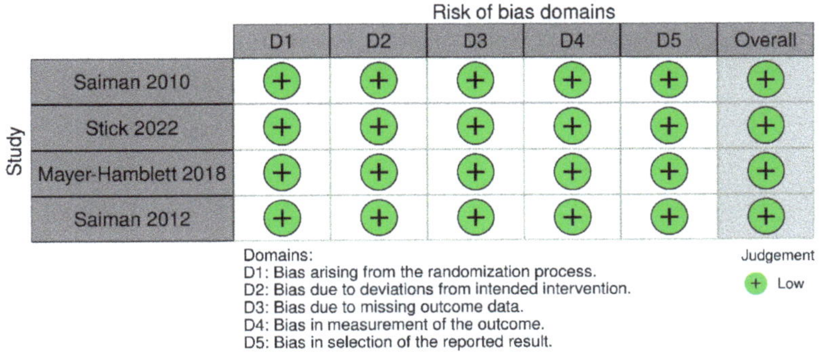

Figure 2. Risk of bias assessment of randomized controlled trials using Rob-2 [13,21,24,26].

Table 1. Quality assessment of cohort studies using the NOS.

Study Name	Representativeness of the Exposed Cohort (★)	Selection of the Non-Exposed Cohort (★)	Ascertainment of Exposure (★)	Demonstration That Outcome of Interest Was Not Present at Start of Study (★)	Comparability of Cohorts Based on the Design or Analysis (Max.: ★★)	Was Follow-Up Long Enough for Outcomes to Occur? (★)	Assessment of Outcome (★)	Adequacy of Follow-Up of Cohorts (★)	Quality Level
Shmarina 2017 [23]	☆	☆	☆	☆	☆	☆	☆	☆	High
Klingel 2019 [25]	☆	☆	☆	☆	☆	☆	☆	-	High
Abdul Aziz 2020 [22]	☆	-	☆	☆	☆	☆	☆	☆	High

3.3. Baseline Characteristics

We included seven studies in the present systematic review and meta-analysis, comparing the use of azithromycin against a control group (no azithromycin) or a placebo in pediatric patients with CF, who either experienced or did not experience *Pseudomonas aeruginosa* infection. Four studies were RCTs, while the other three were cohort studies. Follow-up ranged from 5.6 to 36 months. The mean age of the patients ranged from 3.6 months to 18 years old. Baseline characteristics are shown in Table 2.

Table 2. Baseline characteristics of the included patients.

Study ID	Design	Population	Follow-Up (Months)	Sample Size		Age, Mean (SD) Years		Male, n (%)		Other Drugs
				AZN	No AZN	AZN	No AZN	AZN	No AZN	
Saiman 2010 [13]	RCT	Patients with cystic fibrosis uninfected with *Pseudomonas aeruginosa*	5.6	131	129	10.7 (3.25)	10.6 (3.1)	77 (59)	70 (71)	Dornase alfa, tobramycin, ibuprofen, and hypertonic saline
Stick 2022 [24]	RCT	Infants with cystic fibrosis	36	68	62	3.6 (1.2) months	3.6 (1.3) months	38 (56)	40 (65)	NR
Mayer-Hamblett 2018 [21]	RCT	Early *Pseudomonas* infection in cystic fibrosis	11	110	111	7.1 (5.1)	6.8 (5)	55 (50)	62 (55.9)	Ivacaftor/lumacaftor
Shmarina 2017 [23]	Cohort	Pediatric patients with cystic fibrosis	12	59	102	14.3 (0.4)	13 (0.4)	28 (47.5)	59 (57.8)	NR
Klingel 2019 [25]	Cohort	Children with cystic fibrosis with exacerbations who are on tobramycin	12	31	36	13.6 (10.6 to 15.4) median (IQR)	14.9 (12.3 to 16.1)	NR	NR	Tobramycin, colistimethate, amikacin, and aztreonam
Abdul Aziz 2020 [22]	Cohort	Children with cystic fibrosis with exacerbations who are on tobramycin	12	30	33	14.4 (3)	9.96 (3.57)	18 (60%)	21 (63.6)	NR
Saiman 2012 [26]	RCT	Patients with cystic fibrosis uninfected with *Pseudomonas aeruginosa*	5.6	77	69	6–18 years		NR	NR	NR

AZN: azithromycin, RCT: randomized controlled trial, NR: not reported, SD: standard deviation.

3.4. Statistical Analysis

Azithromycin was observed to be associated with increased FEV1 compared with the control, showing an MD of 1.91 (95% CI: 1.09, 2.74, $p < 0.00001$) and non-significant heterogeneity. However, no significant difference was observed between the azithromycin and control groups regarding FVC, with an MD = 0.62 (95% CI: −0.01, 1.25, $p = 0.06$) (Figures 3 and 4).

Compared with the control group, azithromycin was significantly associated with a lower risk and a lower number of exacerbations, with an OR = 0.48 (95% CI: 0.34, 0.67, $p < 0.0001$) and an MD = −0.82 (95% CI: −1.32, −0.33, $p = 0.001$), respectively, with non-significant heterogeneity (Figures 5 and 6).

Study or Subgroup	Azithromycin Mean	SD	Total	Control Mean	SD	Total	Weight	Mean Difference IV, Fixed, 95% CI
Klingel 2019	21.3	22.1	31	23.5	13.1	36	0.9%	-2.20 [-11.08, 6.68]
Saiman 2010	-0.5	11.7	125	-1.9	11.5	124	8.3%	1.40 [-1.48, 4.28]
Shmarina 2017	1.7	2.3	59	-0.3	3.3	102	90.9%	2.00 [1.13, 2.87]
Total (95% CI)			**215**			**262**	**100.0%**	**1.91 [1.09, 2.74]**

Heterogeneity: Chi² = 0.98, df = 2 (P = 0.61); I² = 0%
Test for overall effect: Z = 4.53 (P < 0.00001)

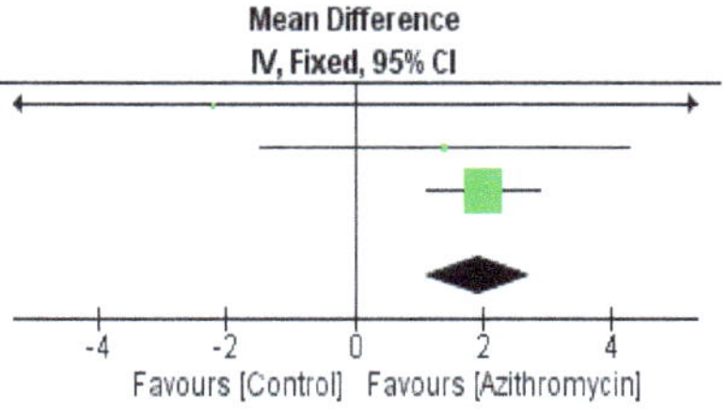

Figure 3. A comparison between the azithromycin and control groups regarding FEV1 change from baseline. The diamond shape is the forest plot, and the squares represent the effect size of each study [13,23,25].

Study or Subgroup	Azithromycin Mean	SD	Total	Control Mean	SD	Total	Weight	Mean Difference IV, Random, 95% CI
Saiman 2010	-2.5	1.1	125	-2.54	0.983	124	36.5%	0.04 [-0.22, 0.30]
Saiman 2012	0.12	0.22	77	0.04	0.31	69	38.6%	0.08 [-0.01, 0.17]
Shmarina 2017	4.8	1.9	59	2.5	3	102	25.0%	2.30 [1.54, 3.06]
Total (95% CI)			**261**			**295**	**100.0%**	**0.62 [-0.01, 1.25]**

Heterogeneity: Tau² = 0.27; Chi² = 32.79, df = 2 (P < 0.00001); I² = 94%
Test for overall effect: Z = 1.92 (P = 0.06)

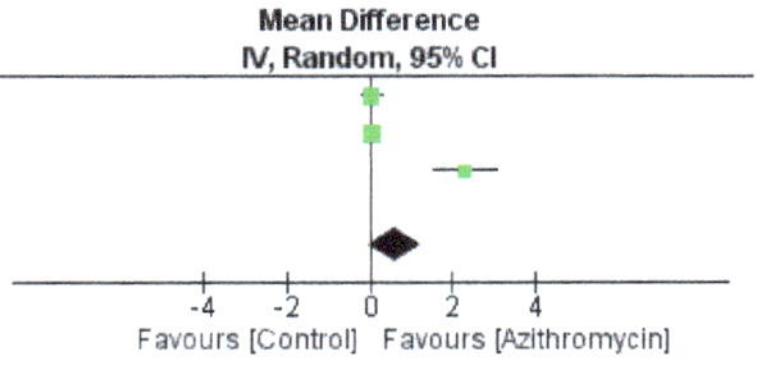

Figure 4. A comparison between the azithromycin and control groups regarding FVC change from baseline. The diamond shape is the forest plot, and the squares represent the effect size of each study [13,23,26].

Study or Subgroup	Azithromycin Events	Total	Control Events	Total	Weight	Odds Ratio M-H, Fixed, 95% CI
Mayer-Hamblett 2018	43	110	58	111	36.3%	0.59 [0.34, 1.00]
Saiman 2010	28	131	50	129	40.9%	0.43 [0.25, 0.74]
Saiman 2012	15	77	26	69	22.8%	0.40 [0.19, 0.84]
Total (95% CI)		**318**		**309**	**100.0%**	**0.48 [0.34, 0.67]**
Total events	86		134			

Heterogeneity: Chi² = 0.93, df = 2 (P = 0.63); I² = 0%
Test for overall effect: Z = 4.24 (P < 0.0001)

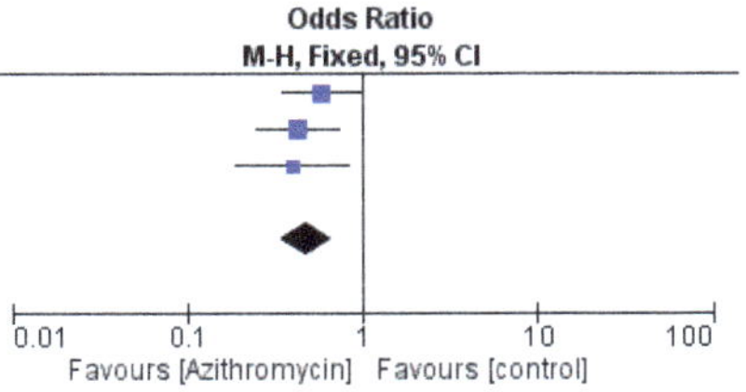

Figure 5. A comparison between the azithromycin and control groups regarding the risk of exacerbations. The diamond shape is the forest plot, and the squares represent the effect size of each study [13,21,26].

Study or Subgroup	Azithromycin Mean	SD	Total	Control Mean	SD	Total	Weight	Mean Difference IV, Fixed, 95% CI
Abdul Aziz 2020	2.7	1.72	30	3.81	1.4	33	40.2%	-1.11 [-1.89, -0.33]
Stick 2022	1.92	1.71	68	2.55	1.98	62	59.8%	-0.63 [-1.27, 0.01]
Total (95% CI)			**98**			**95**	**100.0%**	**-0.82 [-1.32, -0.33]**

Heterogeneity: Chi² = 0.87, df = 1 (P = 0.35); I² = 0%
Test for overall effect: Z = 3.27 (P = 0.001)

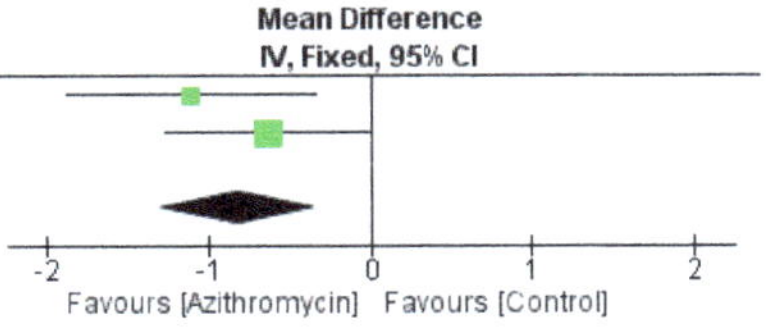

Figure 6. A comparison between the azithromycin and control groups regarding number of exacerbations. The diamond shape is the forest plot, and the squares represent the effect size of each study [22,24].

Regarding the need to use additional antibiotics, azithromycin resulted in a significantly lower need, with an OR = 0.35 (95% CI: 0.13, 0.94, p = 0.04), I^2 = 75%, p = 0.02 (Figure 7). No significant difference was observed between both groups regarding hospitalization rates, with an OR = 0.88 (95% CI: 0.55, 1.4, p = 0.59) (Figure 8).

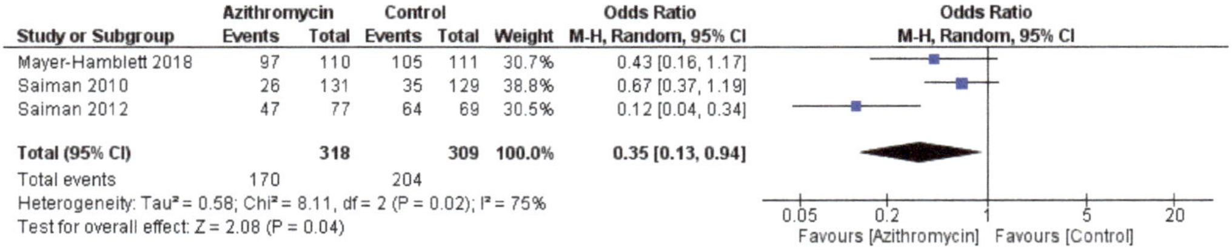

Figure 7. A comparison between the azithromycin and control groups regarding additional antibiotic usage. The diamond shape is the forest plot, and the squares represent the effect size of each study [13,21,26].

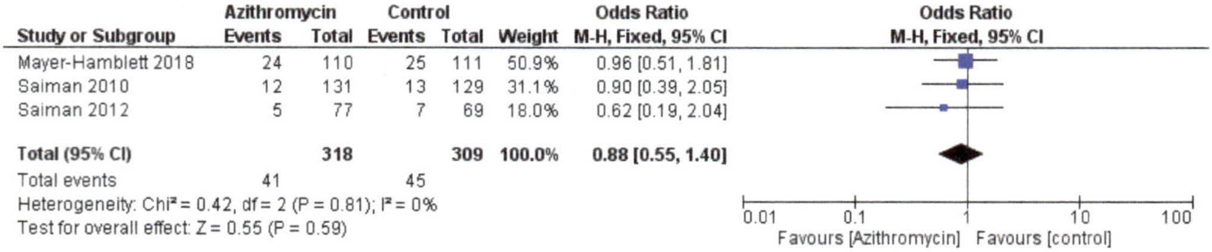

Figure 8. A comparison between the azithromycin and control groups regarding hospitalization rates. The diamond shape is the forest plot, and the squares represent the effect size of each study [13,21,26].

4. Discussion

The current systematic review and meta-analysis aimed to evaluate the efficacy of azithromycin use in pediatric patients with CF. The present analysis showed the efficacy of azithromycin in increasing the FEV1, which indicates improved pulmonary function, in decreasing exacerbations, which is the main complaint of patients with CF, and in decreasing the need to use additional antibiotics, which is an important parameter to avoid associated adverse events, mainly antibiotic resistance.

The mechanism of action of azithromycin in CF remains unclear. Previous research [12,27,28] has indicated that azithromycin does not eliminate CF germs. Previous in vitro investigations indicated that azithromycin reduced the expression of proinflammatory cytokines, while exhibiting inconsistent effects on anti-inflammatory cytokines and modifying bacterial traits, including the pili, flagella, exoproducts, and the quorum-sensing ability of *Pseudomonas aeruginosa* [29,30]. Azithromycin has demonstrated efficacy in diminishing neutrophil recruitment in non-CF animal models [31] infected with *Pseudomonas aeruginosa* and in reducing neutrophilia and interleukin (IL)-8 levels in people with bronchiolitis obliterans syndrome [32]. In CF airway epithelial cells, azithromycin decreased IL-8 transcription and protein production while decreasing the DNA binding of the IL-8 transcriptional regulators nuclear factor-kappa B (NF-κB) and activator protein-1 (AP-1) [33]. In F508 homozygous CF mice, azithromycin has demonstrated efficacy in diminishing baseline inflammation and inflammation produced by *Pseudomonas aeruginosa* lipopolysaccharide [34]. Nonetheless, empirical evidence regarding the anti-inflammatory properties of azithromycin in CF is limited.

The impact of prolonged low-dose azithromycin treatment on the airways can be elucidated by many theories. The predominant mode of action examined is the antibacterial efficacy of the medication in both intracellular and extracellular environments. Azithromycin, a 15-membered ring azalide chemical, is produced from erythromycin. Its distinctive structure facilitates improved intracellular penetration and tissue accumulation [35]. Azithromycin is recognized for its anti-inflammatory and tissue reparative properties. Reported additional effects of macrolides include the inhibition of proinflammatory mediator release, reduced neutrophil infiltration in the lungs, the modulation of mucus secretion, and the modification of the biofilm matrix [36]. This demonstrates that macrolides significantly advantage the azithromycin group by suppressing the proliferation of *Pseudomonas aeruginosa*, altering host defenses, and interacting with several cell types in the airways to diminish inflammation [35]. Saiman and colleagues [12] observed that sputum neutrophil elastase activity escalated in the placebo group after six months, but it remained unchanged in the azithromycin group. In contrast, Equi and colleagues [27] were unable to record any alterations in airway IL-8 and neutrophil elastase levels in the subgroup of patients who underwent sputum testing. This gap can be attributed to the challenges of acquiring valid measures of inflammatory mediators in the sputum of patients with CF. Future studies should implement standardized sputum collection and processing protocols to ensure consistency, use biomarker normalization techniques (e.g., expressing inflammatory mediator levels relative to total protein content or sputum volume) to account for dilution effects, and adopt longitudinal sampling to capture fluctuations in inflammation over time. Additionally, employing advanced analytical techniques, such as high-sensitivity assays or mass spectrometry, can enhance biomarker detection and quantification. Exploring alternative biofluids, like exhaled breath condensate or bronchoalveolar lavage fluid, may also provide complementary insights into airway inflammation. These refinements can help improve the reliability of inflammatory mediator measurements and clarify the effects of azithromycin on CF airway inflammation. Culic et al. [37] discovered that the immunomodulatory effect of azithromycin is contingent upon the duration and stages of inflammation experienced. Research conducted on both human and animal models indicates that azithromycin exerts a beneficial immunomodulatory effect when administered early during bacterial infection; however, its efficacy diminishes significantly when used later in the inflammatory process, resulting in an elevation of inflammatory mediators. This elucidates why pre-treatment is a superior technique for preventing exacerbations [22].

In addition to its well-documented anti-inflammatory and antimicrobial effects in cystic fibrosis, azithromycin has been investigated for its impact on gastrointestinal motility. Patients with CF frequently experience gastrointestinal dysfunction, including delayed gastric emptying and small bowel dysmotility, which can contribute to malabsorption and nutritional challenges [38]. Emerging evidence suggests that azithromycin may modulate gastrointestinal motility, as demonstrated by Shakir and Altaf [39], who reported that azithromycin induces migrating motor complexes in pediatric patients undergoing antroduodenal motility studies. This prokinetic effect could have clinical relevance for patients with CF and gastroparesis or small bowel dysmotility. Altered motility patterns may influence the timing and efficiency of nutrient absorption, potentially impacting the overall nutritional status of patients with CF who are already at risk of malnutrition. Furthermore, changes in gastrointestinal transit time could interfere with the effectiveness of pancreatic enzyme replacement therapy (PERT), which requires appropriate timing relative to food intake for optimal digestion and nutrient absorption. If azithromycin significantly alters small bowel transit, adjustments of PERT dosing or timing may be necessary to maintain adequate digestion and absorption.

Azithromycin use has been reported to have an impact on the gut microbiome. A meta-analysis by McDonnell et al. [40] highlighted the significant impact of macrolide antibiotics on the gut microbiome in children, particularly in reducing alpha-diversity and microbial richness. Significant reductions were seen in Bifidobacteria and Lactobacillus, and significant increases in Proteobacteria such as E. coli were also observed. This reduction can have substantial downstream effects on immune function and metabolic processes. The findings suggest that macrolide-induced gut dysbiosis may contribute to long-term alterations in host immunity, potentially increasing susceptibility to inflammatory conditions, allergies, and metabolic disorders. Therefore, this should be adequately monitored. Azithromycin has a prolonged half-life, allowing it to persist in tissues for an extended period. This pharmacokinetic property contributes to its long-term side effects including its effects on the gut microbiome, even after the discontinuation of treatment. Further research is necessary to determine the optimal strategies for mitigating these effects, such as probiotic co-administration or microbiome monitoring during prolonged azithromycin use [41].

Saiman et al. [13] reported that azithromycin was well tolerated in terms of safety. No rise in serious or nonserious adverse events was seen among subjects administered azithromycin. Nausea, diarrhea, and wheezing, previously noted to occur more frequently in the azithromycin group [12], manifested with comparable frequency in both the azithromycin and placebo groups in the current trial, affecting fewer than 10% of patients in each cohort. Conversely, cough and productive cough were less prevalent in the azithromycin group, aligning with the decrease in pulmonary exacerbations, as delineated in the current meta-analysis.

Prior research in adults has indicated a heightened risk of hearing loss [42,43] and a possible extension of the corrected QT interval (QTc) interval in patients with chronic cardiovascular illnesses [44] associated with azithromycin. While analogous findings have not been observed in the CF population [12,13,27], the extended duration of OPTIMIZE [21] facilitated a more thorough identification of potential cardio- or ototoxicity in this young, susceptible demographic via meticulous audiologic and Electrocardiogram (ECG) surveillance. The randomized, controlled segment of OPTIMIZE demonstrated no instances of temporary or permanent hearing loss or clinically significant QTc prolongation, so further affirming the safety of macrolides in this demographic. The recent literature indicates a detrimental interaction between tobramycin inhalation solution and azithromycin, both in vitro [45] and in vivo [46], as evidenced by retrospective investigations involving persons with CF chronically infected with *Pseudomonas aeruginosa*. The OPTIMIZE [21] experiment assessed a possible interaction when both medications were administered concurrently. Tobramycin inhalation solution was prescribed solely in reaction to a *Pseudomonas aeruginosa*-positive culture during the subsequent 15-month follow-up period following the initial medication. Consequently, a potential interaction may be most effectively assessed at the beginning phase of treatment for the eradication of *Pseudomonas aeruginosa*. At the conclusion of the first quarter of therapy, no significant disparity was observed in eradication rates or clinical outcomes, including lung function, between patients administered tobramycin inhalation solution with azithromycin and those receiving tobramycin inhalation solution with placebo. Consequently, in this context, they were unable to identify any adverse interaction; nonetheless, this study may not have permitted adequate time to explore a possible antagonism. Consequently, further exploration remains necessary [21].

Despite the efficacy provided by azithromycin in the long-term management of CF in pediatrics, the resistance to macrolides remains a problem. A prior meta-analysis [47] showed that the long-term use of azithromycin in chronic lung diseases was significantly associated with increased risk of resistance. Therefore, strategies to manage this risk are still needed due to the lack of data concerning this finding.

In the evolving landscape of CF management, the introduction of disease-modifying drugs (DMDs) has fundamentally altered treatment paradigms. While azithromycin has demonstrated efficacy in reducing exacerbations and improving lung function, its long-term use must be re-evaluated in light of emerging therapies that directly target the underlying CFTR dysfunction. The potential impact of DMDs on airway inflammation, infection burden, and overall disease trajectory raises important questions about the necessity and optimal duration of adjunctive macrolide therapy. Notably, the current body of literature, as included in this meta-analysis, lacks substantial data on the interplay between long-term azithromycin use and DMD therapy. Future research should focus on defining patient subgroups who may continue to benefit from azithromycin in the DMD era, ensuring a more tailored and evidence-based approach to CF management [48].

Although the current systematic review and meta-analysis have several methodological advantages, such as investigating different outcomes regarding the pulmonary function and signs and symptoms of CF, in addition to the inclusion of all available RCTs and cohort studies conducted on children with CF receiving azithromycin, some limitations still exist which warrant further investigation. These include the small number of studies for most of the outcomes and, therefore, the small sample size for these outcomes; the inadequate investigation of adverse events in the published articles; the lack of comparisons made between patients with CF and *Pseudomonas aeruginosa* and those without, which may affect the efficacy of azithromycin; and the absence of investigation of confounding factors that affect treatment results such as the use of other drugs, associated comorbidities, and the duration of treatment. Therefore, we recommend that future large-scale RCTs be conducted to investigate the risk of adverse events, the effect of *Pseudomonas aeruginosa* infection, and the role of confounding factors on the treatment outcomes. We also recommend further trials to investigate the risk of macrolide resistance and how to overcome it.

5. Conclusions

This systematic review and meta-analysis showed the efficacy of azithromycin in pediatric patients with CF; it improved lung function by increasing FEV1, reduced exacerbations of CF, which is the most common symptom of CF that leads to mortality, and reduced the number of additional antibiotics that needed to be administered to patients with CF, which reduces the risk of antibiotic resistance. Therefore, the long-term use of azithromycin is recommended for pediatric patients with CF as part of their treatment regimen; however, future RCTs are still warranted to determine the duration of treatment and the effect of other factors in the process of management.

Supplementary Materials: The following supporting information can be downloaded at: https://www.mdpi.com/article/10.3390/medicina61040653/s1. File S1. Prisma 2020 checklist.

Author Contributions: H.A.-s. and D.A. contributed equally to this work. Both authors participated in the conceptualization and design of the study, conducted the systematic literature search, performed data extraction and statistical analyses, and contributed to drafting and revising the manuscript. All authors have read and agreed to the published version of the manuscript.

Funding: This work was supported and funded by the Deanship of Scientific Research at Imam Mohammad Ibn Saud Islamic University (IMSIU) (grant number IMSIU-DDRSP2501).

Data Availability Statement: The datasets analyzed during the current study are available from the corresponding author upon reasonable request.

Conflicts of Interest: The authors declare no conflicts of interest.

References

1. Cogen, J.D.; Oron, A.P.; Gibson, R.L.; Hoffman, L.R.; Kronman, M.P.; Ong, T.; Rosenfeld, M. Characterization of Inpatient Cystic Fibrosis Pulmonary Exacerbations. *Pediatrics* **2017**, *139*, e20162642. [CrossRef] [PubMed]
2. Aziz, D.A.; Billoo, A.G.; Qureshi, A.; Khalid, M.; Kirmani, S. Clinical and laboratory profile of children with Cystic Fibrosis: Experience of a tertiary care center in Pakistan. *Pak. J. Med. Sci.* **2017**, *33*, 554–559. [CrossRef] [PubMed]
3. Sanders, D.B.; Fink, A.K. Background and Epidemiology. *Pediatr. Clin. N. Am.* **2016**, *63*, 567–584. [CrossRef]
4. Cant, N.; Pollock, N.; Ford, R.C. CFTR structure and cystic fibrosis. *Int. J. Biochem. Cell Biol.* **2014**, *52*, 15–25. [CrossRef]
5. Berkebile, A.R.; McCray, P.B., Jr. Effects of airway surface liquid pH on host defense in cystic fibrosis. *Int. J. Biochem. Cell Biol.* **2014**, *52*, 124–129. [CrossRef]
6. Stoltz, D.A.; Meyerholz, D.K.; Welsh, M.J. Origins of cystic fibrosis lung disease. *N. Engl. J. Med.* **2015**, *372*, 351–362. [CrossRef] [PubMed]
7. Cantin, A.M.; Hartl, D.; Konstan, M.W.; Chmiel, J.F. Inflammation in cystic fibrosis lung disease: Pathogenesis and therapy. *J. Cyst. Fibros.* **2015**, *14*, 419–430. [CrossRef]
8. Nichols, D.P.; Chmiel, J.F. Inflammation and its genesis in cystic fibrosis. *Pediatr. Pulmonol.* **2015**, *50* (Suppl. 40), S39–S56. [CrossRef]
9. Goss, C.H.; Burns, J.L. Exacerbations in cystic fibrosis. 1: Epidemiology and pathogenesis. *Thorax* **2007**, *62*, 360–367. [CrossRef]
10. Boucher, R.C. New concepts of the pathogenesis of cystic fibrosis lung disease. *Eur. Respir. J.* **2004**, *23*, 146–158. [CrossRef]
11. Bonfield, T.L.; Panuska, J.R.; Konstan, M.W.; Hilliard, K.A.; Hilliard, J.B.; Ghnaim, H.; Berger, M. Inflammatory cytokines in cystic fibrosis lungs. *Am. J. Respir. Crit. Care Med.* **1995**, *152 Pt 1*, 2111–2118. [CrossRef] [PubMed]
12. Saiman, L.; Marshall, B.C.; Mayer-Hamblett, N.; Burns, J.L.; Quittner, A.L.; Cibene, D.A.; Macrolide Study Group. Azithromycin in patients with cystic fibrosis chronically infected with Pseudomonas aeruginosa: A randomized controlled trial. *JAMA* **2003**, *290*, 1749–1756. [CrossRef] [PubMed]
13. Saiman, L.; Anstead, M.; Mayer-Hamblett, N.; Lands, L.C.; Kloster, M.; Hocevar-Trnka, J.; AZ0004 Azithromycin Study Group. Effect of azithromycin on pulmonary function in patients with cystic fibrosis uninfected with Pseudomonas aeruginosa: A randomized controlled trial. *JAMA* **2010**, *303*, 1707–1715. [CrossRef] [PubMed]
14. Ratjen, F.; Saiman, L.; Mayer-Hamblett, N.; Lands, L.C.; Kloster, M.; Thompson, V.; Anstead, M. Effect of azithromycin on systemic markers of inflammation in patients with cystic fibrosis uninfected with Pseudomonas aeruginosa. *Chest* **2012**, *142*, 1259–1266. [CrossRef]
15. Ichimiya, T.; Takeoka, K.; Hiramatsu, K.; Hirai, K.; Yamasaki, T.; Nasu, M. The influence of azithromycin on the biofilm formation of Pseudomonas aeruginosa in vitro. *Chemotherapy* **1996**, *42*, 186–191. [CrossRef]
16. Moher, D.; Liberati, A.; Tetzlaff, J.; Altman, D.G. Preferred reporting items for systematic reviews and meta-analyses: The PRISMA statement. *BMJ* **2009**, *339*, b2535. [CrossRef]
17. Rayyan. Available online: https://rayyan.ai/ (accessed on 1 September 2024).
18. Goebell, P.J.; Kamat, A.M.; Sylvester, R.J.; Black, P.; Droller, M.; Godoy, G.; Hudson, M.A.; Junker, K.; Kassouf, W.; Knowles, M.A.; et al. Assessing the quality of studies on the diagnostic accuracy of tumor markers. *Urol Oncol.* **2014**, *32*, 1051–1060. [CrossRef] [PubMed] [PubMed Central]
19. Flemyng, E.; Moore, T.H.; Boutron, I.; Higgins, J.P.; Hróbjartsson, A.; Nejstgaard, C.H.; Dwan, K. Using Risk of Bias 2 to assess results from randomised controlled trials: Guidance from Cochrane. *BMJ Evid. Based Med.* **2023**, *28*, 260–266. [CrossRef]
20. RevMan: Systematic Review and Meta-Analysis Tool for Researchers Worldwide | Cochrane RevMan. Available online: https://revman.cochrane.org/info (accessed on 1 September 2024).
21. Mayer-Hamblett, N.; Retsch-Bogart, G.; Kloster, M.; Accurso, F.; Rosenfeld, M.; Albers, G.; Ramsey, B.W. Azithromycin for Early Pseudomonas Infection in Cystic Fibrosis. The OPTIMIZE Randomized Trial. *Am. J. Respir. Crit. Care Med.* **2018**, *198*, 1177–1187. [CrossRef]
22. Aziz, D.A.; Shahid, S.; Iftikhar, H.; Mir, F. Role of Long-Term Intermittent Use of Oral Azithromycin On Pulmonary Exacerbations In Cystic Fibrosis Children. *J. Ayub Med. Coll. Abbottabad* **2020**, *32*, 429–434.
23. Shmarina, G.; Pukhalsky, A.; Avakian, L.; Semykin, S.; Pukhalskaya, D.; Alioshkin, V. Steady-State Therapy with Azithromycin or Low-Dose Prednisolone in Paediatric Cystic Fibrosis Patients: Inflammatory Markers and Disease Progression. *Int. Arch. Allergy Immunol.* **2017**, *172*, 45–54. [CrossRef] [PubMed]
24. Stick, S.M.; Foti, A.; Ware, R.S.; Tiddens, H.A.; Clements, B.S.; Armstrong, D.S.; Sly, P.D. The effect of azithromycin on structural lung disease in infants with cystic fibrosis (COMBAT CF): A phase 3, randomised, double-blind, placebo-controlled clinical trial. *Lancet Respir. Med.* **2022**, *10*, 776–784. [CrossRef] [PubMed]
25. Klingel, M.; Stanojevic, S.; Tullis, E.; Ratjen, F.; Waters, V. Oral Azithromycin and Response to Pulmonary Exacerbations Treated with Intravenous Tobramycin in Children with Cystic Fibrosis. *Ann. Am. Thorac. Soc.* **2019**, *16*, 861–867. [CrossRef]

26. Saiman, L.; Mayer-Hamblett, N.; Anstead, M.; Lands, L.C.; Kloster, M.; Goss, C.H.; AZ0004 Macrolide Study Team. Open-label, follow-on study of azithromycin in pediatric patients with CF uninfected with Pseudomonas aeruginosa. *Pediatr. Pulmonol.* **2012**, *47*, 641–648. [CrossRef]
27. Equi, A.; Balfour-Lynn, I.M.; Bush, A.; Rosenthal, M. Long term azithromycin in children with cystic fibrosis: A randomised, placebo-controlled crossover trial. *Lancet* **2002**, *360*, 978–984. [CrossRef]
28. Clement, A.; Tamalet, A.; Leroux, E.; Ravilly, S.; Fauroux, B.; Jais, J.P. Long term effects of azithromycin in patients with cystic fibrosis: A double blind, placebo controlled trial. *Thorax* **2006**, *61*, 895–902. [CrossRef]
29. Saiman, L. The use of macrolide antibiotics in patients with cystic fibrosis. *Curr. Opin. Pulm. Med.* **2004**, *10*, 515–523. [CrossRef]
30. Tateda, K.; Ishii, Y.; Kimura, S.; Horikawa, M.; Miyairi, S.; Yamaguchi, K. Suppression of Pseudomonas aeruginosa quorum-sensing systems by macrolides: A promising strategy or an oriental mystery? *J. Infect. Chemother.* **2007**, *13*, 357–367. [CrossRef] [PubMed]
31. Tsai, W.C.; Rodriguez, M.L.; Young, K.S.; Deng, J.C.; Thannickal, V.J.; Tateda, K.; Standiford, T.J. Azithromycin blocks neutrophil recruitment in Pseudomonas endobronchial infection. *Am. J. Respir. Crit. Care Med.* **2004**, *170*, 1331–1339. [CrossRef]
32. Verleden, G.M.; Vanaudenaerde, B.M.; Dupont, L.J.; Van Raemdonck, D.E. Azithromycin reduces airway neutrophilia and interleukin-8 in patients with bronchiolitis obliterans syndrome. *Am. J. Respir. Crit. Care Med.* **2006**, *174*, 566–570. [CrossRef]
33. Cigana, C.; Nicolis, E.; Pasetto, M.; Assael, B.M.; Melotti, P. Anti-inflammatory effects of azithromycin in cystic fibrosis airway epithelial cells. *Biochem. Biophys. Res. Commun.* **2006**, *350*, 977–982. [CrossRef]
34. Legssyer, R.; Huaux, F.; Lebacq, J.; Delos, M.; Marbaix, E.; Lebecque, P.; Leal, T. Azithromycin reduces spontaneous and induced inflammation in DeltaF508 cystic fibrosis mice. *Respir. Res.* **2006**, *7*, 134. [CrossRef]
35. Parnham, M.J.; Haber, V.E.; Giamarellos-Bourboulis, E.J.; Perletti, G.; Verleden, G.M.; Vos, R. Azithromycin: Mechanisms of action and their relevance for clinical applications. *Pharmacol. Ther.* **2014**, *143*, 225–245. [CrossRef] [PubMed]
36. Venditto, V.J.; Haydar, D.; Abdel-Latif, A.; Gensel, J.C.; Anstead, M.I.; Pitts, M.G.; Feola, D.J. Immunomodulatory Effects of Azithromycin Revisited: Potential Applications to COVID-19. *Front. Immunol.* **2021**, *12*, 574425. [CrossRef]
37. Čulić, O.; Eraković, V.; Čepelak, I.; Barišić, K.; Brajša, K.; Ferenčić, Ž.; Parnham, M.J. Azithromycin modulates neutrophil function and circulating inflammatory mediators in healthy human subjects. *Eur. J. Pharmacol.* **2002**, *450*, 277–289. [CrossRef]
38. Davis, T.A.; Miller, A.; Hachem, C.; Velez, C.; Patel, D. The current state of gastrointestinal motility evaluation in cystic fibrosis: A comprehensive literature review. *Transl. Gastroenterol. Hepatol.* **2024**, *9*, 10. [CrossRef] [PubMed]
39. Shakir, A.K.; Altaf, M.A. Azithromycin Induces Migrating Motor Complexes in Pediatric Patients Undergoing Antroduodenal Motility Studies. *J. Pediatr. Pharmacol. Ther.* **2018**, *23*, 390–394. [CrossRef]
40. McDonnell, L.; Gilkes, A.; Ashworth, M.; Rowland, V.; Harries, T.H.; Armstrong, D.; White, P. Association between antibiotics and gut microbiome dysbiosis in children: Systematic review and meta-analysis. *Gut Microbes* **2021**, *13*, 1–18. [CrossRef]
41. Heidary, M.; Ebrahimi Samangani, A.; Kargari, A.; Kiani Nejad, A.; Yashmi, I.; Motahar, M.; Khoshnood, S. Mechanism of action, resistance, synergism, and clinical implications of azithromycin. *J. Clin. Lab. Anal.* **2022**, *36*, e24427. [CrossRef]
42. Albert, R.K.; Connett, J.; Bailey, W.C.; Casaburi, R.; Cooper, J.A.D., Jr.; Criner, G.J.; Anthonisen, N.R. Azithromycin for prevention of exacerbations of COPD. *N. Engl. J. Med.* **2011**, *365*, 689–698. [CrossRef]
43. Grayston, J.T.; Kronmal, R.A.; Jackson, L.A.; Parisi, A.F.; Muhlestein, J.B.; Cohen, J.D.; Knirsch, C. Azithromycin for the secondary prevention of coronary events. *N. Engl. J. Med.* **2005**, *352*, 1637–1645. [CrossRef] [PubMed]
44. Ray, W.A.; Murray, K.T.; Hall, K.; Arbogast, P.G.; Stein, C.M. Azithromycin and the risk of cardiovascular death. *N. Engl. J. Med.* **2012**, *366*, 1881–1890. [CrossRef] [PubMed]
45. Nichols, D.P.; Happoldt, C.L.; Bratcher, P.E.; Caceres, S.M.; Chmiel, J.F.; Malcolm, K.C.; Nick, J.A. Impact of azithromycin on the clinical and antimicrobial effectiveness of tobramycin in the treatment of cystic fibrosis. *J. Cyst. Fibros.* **2017**, *16*, 358–366. [CrossRef]
46. Nick, J.A.; Moskowitz, S.M.; Chmiel, J.F.; Forssén, A.V.; Kim, S.H.; Saavedra, M.T.; Nichols, D.P. Azithromycin may antagonize inhaled tobramycin when targeting Pseudomonas aeruginosa in cystic fibrosis. *Ann. Am. Thorac. Soc.* **2014**, *11*, 342–350. [CrossRef] [PubMed]
47. Li, H.; Liu, D.H.; Chen, L.L.; Zhao, Q.; Yu, Y.Z.; Ding, J.J.; Xie, C.M. Meta-analysis of the adverse effects of long-term azithromycin use in patients with chronic lung diseases. *Antimicrob. Agents Chemother.* **2014**, *58*, 511–517. [CrossRef]
48. Harman, K.; Dobra, R.; Davies, J.C. Disease-modifying drug therapy in cystic fibrosis. *Paediatr. Respir. Rev.* **2018**, *26*, 7–9. [CrossRef]

medicina

MDPI

Review

The Adverse Effects of Tuberculosis Treatment: A Comprehensive Literature Review

Rūta Mereškevičienė * and Edvardas Danila

Institute of Clinical Medicine, Clinic of Chest Diseases, Immunology and Allergology, Faculty of Medicine, Vilnius University, LT-03101 Vilnius, Lithuania; edvardas.danila@santa.lt
* Correspondence: ruta.mereskeviciene@santa.lt

Abstract: Tuberculosis remains a significant public health challenge globally. The emergence of multidrug-resistant Mycobacterium tuberculosis strains presents one of the biggest hurdles in tuberculosis management. Both first- and second-line tuberculosis drugs are associated with common adverse reactions, which can lead to treatment interruptions and decreased adherence. In this article, we review the most commonly used drugs for the treatment of tuberculosis, focusing on the adverse reactions they may cause. We will examine the frequency and timeline of adverse drug reactions involving gastrointestinal, cardiac, neurological, nephrological, and cutaneous systems. Identifying patients at risk of developing those reactions is crucial for healthcare providers to implement monitoring strategies and manage complications effectively. In the review, we present the data about risk factors, management recommendations, and drug discontinuation rates as a result of side effects.

Keywords: tuberculosis; adverse drug reactions; first-line drugs; second-line drugs; drug-susceptible tuberculosis; drug-resistant tuberculosis

1. Introduction

Tuberculosis remains a significant public health challenge on a global scale. In 2023, it was estimated that approximately 10.8 million individuals fell ill with tuberculosis, a disease that affects populations in all countries worldwide. Of the 10.8 million cases, 6 million were men, 3.6 million were women, and 1.3 million were children [1]. Tuberculosis has been reaffirmed as the leading cause of death attributed to a single infectious agent, with a staggering 1.25 million fatalities reported in 2023. Among these, 161,000 deaths occurred in individuals co-infected with HIV [1].

The main causative agent of tuberculosis is Mycobacterium tuberculosis. It is a rod-shaped obligate aerobe that can be inhaled into the lungs, where it inhabits and slowly multiplies within macrophages. Despite being an ancient disease, tuberculosis still poses difficulties for healthcare professionals who are treating it. First-line antituberculosis drugs that are used widely for drug-susceptible tuberculosis treatment are rifampicin, isoniazid, ethambutol, and pyrazinamide. Meanwhile, the second-line drugs are prescribed for drug-resistant tuberculosis treatment. They must be carefully selected from a seemingly long list of drugs and regimens. However, patients with multidrug- or extensively drug-resistant tuberculosis prove that this list is still too short.

Drug-resistant Mycobacterium tuberculosis strains complicate treatment protocols, requiring more extensive use of second-line antituberculosis drugs that often involve complex, multi-drug regimens. While necessary for effective treatment, these regimens are linked to a higher incidence of adverse drug reactions [2]. Such reactions can lead to treatment interruption and poorer adherence [3].

Effective management of the side effects associated with antituberculosis therapy requires an understanding of the pharmacodynamics and pharmacokinetics involved, including the mechanisms of drug action and side effects. Clinicians must be able to identify both the common and rare adverse reactions, along with the risk factors that may predispose certain individuals to a heightened risk of these side effects [4].

There have been excellent reviews [2,5,6] published on the topic of adverse drug reactions. Most of them were published some time ago, and new data emerged regarding some of the drugs. There are also new antituberculosis drugs, like bedaquiline, delamanid, and pretomanid, that were unavailable before some of the previously published reviews. We aim to focus on the prevalence of adverse effects in different studies and the risk factors for their development. We also include management and prevention recommendations.

2. Adverse Drug Reactions of First-Line Antituberculosis Drugs

Isoniazid, also named isonicotinic acid hydrazide, was synthesized in Prague in 1912 and has been used as an antitubercular drug since 1952. It remains one of the essential components for drug-susceptible and latent tuberculosis treatment to this day. It has recently started to be used in some regimens for drug-resistant tuberculosis [7–10]. Isoniazid is a nicotinic acid derivative. It passively diffuses into the bacterial cytoplasm and is activated by the enzyme KatG. During activation, isoniazid forms free radical species that disrupt many cellular processes. The isonicotinyl radical binds with the InhA enzyme and NADH. Since the InhA enzyme participates in mycobacteria's mycolic acid synthesis, this process is blocked, and the cell wall cannot form normally. Radical species also affect nucleic acid, protein, carbohydrate, and lipid synthesis [11,12]. Isoniazid is most effective against actively dividing bacteria [12].

Isoniazid is metabolized in the liver and forms toxic metabolites (e.g., acetyl hydrazine), which are most likely the cause of liver damage [12,13]. Pyridoxine (vitamin B6) metabolism can be disrupted when taking isoniazid, causing reversible neuropathy. While hepatotoxicity is most common within the first few weeks, peripheral neuropathy occurs gradually after several weeks or months [14–18]. The severity of those adverse drug reactions can vary, the most common being elevated liver enzymes and gastrointestinal disturbances [5,15], and the relatively common and more severe—peripheral neuropathy [15]. Severe but less common reactions are symptomatic hepatotoxicity and skin reactions like Stevens–Johnson syndrome and drug-induced lupus [5]. Psychosis, optic neuritis, and pancreatitis are rare, severe adverse reactions [5,19,20]. Through several CYP enzymes, isoniazid can potentially increase concentrations of phenytoin, carbamazepine, warfarin, theophylline, and benzodiazepines [5]. The risk factors for adverse drug reactions due to isoniazid include older age, daily alcohol consumption, and pre-existing liver disease, particularly hepatitis C [21]. However, findings on the relationship between age and hepatitis vary; some studies indicate that neither age nor hepatitis is linked to an increased risk of liver damage [22,23]. It is commonly agreed that the genetic slow acetylator phenotype is a significant risk factor for isoniazid-induced adverse drug reactions to develop [7,15,23,24]. There is a more significant risk for drug-induced peripheral neuropathy in the presence of diabetes, HIV infection, uremia, malnutrition, and alcoholism [14].

Since hepatotoxicity is one of the most common adverse drug reactions, liver enzyme monitoring every 2–4 weeks during the intensive phase should be conducted for those with higher risk and/or baseline abnormalities. To prevent peripheral neuropathy, pyridoxine 50–100 mg daily supplementation needs to be administered. In the case of skin reactions, the first choice of treatment could be ointments with antihistamines and corticosteroids; in severe cases, desensitization may be attempted [4,5,14,24]. When isoniazid-induced mania manifests, the drug should be discontinued; in the more serious cases, psychiatric medications are needed [20].

Imam et al. conducted an observational study involving patients with active tuberculosis who were being treated with first-line antituberculosis drugs. The study revealed a 0.99% discontinuation prevalence of isoniazid as a result of hepatotoxicity, 0.89%—fever; 0.79%—peripheral neuropathy; 0.69%—skin reactions; 0.49%—hypersensitivity; and 0.18%—psychiatric changes [18].

In the studies where isoniazid for latent tuberculosis treatment was used, the prevalence of total adverse drug reactions to isoniazid ranged from 9.2% to 12.8% [25–30]. Two studies with the widest participant samples were conducted in the USA and Italy, although many patients were migrants and refugees from South America, Africa, and Asia. Liver enzyme elevation was seen in the USA study for 1.0% and in the Italy study for 5.5% of cases, with hepatotoxicity and severe hepatitis in 1.8% and 0.4%, respectively [29,30].

When used to treat latent tuberculosis, isoniazid caused gastrointestinal disturbances in 1.2–2.8%, skin reactions in 0.4–2.1%, neurological disorders in 1.4–2.5%, peripheral neuropathy in 0.1–0.8%, and psychiatric disorders in 0.7% of cases [15,25–30].

Rifampicin (rifampin) was synthesized in 1965 and started to be used in 1968. It belongs to the antibiotic class rifamycin [31]. This antibiotic enters the cytoplasm of bacteria and binds with RNA polymerase, inhibiting RNA synthesis [32]. Rifampicin has high sterilizing activity in bacteria recovering from dormancy and in the case of a spurt of metabolism (actively dividing and semi-dormant bacteria) [33]. Despite the drug's short half-life, the antibiotic effect remains active through its metabolites [34].

Liver injury caused by rifampicin is uncommon but can occur due to hypersensitivity reactions. In combination with isoniazid, hepatotoxicity is more frequent, since rifampicin activates the CYP3A4 enzyme and thus accelerates the metabolism of isoniazid, resulting in higher rates of hydrazine [13].

The most common reactions are rash, gastrointestinal disturbances, and elevated liver enzymes [5,15]. Less common but more severe adverse drug reactions—hepatotoxicity; thrombocytopenia; acute renal failure; flu-like syndrome; rare hemolytic anemia; and pseudomembranous colitis [2,5]. Gastrointestinal disturbances manifest mainly during the first month of the treatment [13].

Since rifampicin strongly induces cytochrome P450 enzymes and UDP-glucuronosyltransferases and drug transporters, it can lead to decreased plasma concentrations of other drugs [5,34,35]. Caution is needed with antiretrovirals, anticoagulants, anticonvulsants, some antifungals, immunosuppressants, digoxin, beta-blockers, calcium channel blockers, oral hypoglycemics, theophylline, methadone, and others [2,5,36].

Risk factors for rifampicin-induced adverse reactions are not very clear since the drug is seldom used alone [21]. Yee et al. found that age over 60 years and HIV infection were associated with higher rates of adverse drug reactions [37]. Mild gastrointestinal disturbances can be managed symptomatically, but monitoring of liver enzymes is needed to detect hepatotoxicity in time [5]. In the case of thrombocytopenia, the drug should be discontinued; corticosteroids and platelet transfusions, in some cases, are needed [38]. Mild hypersensitivity reactions might need antihistamines or corticosteroids; in severe cases, desensitization may be attempted [39]. The frequency of treatment discontinuation due to adverse drug reactions varies among studies, in 0.6–1.19% [15,18].

In a study of latent tuberculosis treatment, rifampicin showed a lower prevalence of adverse drug reactions as compared to isoniazid. Elevated liver enzymes were seen in 0.8%, hepatotoxicity in 0.08%, gastrointestinal disturbances in 2.4%, and rash and skin reactions in 1.6% of cases. A rare but significant adverse drug reaction was thrombocytopenia, which was seen in 0.2% of cases [29]. Another latent tuberculosis treatment study showed a much higher prevalence of adverse drug reactions: gastrointestinal disturbances in 22.7%, skin reactions in 5.1%, and neurological symptoms in 9.6% of cases [26].

When used in combination, data on adverse risk factors attributed to rifampicin vary. Castro et al. report only rash and gastrointestinal disturbances due to rifampicin, both as frequent as 1.6% [40]. Another study found that rifampicin was a culprit of hepatotoxicity in 0.2%, cutaneous reactions in 0.1%, flu-like syndrome in 0.26%, hemolytic reaction in 0.1%, and change in glucose tolerance in 0.1% of cases [15]. Yee et al. found that rifampicin was the cause of a rash in 2% and gastrointestinal disturbances in 1% of cases [37].

Pyrazinamide, as a chemical compound, has been known since 1931. Still, its role in tuberculosis treatment was only recognized in 1952 when other nicotinamide derivatives were recognized as effective drugs against *M. tuberculosis* [41]. Pyrazinamide is a prodrug that is converted into pyrazinoic acid by the intracellular enzyme of *M. tuberculosis*, which damages cellular walls by inhibiting fatty acid synthesis [41–45]. Its activity against dormant, nongrowing mycobacteria in tuberculosis treatment is irreplaceable, though perplexing—the mechanism of action is still poorly understood [41].

It is widely accepted that pyrazinamide is hepatotoxic. At the same time, the mechanisms of its toxicity are not precisely known, and there is a lack of studies that could collect prevalence data on pyrazinamide toxicity since it is mainly used together with other drugs. However, data shows that pyrazinamide hepatotoxicity is a direct toxic effect through its metabolites, not related to hypersensitivity or immune response [46,47]. Results on dose dependency differ throughout studies [46,48]. Pyrazinamide can inhibit urine acid transporters in the kidneys, resulting in the reuptake of uric acid back into the bloodstream. This causes hyperuricemia, joint pain, and kidney stones if oxalates are formed [49,50].

Hepatotoxicity can occur at any time during treatment, but it is most common during the first 2–9 weeks, as is hyperuricemia [15,24,50]. Adverse reactions due to pyrazinamide can vary from mild to severe. More common are hyperuricemia, arthralgia, elevated liver enzymes, exanthema, and gastrointestinal disorders; less common but more severe are hepatotoxicity, gout, and rhabdomyolysis [5,24,50]. Rarely, toxic epidermal necrolysis can develop [51].

Not much is known about drug interactions—pyrazinamide can reduce the effectiveness of allopurinol by increasing uric acid levels [52]. It antagonizes the effects of probenecid and decreases the serum concentration of cyclosporine [5].

Older age and diabetes mellitus were found as risk factors for pyrazinamide-induced hepatotoxicity in one study [48], but in others, it was not confirmed [15]. As the half-life of pyrazinamide is significantly prolonged in patients with pre-existing liver or kidney disease [46], one could account for those as risk factors for adverse drug reactions to develop. Risk factors for uricemia include gout or elevated uric acid levels before antituberculosis treatment [53].

In the case of hyperuricemia and related symptoms, allopurinol should be administered [5,52]. Arthralgia can be managed with analgesics [21,24]. If significant liver injury is present, pyrazinamide should be discontinued [5,21,24].

Pyrazinamide discontinuation rates vary. Some studies report rates of 2–5% [37]. However, in elderly patients, early discontinuation of pyrazinamide is frequent, 20.6% [48]. In a study from Turkey, pyrazinamide had to be stopped due to severe hepatotoxicity in 7 cases (0.6%) [15].

Borisov et al. reported adverse drug reactions due to pyrazinamide in 13.2% of cases, most of which were mild (11.3%) [54]. In a South Korean study, the prevalence of hepatotoxicity was 5.13%, and 10 out of 12 drug-induced hepatotoxicity cases were pyrazinamide-related [55]. In the study of Shin et al., which had a significant sample of participants with a wide range of concomitant diseases, 87% of participants treated with pyrazinamide had hyperuricemia [56]. Smaller sample studies showed a prevalence of 58–60% [50,53], and one study from India showed 28.57% [57].

Ethambutol was mentioned for the first time in 1961 by the Lederle Company (New York, NY, USA) when they announced the discovery of a new synthetic compound that protects mice from the lethal *M. tuberculosis* strain [36]. Ethambutol targets Emb proteins, competing for binding to the EmbB and EmbC subunits. These enzymes are important in cell wall biosynthesis [58].

Optic neuropathy is the primary concern when prescribing ethambutol. The precise mechanism is unclear, possibly involving mitochondrial toxicity and disruption of axonal transport in the optic nerve. Optic neuropathy develops after several weeks or months and is rarely seen earlier in treatment [59]. Other less common adverse drug reactions include peripheral neuropathy, rash, and gastrointestinal disturbances. It is known that aluminum-containing antacids may decrease ethambutol absorption [60]. Ethionamide can exacerbate the toxic effects of ethambutol [5].

Risk factors for developing optic neuropathy are high doses of ethambutol, long treatment duration, renal impairment (causing higher levels of ethambutol in the blood), older age, and pre-existing optic nerve disease [5,36,59]. Although optic neuropathy due to ethambutol is reversible in most cases, the drug should be immediately discontinued if signs of this adverse drug reaction occur [21,24]. Visual acuity and fields should be monitored, and ophthalmologist consultation is needed [4,59]. Discontinuation rates due to ethambutol-related adverse reactions are variable, 0.2–1% when 15 mg/kg doses are prescribed [5,21] and 15–18% at a 35 mg/kg dosage [5,36].

The most common drug combination for drug-susceptible tuberculosis treatment includes two months of rifampicin, isoniazid, pyrazinamide, and ethambutol for the intensive phase, followed by four months of rifampicin and isoniazid alone [9]. The prevalence of adverse drug reactions with combined drug regimens varies significantly between studies, ranging between 8 and 83 percent of patients who were treated with first-line antituberculosis drugs using the Directly Observed Treatment and Short-course chemotherapy strategy [2,61–63]. There is an even more significant difference if you take studies that did not use those strategies into account [64]. The absolute majority of adverse drug reactions were reported in the intensive treatment phase [65–67]. Most of them, during the first month of treatment [68], and some even in the first week [67].

A recent retrospective study used data from a spontaneous adverse event reporting system in Korea; there were almost 18 thousand cases with a prevalence of adverse drug reactions to first-line antituberculosis drugs of 1.14%. All four drugs were similarly common causes of those reactions, with 28.7% for rifampicin, 24.0% for isoniazid, 23.4% for ethambutol, and 23.9% for pyrazinamide. Approximately 80.37% of adverse drug reactions were possible, 17.54% probable, and 2.09% certain. Nausea and liver enzyme elevation were most common, with a prevalence of 14.6% and 14.2%, respectively. Rash (11.7%), pruritus (9.1%), and vomiting (8.9%) were also among the most commonly reported reactions [68].

However, a prospective cohort study in Brazil showed a 78.8% prevalence of adverse drug reactions to first-line antituberculosis drugs [65]. In another prospective observational study from India, a prevalence of 34.72% of adverse drug reactions was found; 10.09% of them were definite, 5.83% probable, 12.17% possible, and 6.63% doubtful [18].

Significant variation in adverse drug reaction prevalence shows the importance of study design, sample size, terminology, and characteristics of participants.

Moxifloxacin- and rifapentine-based treatment combinations are now available for drug-susceptible tuberculosis treatment [9]. In a multicenter randomized controlled trial, the significant difference between the rifapentine–moxifloxacin group and the control group according to grade 3 and higher adverse drug reaction prevalence was not found; it was 18.8% and 19.3%, respectively [69].

Mechanisms of drug action and adverse drug reactions, drug interactions, and risk factors for adverse drug reactions to develop are summarized in Table 1.

Table 1. Mechanism of drug action and adverse drug reaction, drug interactions, and risk factors for adverse drug reactions (additional information adopted from [4–6,70]).

Drug	Mechanism of Action	Mechanism of Adverse Drug Reaction	Drug Interactions	Risk Factors for Adverse Drug Reactions
		First-line antituberculosis drugs		
Isoniazid	Diffuses into the bacterial cytoplasm and disrupts mycobacteria's mycolic acid synthesis	Toxic metabolites cause liver damage. Disrupts the metabolism of pyridoxine.	Foods, antacids/aluminum hydroxide, corticosteroids (decreased absorption and/or serum levels of isoniazid) Valproic acid, oral anticoagulants, benzodiazepines, carbamazepine, diazepam, levodopa, phenytoin, and theophylline (increased serum levels of those drugs or their effectiveness) Enflurane (possibility of nephrotoxicity) Ketoconazole (decreased serum concentration of ketoconazole) Cycloserine (greater neurotoxicity) Disulfiram (possibility of psychotic events) Paracetamol, rifampin (greater hepatotoxicity)	Older age, daily alcohol consumption, pre-existing liver disease, hepatitis C *. Genetic slow acetylator phenotype. For peripheral neuropathy—diabetes, HIV infection, uremia, malnutrition, and alcoholism.
Rifampicin	Penetrates the cytoplasm and inhibits RNA synthesis	Liver injury due to hypersensitivity reactions. Hepatic porphyria due to protoporphyrin IX toxicity if used in combination with isoniazid.	Foods and para-aminosalicylic acid (decreased absorption of rifampin) Amiodarone, oral anticoagulants, contraceptives, anticonvulsants, tricyclic antidepressants, antipsychotics, barbiturates and benzodiazepines, beta-blockers, cyclosporine, ketoconazole, codeine, corticosteroids, dapsone, digitalis, diltiazem, enalapril, statins, fluconazole, haloperidol, oral hypoglycemic agents, itraconazole, methadone, morphine, narcotics and analgesics, propafenone, nifedipine, quinidine, theophylline, verapamil, efavirenz, indinavir, lopinavir/ritonavir, nelfinavir, saquinavir, zidovudine (decreased serum levels of those drugs or reduced their effectivity) Isoniazid + ketoconazole, ethionamide, phenytoin, isoniazid, sulfonamides (greater hepatotoxicity) Pyrazinamide (greater uric acid excretion)	Age over 60 years and HIV infection
Pyrazinamide	It damages the cellular wall by inhibiting fatty acid synthesis.	Toxic effect on the liver through metabolites. Inhibition of urine acid transporters in the kidneys.	Allopurinol, colchicine (decreased effect of these drugs; pyrazinamide increases the serum levels of uric acid) Cyclosporine (decreased serum concentration of cyclosporine) Ethionamide (the adverse effects of ethionamide can increase) Rifampin, isoniazid, ketoconazole (greater hepatotoxicity)	Older age, diabetes mellitus * Pre-existing liver or kidney disease, elevated uric acid levels.

Table 1. *Cont.*

Drug	Mechanism of Action	Mechanism of Adverse Drug Reaction	Drug Interactions	Risk Factors for Adverse Drug Reactions
Ethambutol	Competes for binding sites to the EmbB and EmbC subunits, disrupting cell wall biosynthesis.	Optic neuropathy mechanisms may involve mitochondrial toxicity and disruption of axonal transport in the optic nerve.	Antacids (decreased absorption of ethambutol) Ethionamide (increased possibility of neurotoxic effects of ethambutol) Pyrazinamide (increased possibility of hepatotoxicity) Didanosine and zalcitabine (peripheral neuritis is potentiated)	High doses of ethambutol, long treatment duration, renal impairment, older age, and pre-existing optic nerve disease.
			Second-line antituberculosis drugs	
Fluoroquinolones	Inhibits DNA gyrase, leaving its ends free. It results in uncontrollable synthesis of mRNAs, exonuclease, and some proteins. Chromosomes degrade.	Block cardiac potassium channels. May involve the production of reactive oxygen species and matrix metalloproteinase activation.	Antacids with cations Ca, Mg, Al, and Fe; sucralfate (decreased absorption of fluoroquinolones) Drugs metabolized by cytochrome P450: cyclosporine, theophylline, warfarin, phenytoin, and sulfonylurea (increased effect of these drugs) Nonsteroidal anti-inflammatory drugs (increased stimulation of the central nervous system and possibility of convulsions) Probenecid (increased serum levels of the fluoroquinolone) Theophylline (increased serum levels of theophylline)	QT prolongation: elderly, female sex, electrolyte imbalance, cardiac diseases, use of other agents that prolong the QTc interval. Tendon rupture: older age, renal insufficiency, corticosteroid therapy.
Linezolid	Disrupts protein synthesis by binding to rRNA and inhibits the initiation process for protein synthesis.	Disrupts mitochondrial function.	Not enough data about interactions with rifampicin. Serotonin reuptake inhibitors.	Thrombocytopenia: low baseline platelet count, minimum concentration, renal insufficiency.
Clofazimine	Increases reactive oxidant species and destabilizes the bacterial membrane. Reverses the inhibition of intracellular phagocyte killing mechanisms and acts synergistically with interferon-gamma.	The drug accumulates in subcutaneous fat. Inhibits hERG cardiac potassium channels.	No data on drug interactions found. Additive QT prolongation can occur when used together with: fluoroquinolones, bedaquiline, delamanid; azoles, macrolides, metoclopramide, efavirenz, furosemide, hydrochlorothiazide, citalopram, escitalopram, methadone, antiarrhythmics, and others.	No data.
Cycloserine/ Terizidone	Inhibits the D-alanyl-D-alanine synthetase, alanine racemase, and alanine permease. These enzymes are involved in the bacterial cell membranes' peptidoglycan formation.	Acts as a partial NMDA receptor agonist, which may contribute to neuropsychiatric effects.	Alcohol (increased effects of alcohol and dizziness) Anticoagulants (increased serum concentration of the anticoagulant) Ethionamide, isoniazid (possibility of increased toxic effects on the central nervous system) Phenytoin (increased serum concentration of phenytoin) Vitamin B6 (increased vitamin B6 clearance)	Higher doses, longer treatment duration
Carbapenems	Enters the bacterial cell and acylate the PBP enzymes, which catalyze peptidoglycan formation, causing autolysis and cell damage due to osmotic pressure. Meropenem acts as a β-lactamase inhibitor.	Can bind to GABA receptors. Disrupts gut flora.	Ganciclovir (elevated risk for convulsions) Imipenem (lower serum concentration of valproate)	History of seizures.

Table 1. *Cont.*

Drug	Mechanism of Action	Mechanism of Adverse Drug Reaction	Drug Interactions	Risk Factors for Adverse Drug Reactions
Amikacin	Bind to the bacterial surfaces, penetrates into the cytoplasm, and interferes with the translation of proteins, damaging the cytoplasmic membrane.	Damage to cranial nerve VIII. Accumulation of the drugs in renal tubules.	Acyclovir, amphotericin, cephalosporins, cisplatin, cyclosporine (increased possibility of nephrotoxicity) Ethacrynic acid (increased possibility of ototoxicity) Oral anticoagulants (greater effect of the anticoagulant) Nonsteroidal anti-inflammatory drugs (increased possibility of ototoxicity and nephrotoxicity) Capreomycin (increased possibility of ototoxicity and nephrotoxicity) Furosemide (increased possibility of ototoxicity) Methotrexate (possible increase in the toxicity of methotrexate) Polymyxins (greater nephrotoxicity) Vancomycin (greater ototoxicity and nephrotoxicity) Neuromuscular blocking agents (additive effect)	Age, long treatment duration, high total accumulated dose, concomitant usage of diuretics, dehydration, and history of hearing impairment.
Ethionamide/ prothionamide	The primary target of ethionamide is InhA, resulting in inhibition of mycolic acid biosynthesis.	No data.	Alcohol (increased possibility of psychotic reactions) Antituberculosis drugs (greater adverse effects) Isoniazid (temporarily increased serum concentration of isoniazid) Para-aminosalicylic acid (increased possibility of hypothyroidism) Dapsone (peripheral neuritis is potentiated)	For hepatotoxicity, history of liver disease and alcoholism. If mental instability in history, administer ethionamide with caution.
Para-aminosalicylic acid	Acts as a competitive inhibitor of para-aminobenzoic acid in folate synthesis by targeting dihydropteroate synthase. This leads to inhibition of dihydrofolate reductase and impaired bacterial growth. Metabolites can inhibit thymidylate synthase, disrupting DNA synthesis.	Immune responses to the drug or its metabolites, thyroid hormone synthesis interference, and the drug's impact on intestinal function (reduces vitamin B12 absorption).	Anticoagulants, sulfonylurea (possibility of increased drug effect) Digoxin, vitamin B12 (decreased serum levels of drug/vitamin) Corticosteroids (possibility of increased adverse effects of the corticosteroid) Ethionamide (increased possibility of hypothyroidism and hepatotoxicity) Isoniazid (possibility of increased serum levels of isoniazid) Probenecid (increased serum concentration of para-aminosalicylic acid) Sulfonylurea (possibility of increasing hypoglycemic effects of sulfonylurea)	No data.
Bedaquiline	Inhibits mycobacteria-specific F-ATP synthase by binding to the c subunit. This halts ATP production.	Inhibits cardiac hERG potassium ion channels. Mitochondrial dysfunction and alterations in cellular signaling pathways (hepatotoxicity).	Rifamycins (decreased serum levels of bedaquiline) Azole antifungals, macrolides (increased serum levels of bedaquiline) Efavirenz, phenytoin, glucocorticoids, metoclopramide, furosemide, hydrochlorothiazide, citalopram, escitalopram, methadone, antiarrhythmics, fluoroquinolones, clofazimine, and delamanid (these drugs may add risk for QTc prolongation)	No data.

Table 1. *Cont.*

Drug	Mechanism of Action	Mechanism of Adverse Drug Reaction	Drug Interactions	Risk Factors for Adverse Drug Reactions
Delamanid	Disrupts the mycobacterial cell wall by inhibiting the synthesis of methoxy-mycolic and keto-mycolic acids. During activation by the enzyme deazaflavin-dependent nitroreductase, delamanid produces reactive nitrogen species.	Probably converted to primary metabolite DM-6705 (toxic).	Fluoroquinolones, clofazimine, bedaquiline, macrolides, metoclopramide, efavirenz, furosemide, hydrochlorothiazide, citalopram, escitalopram, methadone, and antiarrhythmics (these drugs prolong QTc themselves) Rifamycin, carbamazepine, ritonavir, ketoconazole Cycloserine/terizidone (higher risk for neuropsychiatric symptoms)	Hypoalbuminemia *
Pretomanid	In an aerobic setting, it inhibits protein and lipid synthesis, decreasing the availability of mycolic acids; in an anaerobic state, it generates des-nitro metabolites and releases nitric oxide, reducing adenosine triphosphate concentration in cells.	Animal studies show hepatic, ophthalmologic, and reproductive organ damage.	Rifampicin, efavirenz, and other strong CYP3A4 inducers (significantly decreased pretomanid serum concentration) Lopinavir/ritonavir, other mild CYP3A4 inducers (smaller effect)	No data.

* Data varies across studies.

Timing, frequency, monitoring and management, and discontinuation rates due to adverse drug reactions are summarized in Table 2.

Table 2. Timing, frequency, monitoring, and management, discontinuation rates due to adverse drug reactions (additional information adopted from [4–6,70]).

Drug	Timing of Adverse Drug Reactions	Common/Rare Adverse Drug Reactions	Monitoring for Adverse Drug Reactions	Management of Adverse Drug Reactions	Discontinuation Due to Adverse Drug Reaction Rate
Isoniazid	Hepatotoxicity—first few weeks. Peripheral neuropathy—gradually after several weeks or months.	*Common* Elevated liver enzymes and gastrointestinal disturbances. *Less common, more severe* Peripheral neuropathy, hepatotoxicity. *Rare* Severe skin reactions, psychosis, depression, dysphoria, irritability, seizures, optic neuritis, dysarthria, pancreatitis, vasculitis, arthralgia, anemia, and thrombocytopenia.	Mental health/neuropsychiatric assessment, HIV, ALT, creatinine, complete blood count, hepatitis B/C serology, and glycated hemoglobin. Laboratory test monitoring without symptoms or baseline abnormalities may not be needed unless risk factors are present. Rash, if severe, assess for organ dysfunction: LFT/creatinine, eosinophils (DRESS syndrome).	Pyridoxine supplementation. Hypersensitivity skin reactions—antihistamines, corticosteroids, and, in severe cases, desensitization. Psychiatric disorders—administer psychiatric medication; in severe cases, discontinue the drug.	0.99%—hepatotoxicity, 0.89%—fever, 0.79%—peripheral neuropathy, 0.69%—skin reactions, 0.49%—hypersensitivity, and 0.18%—psychiatric changes.
Rifampicin	Gastrointestinal disturbances—during the first month.	*Common* Rash, gastrointestinal disturbances, and elevated liver enzymes. *Less common, more severe* Hepatotoxicity, thrombocytopenia, acute renal failure, and flu-like syndrome. *Rare* Hemolytic anemia, pseudomembranous colitis, pseudoadrenal crisis.	HIV, ALT, creatinine, complete blood count, hepatitis B/C serology, and glycated hemoglobin. Laboratory test monitoring without symptoms or baseline abnormalities may not be needed unless risk factors are present. Rash, if severe, assess for organ dysfunction: LFT/creatinine, eosinophils (DRESS syndrome).	Liver enzyme monitoring. Gastrointestinal disturbances can be managed symptomatically. If thrombocytopenia occurs, discontinue the drug, corticosteroids, and platelet transfusions in some cases.	0.6–1.19%

Table 2. *Cont.*

Drug	Timing of Adverse Drug Reactions	Common/Rare Adverse Drug Reactions	Monitoring for Adverse Drug Reactions	Management of Adverse Drug Reactions	Discontinuation Due to Adverse Drug Reaction Rate
Pyrazinamide	Hepatotoxicity and hyperuricemia—most common during the first 2–9 weeks.	*Common* Hyperuricemia, arthralgia, elevated liver enzymes, exanthema, and gastrointestinal disorders. *Less common, more severe* Hepatotoxicity, gout, rhabdomyolysis. *Rare* Toxic epidermal necrolysis, photosensitivity, thrombocytopenia, and sideroblastic anemia.	Liver function (AST, ALT, and bilirubin) should be monitored at baseline and monthly if possible. Patients should be closely monitored if they are at risk for drug-related hepatitis and if signs or symptoms of hepatotoxicity occur.	If symptomatic hyperuricemia, allopurinol should be administered. Arthralgia can be managed symptomatically.	0.6–5% In elderly patients, 20.6%.
Ethambutol	Optic neuropathy develops after several weeks or months.	*Common* Optic neuropathy. *Rare* Peripheral neuropathy, rash, gastrointestinal disturbances, thrombocytopenia, cutaneous reaction, and acute renal failure	Patients should report any vision changes. Baseline and monthly visual acuity and color discrimination monitoring should be performed; high risk for patients on higher doses or with renal impairment. Each eye must be tested separately, and both eyes tested together.	An ophthalmologist consultation is needed. Visual acuity and fields should be monitored. Immediately discontinue if visual symptoms occur.	0.2–1% at 15 mg/kg dosage. 15–18% at 35 mg/kg dosage.
Fluoroquinolones	Adverse drug reactions to moxifloxacin in a median of 15 days and to levofloxacin in a median of 35 days. Tendon rupture—early during treatment and weeks to months after.	*Common* Gastrointestinal disturbances, nausea, diarrhea, dizziness, insomnia, and skin rash. *Less common, more severe* QT prolongation, arrhythmia, tendon rupture, peripheral neuropathy, hallucinations, delusions, pseudomembranous colitis, urticaria, vasculitis	Symptomatic monitoring. ECG should be carried out before treatment and at least 2, 12, and 24 weeks after starting treatment. More frequent monitoring is required if cardiac conditions, hypothyroidism, or electrolyte disturbances are present.	Correct electrolyte imbalances. Fluoroquinolones should be stopped if the QTc > 500 msec, and ECGs and potassium should be monitored frequently until the QTc returns to normal.	Levofloxacin—3.2%, moxifloxacin—4.5%.
Linezolid	Myelosuppression occurs after 2–4 weeks of treatment, peripheral neuropathy—gradually after several weeks or months, and optic neuropathy—after more than 2 months of treatment.	*Common* Gastrointestinal disorders, peripheral neuropathy, and anemia. *Rare* Optic neuritis, thrombocytopenia, and lactic acidosis.	Monitor for: -peripheral neuropathy and optic neuritis, through visual eye acuity (both eyes) and Ishihara tests every 2 months or, if symptoms develop, clinical examination for peripheral neuropathy monthly; -complete blood count weekly during the initial period, then monthly, and thereafter as needed based on symptoms; -pH, anion gap, and lactate levels in case of suspected lactic acidosis (hyperlactatemia, if lactate >2.0 mmol/L and confirmed lactic acidosis at >4.0 mmol/L), hypotension, lethargy, or clinical worsening without a clear explanation.	If peripheral neuropathy or optic neuritis occurs, the drug should be discontinued. Anemia and thrombocytopenia could be reversed with dosage reduction.	14.1%

Table 2. *Cont.*

Drug	Timing of Adverse Drug Reactions	Common/Rare Adverse Drug Reactions	Monitoring for Adverse Drug Reactions	Management of Adverse Drug Reactions	Discontinuation Due to Adverse Drug Reaction Rate
Clofazimine	Skin discoloration develops within a few weeks.	*Common* Skin discoloration, gastrointestinal disorders, skin dryness, and ichthyosis, QT prolongation *Rare* Hepatitis, hypersensitivity reaction, nephrotoxicity, and acne.	Monitor clinical signs and symptoms. Perform an ECG if other QT interval-prolonging agents are given concomitantly.	Skin discoloration—patient advisement. Gastrointestinal disorders may be managed symptomatically. QT prolongation—analysis and correction of electrolytes, cardiac diseases, and, if severe, discontinuation of the drug.	
Cycloserine/ Terizidone	A median of 71 days.	*Common* Headache, tremors, sleep disturbances, anxiety, depression, confusion, pale skin. *Rare* Visual changes, skin rash, hepatitis, tingling, and numbness in the extremities.	Baseline and monthly monitoring for depression should be carried out using a tool (e.g., the Beck Depression Index). If therapeutic drug monitoring is possible, obtain peak concentrations within the first 1–2 weeks of therapy and monitor them serially during therapy, keeping peak concentrations at <35 mcg/mL. When administering delamanid and cycloserine concurrently, monitor for neuropsychiatric side effects.	If seizures or psychotic symptoms occur, discontinue the drug. Pyridoxine supplementation is recommended.	6.25–66%
Carbapenems	No data.	*Common* Gastrointestinal disturbances. *Less common* Pseudomembranous colitis. *Rare* Seizures (more linked to imipenem). Injection site inflammation.	Monitor clinical signs and symptoms.	Gastrointestinal symptoms—symptomatic management. If diarrhea and fever, test for pseudomembranous colitis.	4.9%
Amikacin		*Common* Pain at the injection site and proteinuria *Less common, more severe* Cochlear, vestibular, nephrotoxicity, peripheral neuropathy, rash, and eosinophilia.	• creatinine at least monthly (more frequently if there is renal or hepatic impairment). • Creatinine clearance if there is baseline renal impairment or any concerns. • Electrolytes: baseline follow-up with monthly minimum potassium, magnesium, and calcium if possible. Audiology examination: baseline and monthly. Vestibular examinations: Question patients regularly about symptoms and perform serial vestibular exams. If possible, in patients aged over 60 years or with altered renal function, peak serum concentrations should be monitored.	If hearing loss occurs, consider discontinuing the drug. If nephrotoxicity occurs, discontinue the drug. Manage electrolyte imbalance.	13.8%

Table 2. *Cont.*

Drug	Timing of Adverse Drug Reactions	Common/Rare Adverse Drug Reactions	Monitoring for Adverse Drug Reactions	Management of Adverse Drug Reactions	Discontinuation Due to Adverse Drug Reaction Rate
Ethionamide/ prothionamide	Hepatic adverse reactions can occur for up to five months after initial treatment.	*Common and severe* Gastrointestinal disturbances. *Less common* Hepatotoxicity, neurological and psychiatric disturbances, hypothyroidism, menstrual irregularity, gynecomastia, arthralgia, and leukopenia. *Rare* Peripheral and optic neuritis, rash, photosensitivity, and thrombocytopenia.	TSH should be monitored for evidence of hypothyroidism requiring replacement therapy. Therapeutic drug monitoring is required if malabsorption is suspected. Liver function tests should be monitored.	Pyridoxine supplementation is recommended. Gastrointestinal disturbances must be managed symptomatically. If psychiatric symptoms, consider specialist consultation. The drug may be stopped, and psychiatric drugs prescribed.	No data.
Para-aminosalicylic acid	Gastrointestinal intolerance occurs after one week of treatment or more.	*Common* Gastrointestinal disturbances, hypothyroidism. *Rare* Hepatitis, allergic reactions, hemolytic anemia, granulocytopenia, polyneuritis, pericarditis, and malabsorption.	Should monitor TSH, electrolytes, blood counts, and liver function tests.	Diarrhea may improve after several weeks of treatment, and nausea and vomiting can be managed symptomatically. Thyroid function normalizes after drug discontinuation; thyroxine therapy may be needed. Splitting the dose or timing with food sometimes alleviates symptoms.	11.6%
Bedaquiline	Most significant QTc prolongation—in 6 or 15 weeks. * 34.2% of reactions were in the first month, and 14.2% were in the second.	*Common* Nausea, vomiting, abdominal pain, anorexia, arthralgia, headache, and QTc prolongation. *Rare* Hyperuricemia, phospholipidosis, elevated transaminases, and pancreatitis.	ECG before treatment and at least 2, 12, and 24 weeks after starting treatment. More frequent monitoring is recommended if cardiac conditions, hypothyroidism, or electrolyte disturbances are present. Liver function tests should be conducted at baseline, then monthly.	Gastrointestinal symptoms and arthralgia can be managed symptomatically and improve after a few weeks of treatment. Bedaquiline should be stopped if the QTc > 500 msec, and ECGs and potassium levels should be monitored regularly until the QTc returns to normal.	1.7%
Delamanid	Changes in ECGs peak at week 8.	*Occasional* QTc prolongation, nausea, vomiting, dizziness, insomnia, anxiety, hallucinations, night terrors, and upper abdominal pain	Before treatment, ensure the albumin level is 2.8 g/dL or higher. ECG and baseline electrolytes should be obtained and repeated if necessary (e.g., documented QTc prolongation or multiple risk factors). When administering delamanid and cycloserine concurrently, monitor for neuropsychiatric side effects.	Gastrointestinal symptoms—symptomatic management.	2.5–3.8%
Pretomanid	No data.	*Common* Nausea and vomiting, acne, headache, musculoskeletal pain, and liver enzyme elevation.	Symptoms of hepatotoxicity should be monitored, and liver function tests should be performed at baseline, at 2 weeks, and then monthly as needed. ECG and baseline electrolytes should be obtained before the initiation of treatment and repeated if needed (e.g., documented QTc prolongation or multiple risk factors).	No data.	No data.

* Data varies across studies.

3. Adverse Drug Reactions of Second-Line Antituberculosis Drugs

Fluoroquinolones are fluorine-containing nalidixic acid derivatives, first synthesized in 1962 [71]. It has broad-spectrum antimicrobial activity by inhibiting DNA gyrase, which is a supercoiling enzyme. This enzyme is essential for DNA expression and replication. When DNA ends are free, mRNAs, exonuclease, and some proteins are produced uncontrollably, and chromosomes start to degrade. This leads to the death of bacteria [6]. In the latest World Health Organization recommendations, levofloxacin (third-generation fluoroquinolone) and moxifloxacin (fourth-generation fluoroquinolone) are in group A of drugs for drug-resistant tuberculosis treatment [10].

Fluoroquinolones can block cardiac potassium channels, leading to prolongation of the QT interval [72]. Due to those drugs, tendon rupture can occur, particularly in the Achilles tendon, but the mechanism is not fully understood. It may involve the production of reactive oxygen species and matrix metalloproteinase activation, weakening tendons [73].

In one study, adverse drug reactions possibly to moxifloxacin occurred in a median of 15 days and to levofloxacin in a median of 35 days [74]. Tendon rupture can occur early during treatment and even weeks to months after treatment [73]. More common adverse drug reactions are gastrointestinal disturbances, nausea, diarrhea, dizziness, insomnia, and skin rash, while less common but more severe reactions are QT prolongation, arrhythmia, tendon rupture, peripheral neuropathy, hallucinations, delusions, pseudomembranous colitis, urticaria, and vasculitis [2,6,73,75].

Possible fluoroquinolone drug interactions include other QT-prolonging drugs (e.g., amiodarone, erythromycin) [76] and drugs and supplements containing multivalent cations—aluminum; magnesium; calcium; and iron (laxatives, some antacids, etc.). Concomitant use of fluoroquinolones can affect oral anticoagulant blood levels. Probenecid and cimetidine can increase levels of fluoroquinolones. When used with analgesics, the possibility of convulsions is higher [6]. Risk factors for QT prolongation are elderly, female sex, electrolyte imbalance, cardiac diseases, and use of other agents that prolong the QTc interval [2,77]. Tendon rupture is more common in patients who are older, have renal insufficiency, and are taking corticosteroid therapy [78].

ECG monitoring is needed to detect adverse drug reactions of fluoroquinolones early, especially in high-risk patients. It is crucial to correct electrolyte imbalances if there are any. If significant QT prolongation or arrhythmia occurs, treatment should be discontinued [2,76].

In a meta-analysis of individual-level patient data of over nine thousand patients, adverse drug reactions that resulted in permanent antituberculosis treatment discontinuation were analyzed. The pooled absolute risk for levofloxacin (3.2%) and moxifloxacin (4.5%) was low [79,80].

In a retrospective study from South Korea, levofloxacin was accountable for slightly more adverse drug reactions than moxifloxacin (11.0% vs. 8.2%). In the levofloxacin group, gastrointestinal disturbances were the most common problem, affecting 5 of 82 participants, followed by musculoskeletal, neurological, and renal adverse reactions; hepatotoxicity; and allergic reactions—each affected one participant. Meanwhile, in the moxifloxacin group, allergic reaction was the main problem, affecting 5 out of 122 participants; gastrointestinal disturbances and neurological problems were seen in 2 participants; in one case, hepatotoxicity was reported [74]. Fluoroquinolones are known to increase the QT interval; moxifloxacin has a more significant effect on ECG changes than levofloxacin [76,81]. Another worldwide study reported opposite results—adverse drug reactions occurred in 6.8% and 10.3% due to levofloxacin and moxifloxacin; respectively [54].

Linezolid belongs to the antimicrobial group called oxazolidinones; they were first used in 1978 for plant diseases. The US Food and Drug Administration approved linezolid in 2000. This drug disrupts protein synthesis by binding to rRNA and inhibits the initiation process for protein synthesis, disrupting protein elongation [82]. Linezolid is in a multidrug-resistant tuberculosis treatment drug group A, according to World Health Organization guidelines [10].

In bone marrow cells, linezolid can disrupt mitochondrial function. Mitochondrial toxicity is the probable cause of peripheral and optic neuropathy, though the mechanism of those adverse drug reactions is not fully understood. The mechanism of myelosuppression is not known. It was thought that it had the same mitochondrial toxicity, but some studies show normal bone marrow, indicating a direct toxic effect on blood cells.

Myelosuppression typically occurs after 2–4 weeks of initial treatment. Peripheral neuropathy develops gradually after several weeks or months. Optic neuropathy can develop after more than 2 months of treatment [82,83]. The most common adverse reactions are gastrointestinal disorders, peripheral neuropathy, and anemia; less common are optic neuritis, thrombocytopenia, and lactic acidosis [2,24]. Optic neuritis due to linezolid is irreversible in most cases [2].

Linezolid has no interactions with most antimicrobials, but there is not enough evidence about interactions with rifampicin. When combined with serotonin reuptake inhibitors, linezolid can cause life-threatening toxicity. It is not contraindicated to prescribe those drugs together, though [82]. Risk factors for thrombocytopenia are baseline platelet count, minimum concentration, and renal insufficiency [84].

Plasma concentrations of linezolid are not dependent on age or mild to moderate hepatic or renal failure [82]. No other risk factors are known for adverse drug reactions. If peripheral neuropathy or optic neuritis occurs, treatment should be discontinued. Meanwhile, anemia and thrombocytopenia could be reversed with a dosage reduction [24].

Individual-level patient data meta-analysis showed that linezolid caused adverse drug reactions, which led to the discontinuation of the drug in 14.1% [79].

Another meta-analysis showed 58.9% of adverse drug reactions were due to linezolid, and 68.4% of them resulted in treatment interruption or dose reduction. The most common were anemia (38.1%) and peripheral neuropathy (47.1%); other adverse reactions were gastrointestinal disorders in 16.7%, optic neuritis in 13.2%, and thrombocytopenia in 11.8% of cases. More adverse drug reactions were seen in daily linezolid dosages >600 mg as compared to ≤600 mg (74.5% vs. 46.7%) [85]. However, another study reported linezolid-induced adverse reactions in 16.2% of patients, most of them (14.6%) were mild [54].

Clofazimine, a hydrophobic riminophenazine, was synthesized in 1954 as an antituberculosis drug. At first, it was thought to be ineffective. However, the drug showed good anti-leprosy results [86–88]. The first theory of the mechanism of action of clofazimine was that the drug binds to the guanine amino acid of bacterial DNA, which results in inhibition of bacterial proliferation [89]. Still, new findings show that the drug increases reactive oxidant species and destabilizes the bacterial membrane. Clofazimine reverses the inhibition of intracellular phagocyte killing mechanisms and acts synergistically with interferon-gamma [90–93].

Skin discoloration develops due to its bioaccumulation and partitioning into subcutaneous fat [94]. Previously, this color was thought to come from crystal-like structures inside macrophages. Clofazimine strongly inhibits hERG cardiac potassium channels, which results in QT prolongation and a higher risk for arrhythmias and sudden cardiac death [95].

Scientific articles cannot be found that report the time of onset of adverse drug reactions. The clofazimine's FDA label says skin discoloration develops within a few weeks.

No clinically significant differences in clofazimine pharmacokinetics have been observed when used concomitantly with bedaquiline, cycloserine/terizidone, dapsone, ethionamide, para-aminosalicylic acid, pyrazinamide, and pyridoxine.

Borisov et al., in their worldwide study, found 7.0% of total adverse reactions due to clofazimine, including 1.4% serious and 5.6% mild [54].

The most common adverse drug reaction caused by clofazimine is yellow to brownish skin discoloration, which occurs in 75–100% of cases [2,24,86,96]. It is reversible, though the drug has a long-lasting effect. In 40–50% of patients, gastrointestinal disturbances occurred. Skin dryness and ichthyosis can also develop in 8–28% [2,86]. QTcF prolongation is another profound side effect of clofazimine, especially important when tuberculosis treatment includes fluoroquinolones, bedaquiline, or delamanid [97]. Less common possible adverse reactions—hepatitis; hypersensitivity reaction; nephrotoxicity; and acne [2].

If skin discoloration occurs, the patient should be advised that this adverse drug reaction will be resolved over a few months or years after discontinuing the drug. Gastrointestinal disturbances can be managed symptomatically in most cases [24]. When QTC prolongation develops, analysis for cardiac diseases and electrolyte imbalance should be performed [2].

In a systematic review by Gopal et al., the prevalence of adverse drug reactions attributable to clofazimine was 11.4%. The drug was discontinued in <1% of patients [86]. Most of the studies in this review were conducted in Asian and South American countries. In a worldwide meta-analysis, the occurrence of discontinuation of clofazimine due to adverse reactions was 1.6% [79].

Cycloserine is one of the oldest antituberculosis drugs, developed around 1955 [88]. It inhibits D-alanyl-D-alanine synthetase, alanine racemase, and alanine permease. These are the enzymes crucial in peptidoglycan formation for the bacterial cell membrane [6,98]. Terizidone is a structural analog of cycloserine; it is a prodrug—each terizidone molecule contains two cycloserine molecules [99].

Cycloserine/terizidone acts as a partial NMDA receptor agonist, which may contribute to its neuropsychiatric effects. The exact mechanism of many CNS and psychiatric cycloserine/terizidone-induced adverse drug reactions is not fully understood [100]. One study found that adverse drug reactions appeared after a median of 71 days [101].

The most common adverse drug reactions due to cycloserine/terizidone are headache and tremors, sleep disturbances, anxiety, depression, confusion, and pale skin. Less common symptoms—visual changes; skin rash; hepatitis; tingling; and numbness in the extremities [2]. In a meta-analysis by Hwang et al., the cycloserine/terizidone pooled estimated prevalence for adverse drug reactions was 9.1%:5.7% psychiatric and 1.1% central nervous system [102]. Borisov et al. reported total adverse events in 6.0% of cases (1.8% serious and 4.4% mild) [54]. Another retrospective study from China showed a 4.3% prevalence of psychiatric adverse drug reactions attributable to cycloserine/terizidone [103].

Risk factors for adverse reactions to develop are higher doses and longer duration [24,104]. When combined with ethionamide and isoniazid, neurotoxic effects can be more frequent. Cycloserine/terizidone can increase serum levels of phenytoin and oral anticoagulants [6].

If seizures or psychotic symptoms develop, the drug should be discontinued. Pyridoxine supplementation in moderate doses is recommended to lower the risk of neuropathy and CNS toxicity [2].

A meta-analysis of individual patient data showed that cycloserine/terizidone was permanently discontinued because of psychiatric adverse drug reactions in 66% of patients [79]. Another study found a discontinuation prevalence of 6.25% [101].

Carbapenems—a class of β-lactam antibiotics; including meropenem and imipenem; that are recommended in some cases of drug-resistant tuberculosis treatment [10]. Thienamycin—the first carbapenem and model for all carbapenems—was discovered in 1976 [105]. There is minimal evidence of carbapenem efficacy, safety, and tolerability in tuberculosis treatment. This group of antibiotics enters the bacterial cell and acylates the PBPs enzymes, which catalyze peptidoglycan formation. This causes continued autolysis and cell damage due to osmotic pressure [105]. *M. tuberculosis* produces the enzyme β-lactamase, which can break down some β-lactam antibiotics, including meropenem. Still, while slowly broken down, it acts as a β-lactamase inhibitor, allowing other antibiotics to work. If combined with clavulanic acid to block β-lactamase, meropenem is more effective [106].

Carbapenems can bind to GABA receptors, causing seizures [107]. As with most broad-spectrum antibiotics, carbapenems disrupt gut flora, elevating the risk of developing pseudomembranous colitis.

There is no data on the timing of adverse drug reactions of carbapenems related to tuberculosis treatment. Considering the mechanism of action and adverse drug reactions, gastrointestinal symptoms and injection site reactions could occur early, while seizures and pseudomembranous colitis should take more time to develop.

The most common adverse drug reactions are gastrointestinal disturbances like nausea, vomiting, and abdominal pain, which occur in up to 20% of patients. Less common—pseudomembranous colitis. Rare reaction—seizures; reported in 1.5% of patients; mostly when given high doses; is more linked to imipenem [70,107]. When administered for a long time, injection site inflammation can occur (in 1.1% of patients) [24,107].

Overall, carbapenems have a low potential for drug interactions. When used with ganciclovir, the risk for convulsions elevates. Imipenem lowers the serum concentration of valproate [70].

There is a higher risk of seizures for those who have a history of them [107]. No specific data on the risk factors of carbapenem-induced adverse drug reactions were found.

Management of gastrointestinal symptoms is symptomatic. When diarrhea and fever occur, patients should be tested for pseudomembranous colitis [70].

Sotgiu et al. found up to 15% prevalence of adverse drug reactions in their systematic review [108]. Meanwhile, the pooled incidence of adverse drug reactions was 7.7% in drug-resistant tuberculosis treatment in a meta-analysis conducted by Lan et al. Meropenem and imipenem were permanently discontinued in 4.9% of cases due to adverse drug reactions [79].

Amikacin is a semi-synthetic derivative of kanamycin A, approved in 1976. Aminoglycosides penetrate into the bacterial cytoplasm and interfere with the translation of proteins, damaging the cytoplasmic membrane [109].

Permanent bilateral hearing loss due to damage to cranial nerve VIII is a severe adverse drug reaction of aminoglycosides; the risk of it increases with age, duration of treatment, and accumulated dose [6,110]. Nephrotoxicity is also a concern because of the accumulation of the drug in renal tubules [6,111].

Most amikacin-induced adverse reactions are duration-dependent when the accumulated dose is high. More frequent adverse events are pain at the injection site and proteinuria; more severe but less common are cochlear, vestibular, and nephrotoxicity; peripheral neuropathy; rash; and eosinophilia [2].

Borisov et al. reported adverse drug reactions due to amikacin in 22.9% of cases in the overall cohort, including 6.9% grades 3–5 and 16.0% grades 1–2 [54]. In the Lan et al. meta-analysis, a pooled incidence of amikacin-related adverse drug reactions was 13.8%.

Ototoxicity was the most common among adverse drug reactions of amikacin, causing drug discontinuation in 87% of those cases [79].

Ototoxicity and nephrotoxicity can be more frequent when amikacin is used with amphotericin B, vancomycin, cephalosporin, cisplatin, and loop diuretics. Concomitant use of neuromuscular blocking agents can cause respiratory depression due to muscle weakness [6].

Risk factors for ototoxicity are age, long treatment duration, high total accumulated dose, concomitant usage of diuretics, dehydration, and history of hearing impairment. Monitoring with audiometry during treatment is needed. If hearing loss is seen, a decision weighing the risks and benefits of the treatment should be made—in some cases; the drug must be discontinued; as it should be if nephrotoxicity develops. Electrolyte imbalance must be corrected [2].

Nephrotoxicity is more common in older patients with a history of kidney disease. Neuromuscular blockades often develop in patients with hypocalcemia, hypokalemia, hypomagnesemia, and in the presence of botulism or myasthenia gravis [6].

Ethionamide was started to be used in medical practice around 1960 [112]. Together with prothionamide, it belongs to the thioamide group of drugs; its structure is similar to that of isoniazid. Thioamides are prodrugs that are activated inside bacterial cells. Like isoniazid, the primary target of ethionamide is InhA, resulting in inhibition of mycolic acid biosynthesis. However, activation of these drugs differs—it was suggested that ethionamide is activated by an enzyme, EthA [80,113,114].

Since ethionamide is similar to isoniazid, adverse drug reactions are similar, too. Hepatic adverse reactions can occur for up to five months after the start of the treatment.

Gastrointestinal disturbances are common and severe when prescribing ethionamide. It includes metallic taste, excessive salivation, nausea, vomiting, loss of appetite, and abdominal pain. Less common are hepatotoxicity, neurological and psychiatric disturbances, hypothyroidism, menstrual irregularity, gynecomastia, arthralgia, and leukopenia. Rare adverse reactions—peripheral and optic neuritis; rash; photosensitivity; and thrombocytopenia [2,6].

When ethionamide is used with terizidone or isoniazid, neurotoxic reactions are more common. When used with para-aminosalicylic acid, hepatotoxicity and risk for hypothyroidism are higher. When used with alcohol, psychotic reactions can develop [6].

Risk factors for hepatotoxicity are a history of liver disease and alcoholism. In the history of mental instability, ethionamide should be administered with caution. Pyridoxine supplementation is recommended when prescribing ethionamide [6].

Symptomatic treatment is needed for gastrointestinal reactions; sometimes, doses of ethionamide can be increased progressively. When psychiatric symptoms occur, specialist consultation may be required. In some cases, drugs can be stopped, and psychiatric medications prescribed [2].

A study showed adverse drug reactions in 17.6% of patients (0.4% serious and 17.2% mild) [54]. In a meta-analysis conducted by Lan et al., the summed pooled incidence of adverse drug reactions was 10.9%. When ethionamide and prothionamide were discontinued, in most cases, it was due to gastrointestinal disorders (48%) [79].

Para-aminosalicylic acid (PAS) has been one of the first antituberculosis drugs since 1946. Despite a long time in clinical use, the mechanism of action remained elusive for a long time. PAS acts as a competitive inhibitor of para-aminobenzoic acid in the folate synthesis by targeting dihydropteroate synthase. This leads to inhibition of dihydrofolate reductase and impaired bacterial growth. Additionally, PAS metabolites can inhibit thymidylate synthase, further disrupting DNA synthesis [115,116].

The mechanism of PAS-induced adverse drug reactions is not fully understood; they can develop due to immune responses to the drug or its metabolites, thyroid hormone synthesis interference, and drug impact on intestinal function (reduces vitamin B12 absorption) [70,117,118].

Gastrointestinal intolerance occurs after one week of treatment or more [119].

The prevalence of adverse drug reactions attributed to PAS varies from 10 to 30% [118]. Common reactions are gastrointestinal disturbances and hypothyroidism. The prevalence of gastrointestinal disturbances when using PAS was reported in 12–58% of cases and was dose-dependent. Hypothyroidism may develop in 40% of the patients. Less common are reactions—hepatitis (0.3–0.5%); allergic reactions (fever, rash, pruritus) (5–10%); hemolytic anemia; granulocytopenia; polyneuritis; pericarditis; malabsorption; etc. [6,24,118,120]. Most of those findings are from studies conducted many years ago, which reflects the need for newer data.

When PAS is prescribed with rifampicin, the level of rifampicin in the blood can fall by about half [121]. Caution is needed when using PAS with probenecid, sulfonylurea, oral anticoagulants, thrombolytics, and salicylates [116].

There is not enough data on risk factors for adverse drug reactions, precisely due to PAS development. Concomitant use of PAS with ethionamide, prothionamide, and some nonselective NSAIDs can lead to more frequent gastrointestinal disturbances. These reactions are also more frequent when higher doses of PAS are prescribed—12%; 15%; and 52% of patients experienced some symptoms when given 5 g; 10 g; or 20 g of PAS per day; respectively [118,120,122].

Occasionally, diarrhea improves after several weeks of treatment, and nausea and vomiting can be managed symptomatically. Thyroid function normalizes after drug discontinuation [24]. Until then, thyroxine therapy should be initiated. Sometimes, splitting the dose or timing with food alleviates symptoms [2].

Severe adverse drug reactions occurred in 0.5% of cases in the worldwide study, with mild reactions in 10.7% [54]. Treatment interruption is needed in 4% [24], and permanent discontinuation—in 11.6% of cases [70].

Bedaquiline is a diarylquinoline group antituberculosis drug discovered in 2005 [123]. It inhibits mycobacteria-specific F-ATP synthase by binding to the c subunit. This halts ATP production and leads to bacterial death [124]. Bedaquiline is active against dormant and actively replicating mycobacteria [125].

Bedaquiline inhibits cardiac hERG potassium ion channels, and this can lead to QTc prolongation [126]. Hepatotoxicity involves mitochondrial dysfunction and alterations in cellular signaling pathways [127].

Concerning timing, the most significant increase in QTc was seen in the first 6 weeks after bedaquiline initiation in a retrospective study by Isralls et al. [128]. Other data shows that QTc increased by 10–15 msec, reaching a maximum at week 15 [70]. Wu et al. analyzed the US Food and Drug Administration's Adverse Event Reporting System's reports about bedaquiline. They found that 34.2% of reactions were seen in the first month and 14.2% in the second month [127].

More common adverse drug reactions include nausea, vomiting, abdominal pain, anorexia, arthralgia, headache, and QTc prolongation. Rarely do hyperuricemia, phospholipidosis, and elevated transaminases occur. Elevated liver enzymes are a sign of an increased risk of pancreatitis [2,70].

When bedaquiline is used with rifamycin, it may cause a significant reduction in bedaquiline concentration. Azole antifungals and macrolides can increase concentration. Caution is also needed when taking bedaquiline together with efavirenz, phenytoin, glucocorticoids, metoclopramide, furosemide, hydrochlorothiazide, citalopram, escitalopram, methadone, antiarrhythmics, and also fluoroquinolones, clofazimine, and delamanid—drugs that are also associated with QTc prolongation [70].

Some authors suggest discontinuing treatment with bedaquiline if liver enzymes are >5 × ULN or >3 × ULN with symptoms. Less likely to cause drugs should be reintroduced when <2 × ULN, adding one drug at a time every 3 days [2,24]. Gastrointestinal symptoms and arthralgia can be managed symptomatically and improve after a few weeks of treatment. Serial monitoring with ECG is recommended [2].

Lan et al. found that bedaquiline has one of the lowest incidences of adverse drug reactions that led to discontinuation of the drug (1.7%) [79].

Bedaquiline-associated reactions developed in 11.1% of cases in the Borisov et al. study (serious—1.0%, mild—10.1%) [54]. Adverse drug reactions that occurred in bedaquiline-containing regimens are hepatotoxicity (pooled rate, 12.6%), renal disorders (pooled rate, 5.9%), optic neuropathy, including blurred vision (pooled rate, 3.9%), ototoxicity, including hearing loss (pooled rate, 7.0%), hematological disorders (pooled rate, 12.5%), gastrointestinal symptoms like nausea or vomiting (pooled rate, 13.8%), peripheral neuropathy (pooled rate, 13.9%), electrolyte disturbances (pooled rate, 6.4%), arthralgia (pooled rate, 10.1%), psychiatric disorders (pooled rate, 4.6%), and dermatological disorders including acne (pooled rate, 9.8%) in Rehman et al.'s meta-analysis. The QTc interval was prolonged in 10.2% of cases when treatment included bedaquiline [129].

In an observational cohort from Guglielmetti et al., gastrointestinal side effects were most common (71.7%), followed by oto-vestibular impairment (55.6%) and peripheral neuropathy (40.9%). No differences were found between standard and prolonged bedaquiline treatment groups [130].

Delamanid was approved in 2014 for the treatment of multidrug-resistant tuberculosis [131]. It is a prodrug that belongs to the dihydro-nitroimidazole class. Delamanid disrupts the mycobacterial cell wall by inhibiting the synthesis of methoxy-mycolic and keto-mycolic acids. During activation by the enzyme deazaflavin-dependent nitroreductase, delamanid produces reactive nitrogen species, which further disrupt bacterial metabolic processes [132–134].

The metabolism of delamanid is not fully understood; the drug is probably converted to the primary metabolite DM-6705. This metabolite is associated with delamanid toxicity, mainly with QTc prolongation [135].

Changes in ECGs peak at week 8; average QTc prolongation is 5–15 ms.

Delamanid is well tolerated; the primary concern when using this drug is QTc prolongation. Other possible reactions are nausea, vomiting, dizziness, insomnia, anxiety, hallucinations, night terrors, and upper abdominal pain [2,24,70].

Caution is recommended when using delamanid together with rifamycin, carbamazepine, ritonavir, ketoconazole, and drugs that tend to prolong QTc themselves—fluoroquinolones, clofazimine, bedaquiline, macrolides, metoclopramide, efavirenz, furosemide, hydrochlorothiazide, citalopram, escitalopram, methadone, antiarrhythmics, etc. When administered with cycloserine/terizidone, there is a higher risk of neuropsychiatric adverse events [70].

At first, it was thought that hypoalbuminemia is linked with an increased risk for QTc prolongation, but recent studies suggest no association [24,70].

In mild cases, a symptomatic approach is recommended for gastrointestinal symptoms. ECG monitoring is recommended [2].

Gler et al. reported similar discontinuation rates in the 100 mg and 200 mg delamanid groups and placebo—2.5%; 3.8%; and 2.5%; respectively. In the 100 mg group, 2 cases were discontinued due to psychiatric side effects, one due to dermatologic side effects, and one due to thrombocytopenia. In the 200 mg group, 1 case was discontinued due to leucopenia, 3 due to psychiatric side effects, and 1 due to dermatologic side effects [132].

Data from the same study showed that in the 200 mg twice daily group, QT interval prolongation occurred more often (13.1%) than at 100 mg twice daily (9.9%). In a placebo group, the prevalence of QT prolongation was 3.8% [132].

Other adverse drug reactions that were common in delamanid treatment groups (lower and higher doses, accordingly) were gastrointestinal disturbances (nausea 36.0–40.6%, vomiting 29.8–36.2%, upper abdominal pain 22.5–25.5%), nervous system (headache 22.4–25.6%, paresthesia 10.6–12.5%, tremor 10.0–11.8%, insomnia 26.1–31.9%), and other (tinnitus 9.9–13.8%, asthenia 12.4–16.9%, malaise 7.5–10.0%, anorexia 14.3–21.2%, hyperuricemia 19.3–23.8%, hypokalemia 12.4–19.4%). Those adverse reactions were also seen in the placebo group; most had a higher prevalence in the high-dose delamanid group [132]. Severe adverse drug reactions were seen in 0.8% of patients and mild in 12.4% [54].

Pretomanid was approved for tuberculosis treatment in 2019 [136]. It is bactericidal against replicating and non-replicating *M. tuberculosis* [123]. Activation of the prodrug is similar to that of delamanid. Pretomanid is transformed into three metabolites after activation. It has two mechanisms of action, depending on conditions in the human body. In an aerobic setting, it inhibits protein and lipid synthesis, decreasing the availability of mycolic acids. In an anaerobic state, pretomanid generates des-nitro metabolites and releases nitric oxide, resulting in a significant reduction of ATP concentrations in cells [137].

Most evidence available about pretomanid toxicity comes from in vitro and preclinical studies; there is no data yet about long-term safety. Animal studies show hepatic, ophthalmologic, and reproductive organ damage when pretomanid is given at the most relevant dose [138].

Common adverse drug reactions are nausea and vomiting, acne, headache, musculoskeletal pain, and liver enzyme elevation [139,140]. The frequency of adverse drug reactions in clinical trials was this: gastrointestinal disturbances in 28.4%, hepatic disorders in 25.5%, liver enzyme elevation in 19.2%, skin reactions in 16.6%, and headache in 11.0% [141]. Pretomanid alone has minimal liver toxicity (2.2%) [138].

When taken with strong CYP3A4 inducers (rifampicin, efavirenz), pretomanid blood levels can be significantly lowered. Meanwhile, with mild inducers (lopinavir/ritonavir), the effect on drug levels is smaller [138].

There is no data about the timing and risk factors of adverse drug reactions. Management recommendations are not put in the WHO operational handbook or other authors' reviews [2,24,70]. The treatment discontinuation rate due to pretomanid is not known.

New regimens for drug-resistant tuberculosis treatment are now in official World Health Organization guidelines: the 6-month bedaquiline, pretomanid, linezolid, and moxifloxacin (BPaLM) and the 9-month all-oral regimen [10].

In an open-label, multicenter, randomized, controlled trial, there were fewer grade 3 or more adverse drug reactions in the BPALM group than in the standard care group (19% vs. 59%). In both groups, the most common reactions were hepatic disorders (4% vs. 11%), QTcF prolongation (1% vs. 14%), peripheral neuropathy (9% vs. 19%), decreased creatinine clearance (1% vs. 7%), anemia (3% vs. 8%), and neutropenia (3% vs. 8%). Ten patients (2%) died; seven of them were in the standard care group. Four of the deaths were considered to be treatment-related, all of them in the standard care group [142].

The 9-month all-oral regimen consists of bedaquiline (6 months), in combination with levofloxacin/moxifloxacin, ethionamide, ethambutol, isoniazid (high-dose), pyrazinamide, and clofazimine (for 4 months, with the possibility of extending to 6 months if the patient remains sputum smear positive at the end of 4 months), followed by treatment with levofloxacin/moxifloxacin, clofazimine, ethambutol, and pyrazinamide (for 5 months). Ethionamide can be replaced by 2 months of linezolid (600 mg daily). Data concerning the adverse drug reactions for a regimen with ethionamide were not collected, which means that it cannot be compared with a regimen containing linezolid [10].

In the Nix-TB trial, 57% of participants had adverse drug reactions. More than 80% had peripheral neuropathy, and 37% had anemia. Moderate or severe liver enzyme elevation was seen in twelve (11%) participants; no participants had QT interval prolongation of more than 480 ms. In the 9-month regimen, the most common adverse drug reactions were anemia (linezolid-containing regimen), hepatotoxicity, QT prolongation, nausea, and vomiting [70].

4. Prevention of Adverse Drug Reactions

There is limited data on the prevention of adverse reactions to tuberculosis medications. Given that alcoholism can lead to liver damage and poses a significant risk for adverse drug reactions, it is crucial to discontinue alcohol consumption as soon as possible. Additionally, pyridoxine supplementation is recommended when prescribing certain antituberculosis drugs. It is essential to meticulously consider drug interactions when selecting medications for tuberculosis treatment, as some drugs can amplify each other's adverse effects (refer to Table 2 for risk factors, management recommendations, and potential drug interactions).

5. Conclusions

Adverse drug reactions are common in tuberculosis treatment with first- and second-line antituberculosis drugs, with a wider variety and more severe reactions seen in the latter. The severity of adverse drug reactions varies considerably; most of them can be managed, and no permanent discontinuation is needed. There is a lack of data on the newest and some old drugs' adverse reaction mechanisms; most of the evidence about risk factors for drug side effects is from a very long time ago. New, less toxic drugs are needed to treat drug-resistant tuberculosis. Healthcare providers' knowledge and vigilance regarding adverse drug reactions are important.

Author Contributions: Conceptualization, Methodology: E.D.; Writing—original draft: R.M.; Writing—review and editing: R.M. and E.D. All authors have read and agreed to the published version of the manuscript.

Funding: This research received no external funding.

Conflicts of Interest: The authors declare no conflicts of interest.

References

1. World Health Organization (WHO). Global Tuberculosis Report. 2024. Available online: https://iris.who.int/bitstream/handle/10665/379339/9789240101531-eng.pdf?sequence=1 (accessed on 1 February 2025).
2. Prasad, R.; Singh, A.; Gupta, N. Adverse Drug Reactions with First-Line and Second-Line Drugs in Treatment of Tuberculosis. *Ann. Natl. Acad. Med. Sci. India* **2021**, *57*, 16–35. [CrossRef]
3. Dela, A.; Tank, N.K.; Singh, A.; Piparva, K. Adverse drug reactions and treatment outcome analysis of DOTS-plus therapy of MDR-TB patients at district tuberculosis centre: A four year retrospective study. *Lung India* **2017**, *34*, 522. [CrossRef] [PubMed]
4. Singh, K.P.; Carvalho, A.C.C.; Centis, R.; D'Ambrosio, L.; Migliori, G.B.; Mpagama, S.G.; Nguyen, B.C.; Aarnoutse, R.E.; Aleksa, A.; Van Altena, R.; et al. Clinical standards for the management of adverse effects during treatment for TB. *Int. J. Tuberc. Lung Dis.* **2023**, *27*, 506–519. [CrossRef]

5. Arbex, M.A.; Varella, M.D.C.L.; Siqueira, H.R.D.; Mello, F.A.F.D. Drogas antituberculose: Interações medicamentosas, efeitos adversos e utilização em situações especiais—Parte 1: Fármacos de primeira linha. *J. Bras. Pneumol.* **2010**, *36*, 626–640. [CrossRef] [PubMed]
6. Arbex, M.A.; Varella, M.D.C.L.; Siqueira, H.R.D.; Mello, F.A.F.D. Drogas antituberculose: Interações medicamentosas, efeitos adversos e utilização em situações especiais—Parte 2: Fármacos de segunda linha. *J. Bras. Pneumol.* **2010**, *36*, 641–656. [CrossRef]
7. Thomas, L.; Raju, A.P.; Mallayasamy, S.; Rao, M. Precision Medicine Strategies to Improve Isoniazid Therapy in Patients with Tuberculosis. *Eur. J. Drug Metab. Pharmacokinet.* **2024**, *49*, 541–557. [CrossRef]
8. McDermott, W. The Story of INH. *J. Infect. Dis.* **1969**, *119*, 678–683. [CrossRef]
9. *WHO Consolidated Guidelines on Tuberculosis. Module 4: Treatment-Drug-Susceptible Tuberculosis Treatment*, 1st ed.; World Health Organization: Geneva, Switzerland, 2022.
10. *WHO Consolidated Guidelines on Tuberculosis. Module 4: Treatment-Drug-Resistant Tuberculosis Treatment*, 1st ed.; World Health Organization: Geneva, Switzerland, 2022.
11. Timmins, G.S.; Deretic, V. Mechanisms of action of isoniazid. *Mol. Microbiol.* **2006**, *62*, 1220–1227. [CrossRef]
12. Unissa, A.N.; Subbian, S.; Hanna, L.E.; Selvakumar, N. Overview on mechanisms of isoniazid action and resistance in Mycobacterium tuberculosis. *Infect. Genet. Evol.* **2016**, *45*, 474–492. [CrossRef]
13. Combrink, M.; Loots, D.T.; Du Preez, I. Metabolomics describes previously unknown toxicity mechanisms of isoniazid and rifampicin. *Toxicol. Lett.* **2020**, *322*, 104–110. [CrossRef]
14. Vilholm, O.J.; Christensen, A.A.; Zedan, A.H.; Itani, M. Drug-Induced Peripheral Neuropathy. *Basic Clin. Pharmacol. Toxicol.* **2014**, *115*, 185–192. [CrossRef] [PubMed]
15. Gülbay, B.E.; Gürkan, Ö.U.; Yıldız, Ö.A.; Önen, Z.P.; Erkekol, F.Ö.; Baççıoğlu, A.; Acıcan, T. Side effects due to primary antituberculosis drugs during the initial phase of therapy in 1149 hospitalized patients for tuberculosis. *Respir. Med.* **2006**, *100*, 1834–1842. [CrossRef]
16. Baghaei, P.; Tabarsi, P.; Chitsaz, E.; Saleh, M.; Marjani, M.; Shemirani, S.; Pooramiri, M.V.; Kazempour, M.; Farnia, P.; Fahimi, F.; et al. Incidence, Clinical and Epidemiological Risk Factors, and Outcome of Drug-Induced Hepatitis Due to Antituberculous Agents in New Tuberculosis Cases. *Am. J. Ther.* **2010**, *17*, 17–22. [CrossRef]
17. Campbell, J.R.; Trajman, A.; Cook, V.J.; Johnston, J.C.; Adjobimey, M.; Ruslami, R.; Eisenbeis, L.; Fregonese, F.; Valiquette, C.; Benedetti, A.; et al. Adverse events in adults with latent tuberculosis infection receiving daily rifampicin or isoniazid: Post-hoc safety analysis of two randomised controlled trials. *Lancet Infect. Dis.* **2020**, *20*, 318–329. [CrossRef]
18. Imam, F.; Sharma, M.; Khayyam, K.U.; Al-Harbi, N.O.; Rashid, M.K.; Ali, M.D.; Ahmad, A.; Qamar, W. Adverse drug reaction prevalence and mechanisms of action of first-line anti-tubercular drugs. *Saudi Pharm. J.* **2020**, *28*, 316–324. [CrossRef] [PubMed]
19. Baral, T.; Sekhar, S.; Thomas, L.; Acharya, R.; Krishnan, K.; Shetty, S.; Rao, M. Isoniazid-induced pancreatitis: A systematic review. *Tuberculosis* **2024**, *148*, 102535. [CrossRef]
20. Samouco, A.I.C.B.; Alves, S.P. Isoniazid-induced mania and the history of antidepressant drugs: Case report and literature review. *Bipolar Disord.* **2023**, *25*, 84–87. [CrossRef] [PubMed]
21. Public Health Agency of Canada and Canadian Lung Association/Canadian Thoracic Society. *Canadian Tuberculosis Standards*, 7th ed.; Public Health Agency of Canada and Canadian Lung Association/Canadian Thoracic Society: Ottawa, ON, Canada, 2014.
22. Shi, C.; Yang, B.; Yang, J.; Song, W.; Chen, Y.; Zhang, S.; Zhan, H.; Xiong, Y.; Rong, P.; Luo, Y.; et al. Evaluation of adverse reactions induced by anti-tuberculosis drugs among hospitalized patients in Wuhan, China: A retrospective study. *Medicine* **2024**, *103*, e38273. [CrossRef]
23. Erwin, E.R.; Addison, A.P.; John, S.F.; Olaleye, O.A.; Rosell, R.C. Pharmacokinetics of isoniazid: The good, the bad, and the alternatives. *Tuberculosis* **2019**, *116*, S66–S70. [CrossRef]
24. Kim, H.Y.; Cho, J.-G.; Akkerman, O.W.; Padanilam, X.; Seaworth, B.; Alffenaar, J.-W.C. Anti-Tuberculosis Drugs and Adverse Events. In *Essential Tuberculosis*; Migliori, G.B., Raviglione, M.C., Eds.; Springer International Publishing: Cham, Switzerland, 2021; pp. 121–129. [CrossRef]
25. Park, S.-J.; Jo, K.-W.; Yoo, B.; Lee, C.-K.; Kim, Y.-G.; Yang, S.-K.; Byeon, J.-S.; Kim, K.-J.; Ye, B.D.; Park, S.-H.; et al. Comparison of LTBI treatment regimens for patients receiving anti-tumour necrosis factor therapy. *Int. J. Tuberc. Lung Dis.* **2015**, *19*, 342–348. [CrossRef]
26. Frésard, I.; Bridevaux, P.; Rochat, T.; Janssens, J. Adverse effects and adherence to treatment of rifampicine 4 months vs isoniazid 6 months for latent tuberculosis. *Swiss Med. Wkly.* **2011**, *141*, w13240. [CrossRef]
27. López, G.; Wood, M.; Ayesta, F.J. 10 Años innovando en el tratamiento de la infección tuberculosa latente: Comparación entre pautas estándar y pautas cortas en tratamiento directamente observado. *Rev. Esp. Sanid. Penit.* **2011**, *13*, 3–14. [CrossRef] [PubMed]

28. Sodré-Alves, B.M.C.; Toledo, M.M.; Zimmermann, I.R.; Araújo, W.N.D.; Tavares, N.U.L. Isoniazid use, effectiveness, and safety for treatment of latent tuberculosis infection: A systematic review. *Rev. Soc. Bras. Med. Trop.* **2024**, *57*, e00402-2024. [CrossRef] [PubMed]
29. Page, K.R.; Sifakis, F.; Montes De Oca, R.; Cronin, W.A.; Doherty, M.C.; Federline, L.; Bur, S.; Walsh, T.; Karney, W.; Milman, J.; et al. Improved Adherence and Less Toxicity With Rifampin vs Isoniazid for Treatment of Latent Tuberculosis: A Retrospective Study. *Arch. Intern. Med.* **2006**, *166*, 1863. [CrossRef]
30. Villa, S.; Ferrarese, M.; Sotgiu, G.; Castellotti, P.F.; Saderi, L.; Grecchi, C.; Saporiti, M.; Raviglione, M.; Codecasa, L.R. Latent Tuberculosis Infection Treatment Completion while Shifting Prescription from Isoniazid-Only to Rifampicin-Containing Regimens: A Two-Decade Experience in Milan, Italy. *J. Clin. Med.* **2019**, *9*, 101. [CrossRef]
31. Grayson, M.L.; Cosgrove, S.E.; Crowe, S.; Hope, W.; McCarthy, J.S.; Mills, J.; Mouton, J.W.; Paterson, D.L. *Kucers' The Use of Antibiotics: A Clinical Review of Antibacterial, Antifungal, Antiparasitic, and Antiviral Drugs, Seventh Edition—Three Volume Set*, 7th ed.; Taylor and Francis: London, UK, 2017.
32. Hartmann, G.R.; Heinrich, P.; Kollenda, M.C.; Skrobranek, B.; Tropschug, M.; Weiß, W. Molecular Mechanism of Action of the Antibiotic Rifampicin. *Angew. Chem. Int. Ed. Engl.* **1985**, *24*, 1009–1014. [CrossRef]
33. Mitchison, D.A. The Diagnosis and Therapy of Tuberculosis During the Past 100 Years. *Am. J. Respir. Crit. Care Med.* **2005**, *171*, 699–706. [CrossRef]
34. Sekaggya-Wiltshire, C.; Dooley, K.E. Pharmacokinetic and pharmacodynamic considerations of rifamycin antibiotics for the treatment of tuberculosis. *Expert Opin. Drug Metab. Toxicol.* **2019**, *15*, 615–618. [CrossRef]
35. Abulfathi, A.A.; Decloedt, E.H.; Svensson, E.M.; Diacon, A.H.; Donald, P.; Reuter, H. Clinical Pharmacokinetics and Pharmacodynamics of Rifampicin in Human Tuberculosis. *Clin. Pharmacokinet.* **2019**, *58*, 1103–1129. [CrossRef]
36. Blumberg, H.M.; Burman, W.J.; Chaisson, R.E.; Daley, C.L. American Thoracic Society/Centers for Disease Control and Prevention/Infectious Diseases Society of America: Treatment of Tuberculosis. *Am. J. Respir. Crit. Care Med.* **2003**, *167*, 603–662. [CrossRef]
37. Yee, D.; Valiquette, C.; Pelletier, M.; Parisien, I.; Rocher, I.; Menzies, D. Incidence of Serious Side Effects from First-Line Antituberculosis Drugs among Patients Treated for Active Tuberculosis. *Am. J. Respir. Crit. Care Med.* **2003**, *167*, 1472–1477. [CrossRef]
38. Garg, R.; Gupta, V.; Mehra, S.; Singh, R.; Prasad, R. Rifampicin induced thrombocytopenia. *Indian J. Tuberc.* **2007**, *54*, 94–96. [PubMed]
39. Koycu Buhari, G.; Oner Erkekol, F.; Koca Kalkan, I.; Ates, H.; Vural Solak, G.T.; Akkale, O.; Aksu, K. Hypersensitivity reactions with first-line antituberculosis drugs and outcomes of rapid desensitizations. *World Allergy Organ. J.* **2024**, *17*, 100862. [CrossRef] [PubMed]
40. Castro, A.T.E.; Mendes, M.; Freitas, S.; Roxo, P.C. Incidence and risk factors of major toxicity associated to first-line antituberculosis drugs for latent and active tuberculosis during a period of 10 years. *Rev. Port. Pneumol. Engl. Ed.* **2015**, *21*, 144–150. [CrossRef] [PubMed]
41. Zhang, Y.; Shi, W.; Zhang, W.; Mitchison, D. Mechanisms of Pyrazinamide Action and Resistance. *Microbiol. Spectr.* **2014**, *2*, MGM2-0023-2013. [CrossRef]
42. Lamont, E.A.; Baughn, A.D. Impact of the host environment on the antitubercular action of pyrazinamide. *EBioMedicine* **2019**, *49*, 374–380. [CrossRef]
43. Wahan, S.K.; Sharma, S.; Chawla, P.A. Anti-Tubercular Activity of Pyrazinamide Conjugates: Synthesis and Structure-Activity Relationship Studies. *Mini-Rev. Med. Chem.* **2023**, *23*, 700–718. [CrossRef]
44. Chen, R.H.; Michael, T.; Kuhlin, J.; Schön, T.; Stocker, S.; Alffenaar, J.-W.C. Is there a need to optimise pyrazinamide doses in patients with tuberculosis? A systematic review. *Int. J. Antimicrob. Agents* **2023**, *62*, 106914. [CrossRef]
45. Stehr, M.; Elamin, A.A.; Singh, M. Pyrazinamide: The importance of uncovering the mechanisms of action in mycobacteria. *Expert Rev. Anti Infect. Ther.* **2015**, *13*, 593–603. [CrossRef]
46. Hussain, Z.; Zhu, J.; Ma, X. Metabolism and Hepatotoxicity of Pyrazinamide, an Antituberculosis Drug. *Drug Metab. Dispos. Biol. Fate Chem.* **2021**, *49*, 679–682. [CrossRef]
47. Xu, A.Y.; Velásquez, G.E.; Zhang, N.; Chang, V.K.; Phillips, P.P.J.; Nahid, P.; Dorman, S.E.; Kurbatova, E.V.; Whitworth, W.C.; Sizemore, E.; et al. Pyrazinamide Safety, Efficacy, and Dosing for Treating Drug-Susceptible Pulmonary Tuberculosis: A Phase 3, Randomized Controlled Clinical Trial. *Am. J. Respir. Crit. Care Med.* **2024**, *210*, 1358–1369. [CrossRef] [PubMed]
48. Kwon, B.S.; Kim, Y.; Lee, S.H.; Lim, S.Y.; Lee, Y.J.; Park, J.S.; Cho, Y.-J.; Yoon, H.I.; Lee, C.-T.; Lee, J.H. The high incidence of severe adverse events due to pyrazinamide in elderly patients with tuberculosis. *PLoS ONE* **2020**, *15*, e0236109. [CrossRef]
49. Lucena, S.D.M.A.; Alberio, C.A.A.; Pinto, A.C.G.; Vieira, J.L.F. Serum pyrazinamide concentrations in patients with pulmonary tuberculosis. *J. Bras. Pneumol.* **2019**, *45*, e20180254. [CrossRef] [PubMed]

50. Putra, O.N.; Purnamasari, T.; Hamami, N.M. Pyrazinamide-induced Hyperuricemia in Pulmonary Tuberculosis Patients. *Int. J. Mycobacteriol.* **2024**, *13*, 282–287. [CrossRef]
51. Datta, A.; Sivasankar, R.; Kar, B.R. Pyrazinamide-induced Toxic Epidermal Necrolysis. *Ann. Afr. Med.* **2024**, *23*, 494–495. [CrossRef] [PubMed]
52. Gerdan, V.; Akkoc, N.; Ucan, E.; Bulac Kir, S. Paradoxical increase in uric acid level with allopurinol use in pyrazinamide-induced hyperuricaemia. *Singap. Med. J.* **2013**, *54*, e125–e126. [CrossRef]
53. Thumamo Pokam, B.; Enoh, J.; Eyo, A.-A.; Umoh, N.; Guemdjom, P. Uric acid levels in patients on antituberculosis drugs in the southwest Region of Cameroon. *Int. J. Mycobacteriol.* **2018**, *7*, 89. [CrossRef]
54. Borisov, S.; Danila, E.; Maryandyshev, A.; Dalcolmo, M.; Miliauskas, S.; Kuksa, L.; Manga, S.; Skrahina, A.; Diktanas, S.; Codecasa, L.R.; et al. Surveillance of adverse events in the treatment of drug-resistant tuberculosis: First global report. *Eur. Respir. J.* **2019**, *54*, 1901522. [CrossRef]
55. Jeong, I.; Park, J.-S.; Cho, Y.-J.; Yoon, H.I.; Song, J.; Lee, C.-T.; Lee, J.-H. Drug-induced Hepatotoxicity of Anti-tuberculosis Drugs and Their Serum Levels. *J. Korean Med. Sci.* **2015**, *30*, 167. [CrossRef]
56. Shin, H.-J.; Yoon, J.-Y.; Na, Y.-O.; Lee, J.-K.; Kho, B.G.; Kim, T.-O.; Kim, Y.-I.; Lim, S.-C.; Jeong, S.-H.; Kwon, Y.-S. Major adverse cardiovascular events and hyperuricemia during tuberculosis treatment. *PLoS ONE* **2023**, *18*, e0294490. [CrossRef]
57. Mohapatra, G.C.; Khan, M.J.; Nayak, S. Incidence of Hyperuricemia and Gouty Arthritis in Patients Taking Pyrazinamide for the Treatment of Tuberculosis. *Ann. Rom. Soc. Cell Biol.* **2021**, *25*, 324–328.
58. Zhang, L.; Zhao, Y.; Gao, Y.; Wu, L.; Gao, R.; Zhang, Q.; Wang, Y.; Wu, C.; Wu, F.; Gurcha, S.S.; et al. Structures of cell wall arabinosyltransferases with the anti-tuberculosis drug ethambutol. *Science* **2020**, *368*, 1211–1219. [CrossRef]
59. Chamberlain, P.D.; Sadaka, A.; Berry, S.; Lee, A.G. Ethambutol optic neuropathy. *Curr. Opin. Ophthalmol.* **2017**, *28*, 545–551. [CrossRef]
60. Peloquin, C.A.; Bulpitt, A.E.; Jaresko, G.S.; Jelliffe, R.W.; Childs, J.M.; Nix, D.E. Pharmacokinetics of Ethambutol under Fasting Conditions, with Food, and with Antacids. *Antimicrob. Agents Chemother.* **1999**, *43*, 568–572. [CrossRef]
61. Singh, A.; Prasad, R.; Balasubramanian, V.; Gupta, N.; Gupta, P. Prevalence of adverse drug reaction with first-line drugs among patients treated for pulmonary tuberculosis. *Clin. Epidemiol. Glob. Health* **2015**, *3*, S80–S90. [CrossRef]
62. Carroll, M.W.; Lee, M.; Cai, Y.; Hallahan, C.W.; Shaw, P.A.; Min, J.H.; Goldfeder, L.C.; Alekseyev, V.; Grinkrug, S.; Kang, H.S.; et al. Frequency of adverse reactions to first- and second-line anti-tuberculosis chemotherapy in a Korean cohort. *Int. J. Tuberc. Lung Dis.* **2012**, *16*, 961–966. [CrossRef]
63. Breen, R.A.M.; Miller, R.F.; Gorsuch, T.; Smith, C.J.; Schwenk, A.; Holmes, W.; Ballinger, J.; Swaden, L.; Johnson, M.A.; Cropley, I.; et al. Adverse events and treatment interruption in tuberculosis patients with and without HIV co-infection. *Thorax* **2006**, *61*, 791–794. [CrossRef]
64. Sivaraj, R.; Umarani, S.; Muralidhar, P.; Parasuraman, S. Revised National Tuberculosis Control Program regimens with and without directly observed treatment, short-course: A comparative study of therapeutic cure rate and adverse reactions. *Perspect. Clin. Res.* **2014**, *5*, 16. [CrossRef] [PubMed]
65. Sant'Anna, F.M.; Araújo-Pereira, M.; Schmaltz, C.A.S.; Arriaga, M.B.; De Oliveira, R.V.C.; Andrade, B.B.; Rolla, V.C. Adverse Drug Reactions Related to Treatment of Drug-Susceptible Tuberculosis in Brazil: A Prospective Cohort Study. *Front. Trop. Dis.* **2022**, *2*, 748310. [CrossRef]
66. Djochie, R.D.A.; Anto, B.P.; Opare-Addo, M.N.A. Determinants of adverse reactions to first-line antitubercular medicines: A prospective cohort study. *J. Pharm. Policy Pract.* **2023**, *16*, 70. [CrossRef]
67. Athira, B.; Manju, C.S.; Jyothi, E. A study on adverse drug reactions to first line antitubercular drugs in DOTS therapy. *Int. J. Pharmacol. Clin. Sci.* **2015**, *4*, 7–11.
68. Chung, S.J.; Byeon, S.; Choi, J.-H. Analysis of Adverse Drug Reactions to First-Line Anti-Tuberculosis Drugs Using the Korea Adverse Event Reporting System. *J. Korean Med. Sci.* **2022**, *37*, e128. [CrossRef]
69. Dorman, S.E.; Nahid, P.; Kurbatova, E.V.; Phillips, P.P.J.; Bryant, K.; Dooley, K.E.; Engle, M.; Goldberg, S.V.; Phan, H.T.T.; Hakim, J.; et al. Four-Month Rifapentine Regimens with or without Moxifloxacin for Tuberculosis. *N. Engl. J. Med.* **2021**, *384*, 1705–1718. [CrossRef] [PubMed]
70. World Health Organization. *WHO Operational Handbook on Tuberculosis Drug-Resistant Tuberculosis Treatment WHO Consolidated Guidelines on Tuberculosis Module 4: Treatment 2022 Update*; World Health Organization: Geneva, Switzerland, 2022.
71. Lesher, G.Y.; Froelich, E.J.; Gruett, M.D.; Bailey, J.H.; Brundage, R.P. 1,8-Naphthyridine Derivatives. A New Class of Chemotherapeutic Agents. *J. Med. Pharm. Chem.* **1962**, *5*, 1063–1065. [CrossRef] [PubMed]
72. Briasoulis, A.; Agarwal, V.; Pierce, W.J. QT Prolongation and Torsade de Pointes Induced by Fluoroquinolones: Infrequent Side Effects from Commonly Used Medications. *Cardiology* **2011**, *120*, 103–110. [CrossRef] [PubMed]

73. European Medicines Agency. *Disabling and Potentially Permanent Side Effects Lead to Suspension or Restrictions of Quinolone and Fluoroquinolone Antibiotics*; European Medicines Agency: Amsterdam, The Netherlands, 2019.
74. Kang, B.H.; Jo, K.-W.; Shim, T.S. Current Status of Fluoroquinolone Use for Treatment of Tuberculosis in a Tertiary Care Hospital in Korea. *Tuberc. Respir. Dis.* **2017**, *80*, 143–152. [CrossRef]
75. Anwar, A.I.; Lu, L.; Plaisance, C.J.; Daniel, C.P.; Flanagan, C.J.; Wenger, D.M.; McGregor, D.; Varrassi, G.; Kaye, A.M.; Ahmadzadeh, S.; et al. Fluoroquinolones: Neurological Complications and Side Effects in Clinical Practice. *Cureus* **2024**, *16*, e54565. [CrossRef]
76. Cho, Y.; Park, H.S. Association of oral ciprofloxacin, levofloxacin, ofloxacin and moxifloxacin with the risk of serious ventricular arrhythmia: A nationwide cohort study in Korea. *BMJ Open* **2018**, *8*, e020974. [CrossRef]
77. Rubinstein, E.; Camm, J. Cardiotoxicity of fluoroquinolones. *J. Antimicrob. Chemother.* **2002**, *49*, 593–596. [CrossRef]
78. Morales, D.R.; Slattery, J.; Pacurariu, A.; Pinheiro, L.; McGettigan, P.; Kurz, X. Relative and Absolute Risk of Tendon Rupture with Fluoroquinolone and Concomitant Fluoroquinolone/Corticosteroid Therapy: Population-Based Nested Case–Control Study. *Clin. Drug Investig.* **2019**, *39*, 205–213. [CrossRef]
79. Lan, Z.; Ahmad, N.; Baghaei, P.; Barkane, L.; Benedetti, A.; Brode, S.K.; Brust, J.C.M.; Campbell, J.R.; Chang, V.W.L.; Falzon, D.; et al. Drug-associated adverse events in the treatment of multidrug-resistant tuberculosis: An individual patient data meta-analysis. *Lancet Respir. Med.* **2020**, *8*, 383–394. [CrossRef] [PubMed]
80. Grosu-Creangă, I.-A.; Trofor, A.C.; Crișan-Dabija, R.A.; Robu-Popa, D.; Ghiciuc, C.M.; Lupușoru, E.C. Adverse effects induced by second-line antituberculosis drugs: An update based on last WHO treatment recommendations for drug-resistant tuberculosis. *Pneumologia* **2021**, *70*, 117–126. [CrossRef]
81. Täubel, J.; Prasad, K.; Rosano, G.; Ferber, G.; Wibberley, H.; Cole, S.T.; Van Langenhoven, L.; Fernandes, S.; Djumanov, D.; Sugiyama, A. Effects of the Fluoroquinolones Moxifloxacin and Levofloxacin on the QT Subintervals: Sex Differences in Ventricular Repolarization. *J. Clin. Pharmacol.* **2020**, *60*, 400–408. [CrossRef]
82. Hashemian, S.M.R.; Farhadi, T.; Ganjparvar, M. Linezolid: A review of its properties, function, and use in critical care. *Drug Des. Devel. Ther.* **2018**, *12*, 1759–1767. [CrossRef] [PubMed]
83. Vinh, D.C.; Rubinstein, E. Linezolid: A review of safety and tolerability. *J. Infect.* **2009**, *59*, S59–S74. [CrossRef]
84. Zou, F.; Cui, Z.; Lou, S.; Ou, Y.; Zhu, C.; Shu, C.; Chen, J.; Zhao, R.; Wu, Z.; Wang, L.; et al. Adverse drug events associated with linezolid administration: A real-world pharmacovigilance study from 2004 to 2023 using the FAERS database. *Front. Pharmacol.* **2024**, *15*, 1338902. [CrossRef] [PubMed]
85. Sotgiu, G.; Centis, R.; D'Ambrosio, L.; Alffenaar, J.-W.C.; Anger, H.A.; Caminero, J.A.; Castiglia, P.; De Lorenzo, S.; Ferrara, G.; Koh, W.-J.; et al. Efficacy, safety and tolerability of linezolid containing regimens in treating MDR-TB and XDR-TB: Systematic review and meta-analysis. *Eur. Respir. J.* **2012**, *40*, 1430–1442. [CrossRef]
86. Gopal, M.; Padayatchi, N.; Metcalfe, J.Z.; O'Donnell, M.R. Systematic review of clofazimine for the treatment of drug-resistant tuberculosis. *Int. J. Tuberc. Lung Dis.* **2013**, *17*, 1001–1007. [CrossRef]
87. Gupta, A.; Kumar, V.; Natarajan, S.; Singla, R. Adverse drug reactions & drug interactions in MDR-TB patients. *Indian J. Tuberc.* **2020**, *67*, S69–S78. [CrossRef]
88. Murray, J.F.; Schraufnagel, D.E.; Hopewell, P.C. Treatment of Tuberculosis. A Historical Perspective. *Ann. Am. Thorac. Soc.* **2015**, *12*, 1749–1759. [CrossRef]
89. Arbiser, J.L.; Moschella, S.L. Clofazimine: A review of its medical uses and mechanisms of action. *J. Am. Acad. Dermatol.* **1995**, *32*, 241–247. [CrossRef]
90. Grant, S.S.; Kaufmann, B.B.; Chand, N.S.; Haseley, N.; Hung, D.T. Eradication of bacterial persisters with antibiotic-generated hydroxyl radicals. *Proc. Natl. Acad. Sci. USA* **2012**, *109*, 12147–12152. [CrossRef]
91. Reddy, V.M.; O'Sullivan, J.F.; Gangadharam, P.R. Antimycobacterial activities of riminophenazines. *J. Antimicrob. Chemother.* **1999**, *43*, 615–623. [CrossRef] [PubMed]
92. Parak, R.B.; Wadee, A.A. The synergistic effects of gamma interferon and clofazimine on phagocyte function: Restoration of inhibition due to a 25 kilodalton fraction from Mycobacterium tuberculosis. *Biotherapy* **1991**, *3*, 265–272. [CrossRef]
93. Wadee, A.A.; Anderson, R.; Rabson, A.R. Clofazimine reverses the inhibitory effect of Mycobacterium tuberculosis derived factors on phagocyte intracellular killing mechanisms. *J. Antimicrob. Chemother.* **1988**, *21*, 65–74. [CrossRef] [PubMed]
94. Murashov, M.D.; LaLone, V.; Rzeczycki, P.M.; Keswani, R.K.; Yoon, G.S.; Sud, S.; Rajeswaran, W.; Larsen, S.; Stringer, K.A.; Rosania, G.R. The Physicochemical Basis of Clofazimine-Induced Skin Pigmentation. *J. Investig. Dermatol.* **2018**, *138*, 697–703. [CrossRef]
95. Stadler, J.A.M.; Maartens, G.; Meintjes, G.; Wasserman, S. Clofazimine for the treatment of tuberculosis. *Front. Pharmacol.* **2023**, *14*, 1100488. [CrossRef] [PubMed]
96. Moore, V.J. A review of side-effects experienced by patients taking clofazimine. *Lepr. Rev.* **1983**, *54*, 327–335. [CrossRef]

97. Lin, C.-J.; Chen, J.-H.; Chien, S.-T.; Huang, Y.-W.; Lin, C.-B.; Lee, J.-J.; Lee, C.-H.; Yu, M.-C.; Chiang, C.-Y. Clofazimine and QT prolongation in the treatment of rifampicin-resistant tuberculosis: Findings of aDSM in Taiwan. *J. Microbiol. Immunol. Infect.* **2024**, *57*, 791–800. [CrossRef]
98. Lambert, M.P.; Neuhaus, F.C. Mechanism of D-Cycloserine Action: Alanine Racemase from *Escherichia coli* W. *J. Bacteriol.* **1972**, *110*, 978–987. [CrossRef]
99. Van Der Laan, L.E.; Garcia-Prats, A.J.; McIlleron, H.; Abdelwahab, M.T.; Winckler, J.L.; Draper, H.R.; Wiesner, L.; Schaaf, H.S.; Hesseling, A.C.; Denti, P. Optimizing dosing of the cycloserine pro-drug terizidone in children with rifampicin-resistant tuberculosis. *Antimicrob. Agents Chemother.* **2023**, *67*, e00611-23. [CrossRef] [PubMed]
100. Schade, S.; Paulus, W. D-Cycloserine in Neuropsychiatric Diseases: A Systematic Review. *Int. J. Neuropsychopharmacol.* **2016**, *19*, pyv102. [CrossRef]
101. Li, Y.; Wang, F.; Wu, L.; Zhu, M.; He, G.; Chen, X.; Sun, F.; Liu, Q.; Wang, X.; Zhang, W. Cycloserine for treatment of multidrug-resistant tuberculosis: A retrospective cohort study in China. *Infect. Drug Resist.* **2019**, *12*, 721–731. [CrossRef] [PubMed]
102. Hwang, T.J.; Wares, D.F.; Jafarov, A.; Jakubowiak, W.; Nunn, P.; Keshavjee, S. Safety of cycloserine and terizidone for the treatment of drug-resistant tuberculosis: A meta-analysis. *Int. J. Tuberc. Lung Dis.* **2013**, *17*, 1257–1266. [CrossRef]
103. Wang, J.; Pang, Y.; Jing, W.; Chen, W.; Guo, R.; Han, X.; Wu, L.; Yang, G.; Yang, K.; Chen, C.; et al. Efficacy and safety of cycloserine-containing regimens in the treatment of multidrug-resistant tuberculosis: A nationwide retrospective cohort study in China. *Infect. Drug Resist.* **2019**, *12*, 763–770. [CrossRef]
104. Court, R.; Centner, C.M.; Chirehwa, M.; Wiesner, L.; Denti, P.; De Vries, N.; Harding, J.; Gumbo, T.; Maartens, G.; McIlleron, H. Neuropsychiatric toxicity and cycloserine concentrations during treatment for multidrug-resistant tuberculosis. *Int. J. Infect. Dis.* **2021**, *105*, 688–694. [CrossRef]
105. Papp-Wallace, K.M.; Endimiani, A.; Taracila, M.A.; Bonomo, R.A. Carbapenems: Past, present, and future. *Antimicrob. Agents Chemother.* **2011**, *55*, 4943–4960. [CrossRef]
106. Hugonnet, J.-E.; Tremblay, L.W.; Boshoff, H.I.; Barry, C.E.; Blanchard, J.S. Meropenem-Clavulanate Is Effective Against Extensively Drug-Resistant *Mycobacterium tuberculosis*. *Science* **2009**, *323*, 1215–1218. [CrossRef] [PubMed]
107. Armstrong, T.; Fenn, S.J.; Hardie, K.R. JMM Profile: Carbapenems: A broad-spectrum antibiotic: This article is part of the JMM Profiles collection. *J. Med. Microbiol.* **2021**, *70*, 001462. [CrossRef]
108. Sotgiu, G.; D'Ambrosio, L.; Centis, R.; Tiberi, S.; Esposito, S.; Dore, S.; Spanevello, A.; Migliori, G. Carbapenems to Treat Multidrug and Extensively Drug-Resistant Tuberculosis: A Systematic Review. *Int. J. Mol. Sci.* **2016**, *17*, 373. [CrossRef]
109. Ramirez, M.S.; Tolmasky, M.E. Amikacin: Uses, Resistance, and Prospects for Inhibition. *Molecules* **2017**, *22*, 2267. [CrossRef] [PubMed]
110. Guthrie, O.W. Aminoglycoside induced ototoxicity. *Toxicology* **2008**, *249*, 91–96. [CrossRef] [PubMed]
111. Wargo, K.A.; Edwards, J.D. Aminoglycoside-Induced Nephrotoxicity. *J. Pharm. Pract.* **2014**, *27*, 573–577. [CrossRef]
112. Riddell, R.W.; Stewart, M.; Somner, A.R. Ethionamide. *BMJ* **1960**, *2*, 1207–1208. [CrossRef]
113. Tan, Y.; Su, B.; Zheng, H.; Song, Y.; Wang, Y.; Pang, Y. Molecular Characterization of Prothionamide-Resistant Mycobacterium tuberculosis Isolates in Southern China. *Front. Microbiol.* **2017**, *8*, 2358. [CrossRef]
114. Wang, F.; Langley, R.; Gulten, G.; Dover, L.G.; Besra, G.S.; Jacobs, W.R.; Sacchettini, J.C. Mechanism of thioamide drug action against tuberculosis and leprosy. *J. Exp. Med.* **2007**, *204*, 73–78. [CrossRef]
115. Zheng, J.; Rubin, E.J.; Bifani, P.; Mathys, V.; Lim, V.; Au, M.; Jang, J.; Nam, J.; Dick, T.; Walker, J.R.; et al. para-Aminosalicylic acid is a prodrug targeting dihydrofolate reductase in Mycobacterium tuberculosis. *J. Biol. Chem.* **2013**, *288*, 23447–23456. [CrossRef] [PubMed]
116. Heo, J.; Koh, D.; Woo, M.; Kwon, D.; De Almeida Falcão, V.C.; Wood, C.; Lee, H.; Kim, K.; Choi, I.; Jang, J.; et al. A combination screening to identify enhancers of para-aminosalicylic acid against Mycobacterium tuberculosis. *Sci. Rep.* **2022**, *12*, 5635. [CrossRef] [PubMed]
117. Macgregor, A.G.; Somner, A.R. The AntiThyroid Action of Para-Aminosalicylic Acid. *Lancet* **1954**, *264*, 931–936. [CrossRef]
118. Abulfathi, A.A.; Donald, P.R.; Adams, K.; Svensson, E.M.; Diacon, A.H.; Reuter, H. The pharmacokinetics of para-aminosalicylic acid and its relationship to efficacy and intolerance. *Br. J. Clin. Pharmacol.* **2020**, *86*, 2123–2132. [CrossRef]
119. Mitchell, R.S. Study of para-aminosalicylic acid intolerance in tuberculosis of lung. *J. Am. Med. Assoc.* **1954**, *156*, 124. [CrossRef] [PubMed]
120. Donald, P.R.; Diacon, A.H. Para-aminosalicylic acid: The return of an old friend. *Lancet Infect. Dis.* **2015**, *15*, 1091–1099. [CrossRef] [PubMed]
121. Boman, G. Serum concentration and half-life of rifampicin after simultaneous oral administration of aminosalicylic acid or isoniazid. *Eur. J. Clin. Pharmacol.* **1974**, *7*, 217–225. [CrossRef]

122. Parvez, M.M.; Shin, H.J.; Jung, J.A.; Shin, J.-G. Evaluation of *para* -Aminosalicylic Acid as a Substrate of Multiple Solute Carrier Uptake Transporters and Possible Drug Interactions with Nonsteroidal Anti-inflammatory Drugs *In Vitro*. *Antimicrob. Agents Chemother.* **2017**, *61*, e02392-16. [CrossRef]
123. Khoshnood, S.; Goudarzi, M.; Taki, E.; Darbandi, A.; Kouhsari, E.; Heidary, M.; Motahar, M.; Moradi, M.; Bazyar, H. Bedaquiline: Current status and future perspectives. *J. Glob. Antimicrob. Resist.* **2021**, *25*, 48–59. [CrossRef]
124. Kundu, S.; Biukovic, G.; Grüber, G.; Dick, T. Bedaquiline Targets the ε Subunit of Mycobacterial F-ATP Synthase. *Antimicrob. Agents Chemother.* **2016**, *60*, 6977–6979. [CrossRef] [PubMed]
125. Chahine, E.B.; Karaoui, L.R.; Mansour, H. Bedaquiline: A Novel Diarylquinoline for Multidrug-Resistant Tuberculosis. *Ann. Pharmacother.* **2014**, *48*, 107–115. [CrossRef]
126. Sarathy, J.P.; Gruber, G.; Dick, T. Re-Understanding the Mechanisms of Action of the Anti-Mycobacterial Drug Bedaquiline. *Antibiotics* **2019**, *8*, 261. [CrossRef]
127. Wu, J.; Pan, H.; Shen, L.; Zhao, M. Assessing the safety of bedaquiline: Insight from adverse event reporting system analysis. *Front. Pharmacol.* **2024**, *15*, 1382441. [CrossRef]
128. Isralls, S.; Baisley, K.; Ngam, E.; Grant, A.D.; Millard, J. QT Interval Prolongation in People Treated With Bedaquiline for Drug-Resistant Tuberculosis Under Programmatic Conditions: A Retrospective Cohort Study. *Open Forum Infect. Dis.* **2021**, *8*, ofab413. [CrossRef]
129. Ur Rehman, O.; Fatima, E.; Ali, A.; Akram, U.; Nashwan, A.; Yunus, F. Efficacy and safety of bedaquiline containing regimens in patients of drug-resistant tuberculosis: An updated systematic review and meta-analysis. *J. Clin. Tuberc. Mycobact. Dis.* **2024**, *34*, 100405. [CrossRef] [PubMed]
130. Guglielmetti, L.; Jaspard, M.; Le Dû, D.; Lachâtre, M.; Marigot-Outtandy, D.; Bernard, C.; Veziris, N.; Robert, J.; Yazdanpanah, Y.; Caumes, E.; et al. Long-term outcome and safety of prolonged bedaquiline treatment for multidrug-resistant tuberculosis. *Eur. Respir. J.* **2017**, *49*, 1601799. [CrossRef]
131. Liu, Y.; Matsumoto, M.; Ishida, H.; Ohguro, K.; Yoshitake, M.; Gupta, R.; Geiter, L.; Hafkin, J. Delamanid: From discovery to its use for pulmonary multidrug-resistant tuberculosis (MDR-TB). *Tuberculosis* **2018**, *111*, 20–30. [CrossRef]
132. Gler, M.T.; Skripconoka, V.; Sanchez-Garavito, E.; Xiao, H.; Cabrera-Rivero, J.L.; Vargas-Vasquez, D.E.; Gao, M.; Awad, M.; Park, S.-K.; Shim, T.S.; et al. Delamanid for Multidrug-Resistant Pulmonary Tuberculosis. *N. Engl. J. Med.* **2012**, *366*, 2151–2160. [CrossRef] [PubMed]
133. Brigden, G.; Hewison, C.; Varaine, F. New developments in the treatment of drug-resistant tuberculosis: Clinical utility of bedaquiline and delamanid. *Infect. Drug Resist.* **2015**, *8*, 367–378. [CrossRef] [PubMed]
134. Rice, A.M.; Long, Y.; King, S.B. Nitroaromatic Antibiotics as Nitrogen Oxide Sources. *Biomolecules* **2021**, *11*, 267. [CrossRef]
135. Khoshnood, S.; Taki, E.; Sadeghifard, N.; Kaviar, V.H.; Haddadi, M.H.; Farshadzadeh, Z.; Kouhsari, E.; Goudarzi, M.; Heidary, M. Mechanism of Action, Resistance, Synergism, and Clinical Implications of Delamanid Against Multidrug-Resistant Mycobacterium tuberculosis. *Front. Microbiol.* **2021**, *12*, 717045. [CrossRef]
136. Stancil, S.L.; Mirzayev, F.; Abdel-Rahman, S.M. Profiling Pretomanid as a Therapeutic Option for TB Infection: Evidence to Date. *Drug Des. Devel. Ther.* **2021**, *15*, 2815–2830. [CrossRef]
137. Occhineri, S.; Matucci, T.; Rindi, L.; Tiseo, G.; Falcone, M.; Riccardi, N.; Besozzi, G. Pretomanid for tuberculosis treatment: An update for clinical purposes. *Curr. Res. Pharmacol. Drug Discov.* **2022**, *3*, 100128. [CrossRef]
138. Fekadu, G.; Tolossa, T.; Turi, E.; Bekele, F.; Fetensa, G. Pretomanid development and its clinical roles in treating tuberculosis. *J. Glob. Antimicrob. Resist.* **2022**, *31*, 175–184. [CrossRef]
139. Deb, U.; Biswas, S. Pretomanid: The latest USFDA-approved anti-tuberculosis drug. *Indian J. Tuberc.* **2021**, *68*, 287–291. [CrossRef] [PubMed]
140. Conradie, F.; Diacon, A.H.; Ngubane, N.; Howell, P.; Everitt, D.; Crook, A.M.; Mendel, C.M.; Egizi, E.; Moreira, J.; Timm, J.; et al. Treatment of Highly Drug-Resistant Pulmonary Tuberculosis. *N. Engl. J. Med.* **2020**, *382*, 893–902. [CrossRef] [PubMed]
141. Nedelman, J.R.; Salinger, D.H.; Subramoney, V.; Woolson, R.; Wade, K.; Li, M.; Everitt, D.; Mendel, C.M.; Spigelman, M. An Exposure-Response Perspective on the Clinical Dose of Pretomanid. *Antimicrob. Agents Chemother.* **2020**, *65*, e01121-20. [CrossRef] [PubMed]
142. Nyang'wa, B.-T.; Berry, C.; Kazounis, E.; Motta, I.; Parpieva, N.; Tigay, Z.; Solodovnikova, V.; Liverko, I.; Moodliar, R.; Dodd, M.; et al. A 24-Week, All-Oral Regimen for Rifampin-Resistant Tuberculosis. *N. Engl. J. Med.* **2022**, *387*, 2331–2343. [CrossRef]

medicina

MDPI

Review

Alternaria Allergy and Asthma in Children

Angela Klain [1], Mattia Giovannini [2,3,*], Stefania Arasi [4], Simona Barni [2], Riccardo Castagnoli [5,6], Lucia Caminiti [7], Mariannita Gelsomino [8], Lucia Liotti [9], Carla Mastrorilli [10], Francesca Mori [2], Luca Pecoraro [11], Francesca Saretta [12], Michele Miraglia del Giudice [1] and Elio Novembre [2,3]

[1] Department of Woman, Child and General and Specialized Surgery, University of Campania Luigi Vanvitelli, 80138 Naples, Italy; angela.klain@studenti.unicampania.it (A.K.); michele.miragliadelgiudice@unicampania.it (M.M.d.G.)
[2] Allergy Unit, Meyer Children's Hospital IRCCS, 50139 Florence, Italy; simona.barni@meyer.it (S.B.); francesca.mori@meyer.it (F.M.); elio.novembre@unifi.it (E.N.)
[3] Department of Health Sciences, University of Florence, 50139 Florence, Italy
[4] Translational Research in Pediatric Specialties Area, Division of Allergy, Bambino Gesù Children's Hospital, IRCCS, 00165 Rome, Italy; stefania.arasi@opbg.net
[5] Department of Clinical, Surgical, Diagnostic and Pediatric Sciences, University of Pavia, 27100 Pavia, Italy; riccardo.castagnoli@unipv.it
[6] Pediatric Clinic, Fondazione IRCCS Policlinico San Matteo, 27100 Pavia, Italy
[7] Pediatric Unit, Department of Human Pathology in Adult and Development Age "Gaetano Barresi", Allergy Unit, AOU Policlinico Gaetano Martino, 98124 Messina, Italy; lcaminiti@unime.it
[8] Pediatric Allergy Unit, Department of Life Sciences and Public Health, University Foundation Policlinico Gemelli IRCCS, Catholic University of the Sacred Heart, 00168 Rome, Italy; mariannita.gelsomino@guest.policlinicogemelli.it
[9] Pediatric Unit, Department of Mother and Child Health, Salesi Children's Hospital, 60123 Ancona, Italy; lucialiotti@ospedaliriuniti.marche.it
[10] Pediatric Hospital Giovanni XXIII, Pediatric and Emergency Department, AOU Policlinic of Bari, 70126 Bari, Italy; carla.mastrorilli@policlinico.ba.it
[11] Pediatric Unit, Ospedale Vito Fazzi, ASL Lecce, 73100 Lecce, Italy
[12] Pediatric Department, Latisana-Palmanova Hospital, Azienda Sanitaria Universitaria Friuli Centrale, 33100 Udine, Italy; francesca.saretta@asufc.sanita.fvg.it
* Correspondence: mattiag88@hotmail.it

Abstract: *Alternaria alternata* is one of the most clinically relevant fungal allergens in pediatric patients with respiratory allergies. Sensitization to this mold has increased in recent decades and is influenced by environmental exposure, geographic location, climate change, and genetic predisposition. In children, *Alternaria* spp. are strongly associated with the development and worsening of asthma and allergic rhinitis, often contributing to severe and difficult-to-control forms of the disease. The major allergen, Alt a 1, plays a central role in the immunopathogenesis of *Alternaria*-induced allergies and exhibits molecular features that allow cross-reactivity with other fungal species. Although *Alternaria* allergy is clinically relevant, its diagnosis remains challenging due to the variability and lack of standardization of fungal extracts. Therefore, it may be necessary to complement traditional diagnostic tools, such as skin prick testing and specific IgE measurement, with component-resolved diagnostics or, in selected cases, nasal provocation tests. Allergen immunotherapy (AIT) has shown promising results in the treatment of *Alternaria* allergy, particularly with the use of standardized Alt a 1-based extracts or chemically modified allergoids, which offer clinical benefits and immunological modulation. However, AIT is still underused in this context, partly because of the lack of widely available commercial products and long-term efficacy data in the pediatric population. This review provides a comprehensive overview of the current knowledge on the epidemiology, mechanisms, clinical implications, and treatment options related to *Alternaria* allergy in children, with the aim of supporting early recognition and tailored therapeutic strategies for this important, yet often underestimated, allergen.

 https://doi.org/10.3390/medicina61091639

Keywords: *Alternaria*; *Alternaria alternata*; pediatric asthma; mold allergy; Alt a 1; allergen immunotherapy; component-resolved diagnostics

1. Introduction

Fungi are a broad kingdom that includes various organisms such as yeasts, mushrooms, and molds. Molds are a specific multicellular type of fungi characterized by their fuzzy, filamentous appearance. They typically thrive on decaying organic matter and reproduce through spores, which can be spread through air or water. They can cause diseases via three main mechanisms: direct infection (mycoses), allergic reactions, and toxin production [1]. Fungi are increasingly being recognized as important contributors to the human exposome, the totality of environmental and biological exposures that influence health. They are present both externally, in outdoor and indoor environments, and internally, as part of the microbiome known as the microbiota, with considerable differences in their composition and health impact [2,3].

Molds are widespread in the environment; however, only a few hundred species act as opportunistic pathogens. Approximately 80 fungal genera induce type I IgE-mediated allergies, leading to conditions such as allergic rhinitis (AR) and asthma [4–6]. The most allergenic fungi belong to *Ascomycota* (e.g., *Alternaria*, *Cladosporium*, *Aspergillus*, *Penicillium*), followed by *Basidiomycota* (e.g., *Malassezia*) and *Zygomycota*. Other notable allergens include *Candida*, *Fusarium*, and *Rhizopus* [7].

Alternaria and *Cladosporium* are major outdoor allergens that disseminate in warm and dry air. Xerophilic species of *Aspergillus* and *Penicillium*, especially those found in indoor environments, contribute to allergic diseases by colonizing the respiratory tract [1]. Unlike pollen grains, *Alternaria* spores are much smaller, typically 3–8 μm in diameter, and can remain airborne for extended periods, allowing them to reach the lower airways upon inhalation [8]. Furthermore, the fungal spore season typically lasts twice as long as the pollen season, prolonging the risk of exposure for sensitized individuals. Despite their lower prevalence in ambient air than other fungal taxa, *Alternaria* spores have been shown to elicit the highest sensitization rates among atopic individuals and are strongly associated with asthma exacerbation, especially in children and during thunderstorm asthma events. Their small size, high allergenic potential, and prolonged presence in the air underline the importance of considering *Alternaria* spp. separately from pollen in allergy assessments and environmental control strategies [8].

Environmental prophylaxis is fundamental in the management of patients with mold allergies. Recommended measures include controlling the indoor moisture through proper building design and maintenance, repairing leaks, using dehumidifiers, and ensuring adequate ventilation. It is also advised to remove mold-contaminated materials, avoid wall-to-wall carpeting in damp areas, and maintain an indoor relative humidity of 30–50% [9,10].

2. Molds and *Alternaria* Sensitization

The prevalence of mold sensitization varies depending on environmental exposure and geographic location. A large-scale analysis conducted by a nationwide clinical laboratory in the United States assessed fungal sensitization in 1651,203 patients aged 0–85 y. Testing for 17 different fungal species indicated that 22% of patients had detectable specific IgE levels (>0.10 kUA/L) for at least one fungal allergen, whereas 13.7% showed sensitivity to more than two fungal allergens. The prevalence of sensitization varied by species, ranging from 7.4% to 18.6%, with the highest rates observed for *Candida albicans* (18.6%), *A. alternata* (16.6%), *Stemphylium herbarum* (14.9%), and *Aspergillus fumigatus* (14.2%). Overall, fungal sensitization is more common in urban areas and regions dominated by grasslands and prairies than in forested and woodland environments [11]. According to skin test results, the estimated prevalence of mold sensitization in Europe is approximately 5%, and *A. alternata* is one of the most common mold allergens in both adults and children [12–14]. Data on the general population are limited as most of the available evidence originates from allergy centers that monitor atopic individuals and/or patients with respiratory diseases. In a study by Mari et al. [15], 19.1% of 4962 patients aged 3–80 y with respiratory allergies were sensitized to at least one fungal species. *Alternaria* had the highest sensitization rate at 66.1%, followed by *Candida* (44.3%), *Trichophyton* (10.2%), *Aspergillus* (12.6%), *Cladosporium* (13.1%), *Penicillium* (8.1%), and *Saccharomyces* (7.4%) [15].

At the beginning of the 2000s, the European Community Respiratory Health Survey (ECRHS), which included 37 centers in 17 countries and approximately 11,355 adults, reported that sensitization to *Alternaria* among adults ranged from 0.2% to 14.4%, whereas *Cladosporium* sensitization varied between 0% and 11.9% [16,17].

In 2009, the Global Asthma and Allergy European Network (GA2LEN) conducted a multicenter, open-label study to assess clinically significant sensitization rates to various allergens across 14 European countries. The study included 3034 adults and children, with a median age of 33 y, suspected of having allergic conditions such as AR, asthma, atopic dermatitis, and food allergies. The prevalence of *Alternaria* sensitization varied across European countries. On a continental scale, the overall sensitization rate in Europe was 8.9% (95% CI: 7.9–9.9). However, substantial regional differences were reported. Greece had the highest prevalence of *Alternaria* sensitization (23.8%), followed by Germany (10.6%), Finland, and France (10.3%). Denmark reported a prevalence of 8.2%, whereas Austria and Hungary reported a prevalence of 6.5%. Belgium recorded 6.2%. At the lower end, the Netherlands, Portugal, and Switzerland had 5.5%, whereas Italy and Poland reported one of the lowest rates at 3.5%. The United Kingdom had the lowest prevalence at only 0.8% [18].

Of 2942 patients from 20 allergology centers in Italy, 10.4% showed sensitivity to *Alternaria*, although the rates varied widely between regions, from 1.8% in Turin to 29.3% in Cagliari. Of those sensitized, 79.7% had rhinitis and 53.3% had asthma. Only 12.1% of *Alternaria*-positive patients were monosensitized, whereas the majority also reacted to other allergens. Sensitization was more common in younger individuals, particularly those under 30 y, with a higher occurrence in males [19]. Similar results were observed in a 2021 study in Spain, in which data from 1156 patients recruited from 15 allergy departments across different bioclimatic regions were analyzed. The results showed that 20.2% of patients were sensitized to at least one of the five fungi tested, with *A. alternata* being the most common; sensitization was more prevalent in children (69.8%) and males (63%); most patients were also polysensitized to other allergens; regional differences were noted, with the highest prevalence observed in the Continental region and the lowest in the Oceanic region [20].

Sensitization to *A. alternata* has been reported in other parts of the world, with prevalence rates varying across populations. In Lima, Peru, 7% of the general adult population were sensitized to *A. alternata* [21]. In Africa, in an urban Gabonese population, 15% of 54 patients sensitized to inhalant allergens tested positive for *Alternaria* [22]. In Iran, a study of 1006 allergic patients found a sensitization rate of 5.3%, whereas in China, the prevalence rates were higher, with 14.9% of 397 asthmatic children showing sensitization, and an even greater rate of 44.9% among 1625 patients with AR [23,24]. Similarly, in Samara,

Russia, 42.2% of 249 children diagnosed with AR and allergic asthma were sensitized to this mold [25] (Table 1).

Table 1. Reported prevalence rates of sensitization to *Alternaria alternata* in various countries and regions. Data reflect studies conducted in general populations or among patients with respiratory allergies, highlighting substantial geographic variability.

Country/Region	Prevalence (%)
USA	16.6% [11]
Europe	~5% (confirmed by skin tests) [12–14]
Greece	23.8% among allergic patients [18]
Germany	10.6% among allergic patients [18]
Finland	10.3% among allergic patients [18]
France	10.3% among allergic patients [18]
Denmark	8.2% among allergic patients [18]
Austria	6.5% among allergic patients [18]
Hungary	6.5% among allergic patients [18]
Belgium	6.2% among allergic patients [18]
Netherlands	5.5% among allergic patients [18]
Portugal	5.5% among allergic patients [18]
Switzerland	5.5% among allergic patients [18]
Italy	3.5% among allergic patients [18]; 10.4% among allergic patients [19]
Poland	3.5% among allergic patients [18]
United Kingdom	0.8% among allergic patients [18]
Spain	20.2% among allergic patients [20]
Peru (Lima)	7% [21]
Gabon (Africa)	15% [22]
Iran	5.3% among allergic patients [23]
China (asthmatic children)	14.9% (with asthma) 44.9% (with AR) [24]
Samara (Russia)	42.2% (children with AR and asthma) [25]

AR: allergic rhinitis.

2.1. Alternaria Characteristics and Allergens

The genus *Alternaria* comprises more than 300 fungal species. The most frequently and widely distributed *Alternaria* species is *A. alternata*, a ubiquitous filamentous fungus belonging to the *Pleosporaceae* family within the *Pleosporales* order. *Alternaria alternata* is a highly adaptable fungus with diverse roles as a saprophyte, plant pathogen, and human allergen [26]. It forms fast-growing black-pigmented colonies due to melanin synthesis, which enhances its resistance to environmental stressors and contributes to its survival and pathogenicity. *Alternaria alternata* produces various secondary metabolites, including mycotoxins, such as tenuazonic acid, alternariol, and alternariol monomethyl ether, which have been implicated in food contamination and pose potential health risks to humans and animals [26,27]. The fungus reproduces asexually via large, elongated, and transversely septate conidia that are produced in chains on the conidiophores [26]. These spores are efficiently dispersed under warm, dry, and windy conditions, reaching peak concentrations in late summer and early autumn, particularly in temperate regions [27].

Typically, airborne outdoor *Alternaria* spores can be detected from May to November, with an allergenic threshold of 100 spores/m^3 [1,28]. Their concentrations are influenced by climate change, with rising temperatures and shifting weather patterns, potentially leading to higher airborne spore levels and extended seasons [28]. A 52-y study in England (1970–2021) indicated a strong link between rising seasonal temperatures and a 44% increase in *Alternaria* spore concentrations. A 1 °C pre-season rise caused a 2% earlier start. The authors suggest that by 2070, projected temperature increases (+1.3 °C to +5.1 °C) could further elevate *Alternaria* levels [29]. Similar findings were reported in a study conducted in Germany, where *Alternaria* sensitization rose substantially from 8.6% (1998–2007) to 11.7% (2008–2017), with a higher prevalence among younger individuals [30]. In contrast, in Korea, over 25 y (1998–2022) there has been a substantial decline in *Alternaria* spore concentrations due to increased rainfall over short periods, leading to longer dry seasons that limit fungal sporulation. Consequently, both spore concentrations and sensitization rates to *Alternaria* spp. decreased [31]. This tendency was also highlighted in Mexico, where over 11 y, *Alternaria* sensitization dropped from 21.4% in 2004 to 14.4% in 2015—a 7% reduction. In contrast, sensitization to other fungi, such as *Candida* and *Penicillium*, has increased [32]. These data suggest limited *Alternaria* adaptation to climate shifts, particularly compared to more adaptable pollen types.

Although *Alternaria* is primarily found outdoors, it can also colonize indoor environments with high humidity, such as damp walls, carpets, and poorly ventilated buildings, contributing to allergic sensitization and "sick building syndrome," which refers to clinical manifestations (headaches, fatigue, and respiratory problems) experienced by building occupants, often due to poor indoor air quality [26,33]. The "Inner-City Asthma Study" analyzed airborne fungal exposure in mold-sensitive children with asthma living in urban areas in the United States. Fungal concentrations were measured in and around 414 homes across seven urban communities; common fungi, such as *Cladosporium*, *Penicillium*, *Aspergillus*, and *Alternaria*, were found. The study showed a strong correlation between indoor and outdoor fungal levels, with 50.5% of outdoor and 30.9% of indoor samples containing *Alternaria* spores. Outdoor spores substantially affected indoor air quality, as indoor fungal concentrations were moderately correlated with outdoor levels ($r = 0.32$, $p < 0.0001$). Homes with moisture issues had 1.9-times higher odds of elevated *Alternaria* levels, whereas cockroach-infested homes had 3.3-times higher odds of increased *Aspergillus* spores. Pet ownership, especially cats, was associated with a 2.3-fold increase in total fungal concentration. Conversely, homes with forced-air heating had 60% lower odds of high fungal levels, and winter sampling reduced *Aspergillus* and *Penicillium* concentrations by 50% [34]. In a study by Soffer et al., *A. alternata* was found in 85% of children's homes in New York City, with higher levels associated with carpeting, wet mopping, and lower-income neighborhoods [35]. Baxi et al. investigated mold exposure in inner-city school classrooms attended by children with asthma. Airborne mold spores were measured in 180 classrooms across 12 schools, indicating the presence of mold in all classrooms, but with substantial variability in concentration and diversity between rooms within the same school. The most commonly detected mold types included *Cladosporium* and *Aspergillus*. *Alternaria* was found in 29% of the classrooms, with higher concentrations observed in rooms with visible mildew. Seasonal variations were also noted, with higher mold concentrations in the fall, highlighting the potential influence of environmental factors on mold growth in classrooms [36]. *Alternaria alternata* is the most common species in the *Alternaria* genus. A total of 16 allergens of *A. alternata* were identified (Alt 1, Alt 3, Alt 4, Alt 5, Alt 6, Alt 7, Alt 8, Alt 10, Alt 12, Alt 13, Alt 14 and Alt 15, Alt a 2, Alt a 9, Alt a NTF2 and Alt a TCTP). However, the World Health Organization (WHO)/International Union of Immunological Societies (IUIS) Allergen Nomenclature Subcommittee includes the first 14 molecules [7,37,38].

Alternaria allergens have various functions and exhibit high cross-reactivity with multiple allergens, including those from both fungal and non-fungal sources. Alt a 1, a major fungal protein of unknown function, shows structural similarities to allergens from *A. brassicola* (Alt b 1), *Ulocladium chartarum* (Ulo c 1), *Embellisia allii* (Emb a 1), *Nimbya celosiae* (Nim c 1), *Sinomyces fusoideus* (Sin fu 1), and *Stemphylium botryosum* (Ste b 1). Minor allergens, such as heat shock proteins (Alt a 3), ribosomal proteins (Alt a 5, 12), enolases (Alt a 6), glutathione transferases (Alt a 13), vacuolar serine protease (Alt a 15), and manganese superoxide dismutase (Alt a 14) exhibit cross-reactivity with homologous proteins from *Penicillium*, *Aspergillus*, *Cladosporium*, *Curvularia*, *Rhodotorula*, and *Malassezia* [7,27,39]. Moreover, Alt a 6, previously known as Alt a 5, shows cross-sensitivity with Hev b 9, the enolase of latex [40] (Table 2). The strong cross-reactivity of *Alternaria* allergens with multiple fungal species is responsible for polysensitization, leading to broader allergic responses and diagnostic challenges, and limiting the efficacy of allergen-specific immunotherapy (AIT).

Table 2. Summary of major and minor *Alternaria alternata* allergens, their functions, and molecular weights.

Allergen	Protein Type/Biological Function	MW (kDa)	Clinical Relevance
Alt a 1	Dimeric β-barrel protein, fungus-specific	15.3/16.4	Major allergen
Alt a 3	Heat shock protein 70	85	Minor allergen
Alt a 4	Disulfide isomerase	57	Minor allergen
Alt a 5	Ribosomal protein P2	11	Minor allergen
Alt a 6	Enolase	45	Minor allergen
Alt a 7	Flavodoxin-like YCP1 protein	22	Minor allergen
Alt a 8	Mannitol dehydrogenase	29	Minor allergen
Alt a 10	Aldehyde dehydrogenase	53	Minor allergen
Alt a 12	Acidic ribosomal protein P1	11	Minor allergen
Alt a 13	Glutathione-transferase	26	Minor allergen
Alt a 14	Manganese superoxide dismutase (Mn-SOD)	24	Minor allergen
Alt a 15	Vacuolar serine protease	58	Minor allergen
Alt a NTF2	Nuclear Transport Factor	14	Minor allergen
Alt a TCTP	Cytokine-like action	ND	Minor allergen

ND: not defined.

2.2. *Alternaria as an Inducer of Allergic Inflammation*

Upon inhalation, *A. alternata* spores penetrate the upper and lower airways, where they come into contact with structural and immune cells, including airway epithelial cells, dendritic cells, and alveolar macrophages. These fungal components are recognized by pattern recognition receptors (PRRs), such as toll-like receptors (TLRs), TLR2, and TLR4, protease-activated receptor 2 (PAR-2), and the organic cation transporter, SLC22A17. This recognition leads to the activation of downstream signaling pathways and rapid release of epithelial-derived alarmins, including interleukin (IL)-33, IL-25, and thymic stromal lymphopoietin (TSLP) [41–43]. These alarmins play a pivotal role in skewing the immune response toward type 2 immunity. They activate group 2 innate lymphoid cells (ILC2s), which secrete IL-5 and IL-13; these are cytokines that respectively promote eosinophilic inflammation and enhance mucus hypersecretion and airway hyperresponsiveness (AHR), which are hallmarks of allergic asthma [44]. TSLP also influences dendritic cells, conditioning them to drive naïve CD4+ T cells toward a Th2 phenotype, thus linking the innate and adaptive immune responses.

Although allergic asthma has traditionally been characterized by Th2-type responses, *A. alternata* exposure may also elicit Th1- and Th17-mediated inflammation, depending on the host immune status and cytokine microenvironment. This is particularly relevant because antifungal immunity is typically dominated by Th1/Th17 responses, whereas allergic responses reflect a dysregulated Th2 axis. IFN-γ and TNF-α, products of Th1 cells, as well as IL-17 from Th17 cells, may contribute to airway inflammation and remodeling, complicating the immune landscape in fungal-induced asthma [44–46]. These immune responses are part of a broader spectrum of fungal-related respiratory conditions. Fungal lung diseases are heterogeneous and can be classified as infectious, toxic, or allergic diseases. Within the allergic domain, two major subtypes have been described [47]. The first involves sensitization to environmental fungi, such as *Alternaria* and *Cladosporium*, which act as seasonal aeroallergens, similar to grass pollen. Exposure correlates with ambient spore concentrations and may provoke acute asthma exacerbations, especially during the peak fungal seasons. The second subtype refers to sensitization to thermotolerant, filamentous fungi, such as *Aspergillus* and *Penicillium*, which are not only aeroallergens, but are also capable of colonizing the lower airways. This colonization creates persistent allergenic and inflammatory stimuli that may cause progressive lung damage.

Alternaria has been implicated in co-sensitization phenomena, acting as an adjuvant for other allergens such as grass pollen and food allergens, such as kiwifruits, peaches, and bananas. In particular, *Alternaria* spp. can act as allergic inducers (e.g., kiwifruit thaumatin-like proteins), further complicating allergy management. When *Alternaria* spores are placed on kiwifruit, they increase the expression of Alt a 1, which binds to kiwi PR5 (Act d 2), a plant defense protein with antifungal properties, and co-localizes within the fruit tissue [48]. This interaction inhibits the enzymatic activity of Act d 2, with several consequences. First, the inhibition of PR5 proteins weakens the plant's natural antifungal defenses, making the fruit more susceptible to infections. Additionally, the interaction increases the risk of co-sensitization, making individuals allergic to *Alternaria* more likely to develop fruit allergies.

In conclusion, the presence of Alt a 1 in the fruit pulp, even in the absence of visible fungal growth, enhances fruit allergenicity and increases the likelihood of allergic reactions in sensitized individuals [42]. This phenomenon complicates allergy diagnosis and management, as patients may experience unexpected allergic responses to eating fruits that they have not previously reacted to.

3. Clinical Manifestations and Natural History of *Alternaria* Sensitization

Asthma and rhinitis are the most common symptoms of *Alternaria* allergy. Because the nasal mucosa represents a primary immunological and anatomical interface with inhaled environmental particulates and allergens, it is a frequent site of fungal deposition. Consequently, fungal species are often identified in nasal secretions [43]. AR affects approximately 40% of the population and is characterized by sneezing, nasal congestion, rhinorrhea, and nasal itching. Ocular symptoms are also common. Despite its benign nature, AR can impair sleep and cognitive function, substantially reducing quality of life [49].

Asthma is a chronic inflammatory airway disease affecting more than 300 million individuals worldwide. It imposes a substantial burden on healthcare systems, both economically and in terms of patient morbidity. The clinical presentation is heterogeneous and characterized by variable airflow limitation, airway inflammation, and symptoms such as dyspnea, wheezing, and chronic cough. The underlying pathophysiological mechanisms include bronchial hyperresponsiveness, smooth muscle contraction, mucus overproduction, and structural changes, such as airway remodeling, fibrosis, and epithelial thickening. These alterations can occur independently or in combination, contributing to the complexity of disease expression. As a result, distinct endotypes have been defined, including allergic asthma, which is closely associated with sensitization to environmental allergens, such as *Alternaria* [43,50,51].

The clinical manifestations of *Alternaria* allergy are best recognized in monosensitized individuals. In a pediatric study, 18 children monosensitized to *Alternaria* in a group of

1057 (1.7%) children seen in an allergy center were identified. Clinical manifestations were asthma in ten (55.5%), recurrent cough in six (33.3%), persistent rhinitis in four (22.2%), dermatitis in four (22.2%), and seasonal oculorhinitis in three (16%) children [52].

These findings were later confirmed by Cantani et al. in a prospective epidemiological study involving 6840 Italian children with asthma or allergic rhinitis. Of these, 213 (3.3%) were sensitized to *A. alternata*, whereas only 89 (1.3%) were monosensitized. Clinically, eighty-three children presented with asthma or allergic rhinitis, and six had atopic dermatitis [53]. Further supporting evidence comes from a population-based French study conducted as part of the ISAAC Phase II (Six Cities) study, which examined the relationship between *Alternaria* sensitization and allergic rhinitis. Of 6726 children (mean age: 10 y), *Alternaria* sensitization was found in 2.8%, with 0.8% being monosensitized. Sensitized children had a substantially higher prevalence of rhinoconjunctivitis. Importantly, even after excluding children with asthma, monosensitization to *Alternaria* remained strongly associated with both past year rhinoconjunctivitis and allergic rhinitis not caused by pollen, suggesting a direct role of *Alternaria* in upper airway disease independent of asthma [54].

Mold sensitization plays a key role in asthma exacerbation, increased emergency room visits, and respiratory distress [55–57]. Soffer et al. [35] found that sensitization to *A. alternata* was linked to a 3.7-fold increased risk of frequent wheezing and other symptoms of asthma. Moreover, *A. alternata* levels in house dust were associated with higher exhaled nitric oxide (FeNO) levels, particularly in areas with high environmental carbon levels, suggesting that combustion byproducts may worsen fungal-induced airway inflammation [35]. Baxi et al. [58] explored the relationship between fungal spore exposure in classrooms and asthma morbidity in inner-city schools as part of the School Inner-City Asthma Study (SICAS). The study involved 280 children (mean age, 7.9 y) with physician-diagnosed asthma, with 9.2% of the participants sensitized to *Alternaria*. *Alternaria* spores were detected in 22% of the classrooms. Children exposed to higher levels of *Alternaria* in the classroom experienced 3.2-times more asthma clinical manifestation days per 2-w period compared to those in low-exposure environments [58].

Geographic location also substantially affects the prevalence of *Alternaria* sensitization. A pediatric study comparing two climatically distinct Chinese cities, Lanzhou (dry and cold) and Wuhan (hot and humid), found higher asthma, AR, and mold exposure rates in Wuhan, particularly in suburban areas and among younger children. Household mold exposure was strongly associated with an increased risk of asthma (OR = 2.399), AR (OR = 1.969), and substance allergies (OR = 1.729) in Wuhan, highlighting the role of regional climate in mold-related health outcomes [59].

Moreover, early-life exposure to *Alternaria* spores has been shown to increase the risk of allergic sensitization and asthma, especially in genetically predisposed children [60]. The results from a high-risk cohort from infancy to 7-y evaluating mold exposure, including *Alternaria*, at both 1-y and 7-y of age, demonstrated that children exposed to high mold levels (high-ERMI homes) at 1 y were more than twice as likely to develop asthma by 7 y compared to children living in low-ERMI homes. Additional substantial risk factors identified included parental asthma and allergic sensitization to house dust mites [60,61]. Similar results were observed in The Isle of Wight birth cohort in the UK, where *Alternaria* sensitization at 4-y of age was associated with long-term risk of asthma, rhinitis, and lung function deficits from 10 to 26 y [62].

Moreover, exposure to airborne *Alternaria* spores was identified as a potential trigger of severe and potentially life-threatening asthma exacerbation, both in outdoor settings and during controlled allergen provocation tests [63]. Of 11 young patients with asthma who experienced sudden respiratory arrest, 91% showed positive skin tests for *Alternaria* versus only 31% of the matched asthma controls. Serum IgE levels to *Alternaria* were also elevated in affected individuals. All respiratory arrest episodes occurred during the peak mold season. After adjusting for age, *Alternaria* sensitization was associated with a nearly 200-fold increase in the risk of respiratory arrest [64].

4. Diagnosis of *Alternaria* Allergy

Diagnosing mold allergies can be challenging due to the variability in mold allergens and the decreasing availability of commercial test solutions. *Alternaria* extract exhibits the highest degree of standardization among mold allergens, meeting international standardization guidelines (Food and Drug Administration, European Medicines Agency, and WHO/IUIS) and ensuring reproducibility in allergy diagnostics and immunotherapy [65]. Some factors must be addressed in the diagnosis of *Alternaria* allergy.

(1) Establishing a clear cause–effect relationship in *Alternaria* allergy is particularly challenging. Unlike other allergens, such as house dust mites or pollen, whose exposure patterns are more easily monitored and temporally linked to symptom onset, *Alternaria* spores exhibit high variability in both time and space. Their concentration in the air can fluctuate rapidly depending on weather conditions, humidity, and local vegetation, making exposure quantification inconsistent. *Alternaria* spores often coexist with other airborne allergens, such as grass or olive pollen, which are prevalent during the same seasons. This co-exposure complicates clinical interpretation, as patients frequently present with polysensitization, and symptoms may not be attributable to a single allergen. Consequently, even in sensitized individuals, it is difficult to definitively associate clinical manifestations with *Alternaria* exposure alone [7]. In addition, traditional environmental monitoring relies on total spore counts, which do not necessarily reflect the actual allergenic load. Symptoms correlate more closely with the levels of specific allergens such as Alt a 1 than with overall spore counts [66]. This discrepancy further impairs the ability to directly link exposure to symptom exacerbation.

(2) In the diagnosis of mold allergy, the skin-prick test (SPT) is more sensitive than specific IgE (sIgE) in detecting mold sensitization, with the exception of *Alternaria* [67]. Kespohl et al. examined 168 patients with mold exposure or mold-induced respiratory symptoms, assessing SPT solutions biochemically, and applying them in duplicate on the patients' arms. The sIgE levels were measured using ImmunoCAP. The SPT identified mold sensitization more frequently (90/168) than sIgE testing (56/168). *Alternaria* represented an exception, showing the highest sensitization prevalence, with 46 patients (27%) testing positive using sIgE and up to 60 (36%) testing positive using SPT, depending on the manufacturer. Concordance among different SPT solutions varied, but for Alt a, the agreement was the highest, with 69% (40 of 58) of sensitized individuals reacting to all tested SPT solutions. The high concordance was between sIgE and SPT for *Alternaria*, with an area under the curve (AUC) of 90.1–91.6% in the receiver operating characteristic analysis, indicating that sIgE for *Alternaria* was as reliable as SPT, unlike other mold allergens, where SPT demonstrated superior sensitivity [68]. Similarly, the study by Fernández et al. demonstrated that both SPT and serum-specific IgE (sIgE) were highly effective in predicting bronchial reactions to *Alternaria* in asthmatic patients; of 74 sensitized individuals, 61% had a positive bronchial challenge. SPT showed excellent predictive accuracy (AUC, 0.957), with a 5.5 mm wheal indicating a 90% likelihood of a positive response and sIgE levels $\geq$16 kUA/L predicting a positive reaction with 99% accuracy [69].

(3) Component-resolved diagnosis (CRD) can differentiate true allergen sensitization from cross-reactions, improving diagnosis and guiding immunotherapy choices. In the

diagnostic process, Alt a 1, the major A. *alternata* allergen, is strongly correlated with clinical manifestations (over 80–90% of patients show sensitivity to this allergen), SPT, and sIgE levels [70,71]. Therefore, SPT and sIgE testing are recommended for patients with suspected allergies, whereas CRD should be reserved for those considered for AIT [72].

(4) The provocation test plays a key role in identifying clinically suspected cases that yield negative skin and laboratory test results. Krouse et al. evaluated the efficacy of epicutaneous and intradermal testing in predicting the nasal response to *Alternaria* antigen in the nasal provocation test (NPT). The sensitivity and specificity of epicutaneous testing were low (42% and 44%, respectively), with intradermal testing only marginally increasing the sensitivity to 58% [73]. Similarly, Kupczyk et al. found that NPT results were not correlated with sIgE levels, SPT results, or seasonal symptoms in children and adolescents allergic to *Alternaria* [74]. Fuiano et al. measured the nasal IgE levels in children with rhinitis during high *Alternaria* spore exposure periods. Of the 56 children studied, 37.5% tested positive on SPT and 80.3% tested positive on nasal IgE testing (NT). A total of 64.3% of the children with negative SPT results had positive NT results, indicating local IgE production. Furthermore, 69.6% of NT-positive cases showed a positive NPT response, compared to only 26.8% of SPT-positive cases ($p < 0.0001$) [75]. This discrepancy suggests that the standard diagnostic tests may not fully capture the complex mechanisms underlying *Alternaria* sensitization, potentially leading to inaccurate or overlooked diagnoses. In particular, *Alternaria* has been identified as a trigger for local AR (LAR), a distinct AR subtype characterized by localized allergic inflammation in the nasal mucosa without systemic sensitization [76]. Unlike classical AR, which is confirmed by detectable allergen-specific IgE in blood tests or positive SPT results, patients with LAR exhibit allergen-specific IgE production exclusively within the nasal mucosa. Utilizing NPT and local sIgE testing can aid in accurately diagnosing cases that may have been misclassified as non-AR (NAR) but are, in fact, indicative of LAR [77–79]. LAR is managed similarly to AR with treatments that include allergen avoidance, medication, and AIT [76,80,81]. The diagnostic and management algorithms for *Alternaria alternata* allergy are shown in Figure 1.

Diagnostic criteria have been suggested for specific clinical conditions, including clinical manifestations and allergological, laboratory, and instrumental tests to direct the diagnosis toward a fungal form. For allergic fungal rhinosinusitis (AFRS), Bent and Kuhn diagnostic criteria have been proposed. These include the presence of chronic rhinosinusitis symptoms lasting for more than 12 w, such as nasal congestion, facial pain, nasal discharge, and anosmia. Bilateral nasal polyps must be observed during nasal endoscopy, and eosinophilic inflammation in the sinus tissue must be observed via histopathological examination. Fungal elements, such as hyphae or spores, must be identified in the sinus tissue through histology, direct culture, or polymerase chain reaction (PCR) testing. Positive allergy tests and CT scan findings of mucosal thickening, sinus opacification, and fungal debris are essential. Finally, other causes of chronic rhinosinusitis, especially non-fungal infections, must be ruled out. A patient must meet all five criteria to be definitively diagnosed with AFRS [82].

Alternaria is a common fungal genus implicated in non-*Aspergillus* allergic bronchopulmonary mycosis (ABPM). A definitive diagnosis of ABPM requires meeting at least six of the established criteria. The patient must have a history of asthma or asthma-like clinical manifestations, with peripheral blood eosinophilia exceeding 500 cells/μL and total IgE levels > 417 IU/mL. Sensitization to filamentous fungi (e.g., *Alternaria, Curvularia, Bipolaris, Cladosporium*) must be confirmed through positive-specific IgE or skin testing, whereas specific IgG or precipitating antibodies further support the diagnosis. Imaging findings should indicate central bronchiectasis and/or high-attenuation mucus on chest CT scans. Additionally, laboratory tests may identify a positive fungal culture from the bronchial mucus or bronchoalveolar lavage. Clinically, the disease often manifests as recurrent expectoration of mucus plugs and migrating pulmonary infiltrates. A definitive diagnosis is confirmed if at least six criteria are met, whereas five criteria suggest a suspected diagnosis [83].

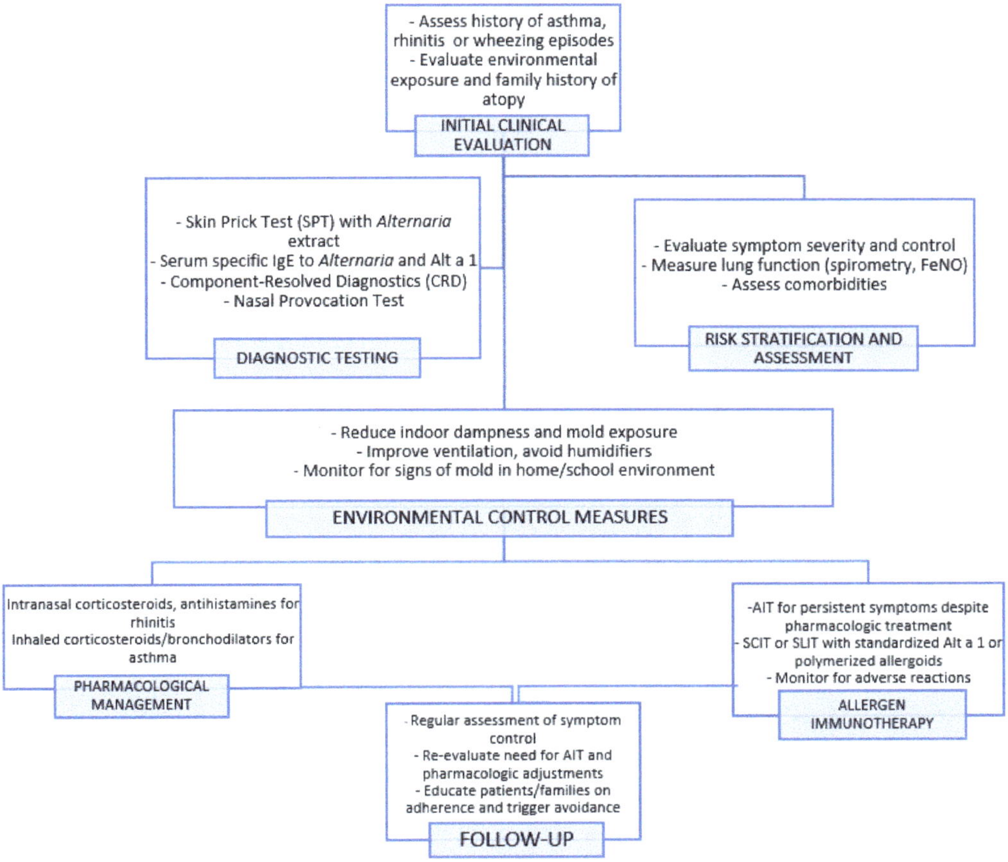

Figure 1. Diagnostic and management algorithm for *Alternaria alternata* allergy. The flowchart outlines steps from initial clinical evaluation and diagnostic testing to environmental control, pharmacological management, and allergen immunotherapy. It emphasizes a personalized approach including symptom monitoring and follow-up.

Finally, the diagnosis of severe asthma with fungal sensitization (SAFS) requires persistent, difficult-to-control asthma with frequent exacerbations despite optimal treatment. These patients typically have a history of poor asthma control and reduced lung function. Fungal sensitization is confirmed by positive allergy tests, such as SPT or serum-specific IgE measurements. Additionally, evidence of fungal exposure, including a history of allergic fungal rhinosinusitis or environmental mold exposure, supports this diagnosis. An elevated eosinophil count in peripheral blood or sputum indicates an underlying eosinophilic inflammatory response. Before confirming SAFS, other potential triggers of asthma exacerbation, such as viral infections or non-fungal allergens, must be ruled out. Treatment strategies typically involve high-dose inhaled corticosteroids, biological therapies, and antifungal medications, depending on the severity and extent of fungal involvement [84] (Table 3).

Table 3. Diagnostic criteria for fungal-associated allergic airway diseases.

Condition	Diagnostic Criteria	Key Notes
AFRS (allergic fungal rhinosinusitis)	1. Symptoms of chronic rhinosinusitis > 12 w (e.g., nasal congestion, facial pain, discharge, anosmia) 2. Bilateral nasal polyps on endoscopy 3. Eosinophilic inflammation on histopathology 4. Fungal elements in sinus tissue (via histology, culture, or PCR) 5. Positive allergy tests + CT findings (e.g., mucosal thickening, opacification, fungal debris)	All five criteria required for definitive diagnosis. Rule out non-fungal causes.
ABPM (allergic bronchopulmonary mycosis)	1. History of asthma or asthma-like symptoms 2. Eosinophils > 500 cells/μL 3. Total IgE > 417 IU/mL 4. Sensitization to filamentous fungi (e.g., *Alternaria*) confirmed by skin test or specific IgE 5. Positive specific IgG or precipitating antibodies 6. Central bronchiectasis and/or high-attenuation mucus on chest CT 7. Positive fungal culture (sputum or BAL) 8. Recurrent mucus plug expectoration 9. History of migrating pulmonary infiltrates 10. Exclusion of other causes	≥Six criteria = definitive diagnosis Five criteria = suspected diagnosis
SAFS (severe asthma with fungal sensitization)	1. Persistent, severe asthma with frequent exacerbations 2. Positive fungal sensitization (SPT or specific IgE) 3. History of poor asthma control and reduced lung function 4. Evidence of fungal exposure (e.g., AFRS or environmental mold) 5. Elevated eosinophil count in blood or sputum 6. Exclusion of non-fungal asthma triggers	Diagnosis is clinical and based on exclusion. Treatment includes high-dose ICS, biologics, antifungals.

ICS: Inhaled Corticosteroids, PCR: Polymerase Chain Reaction, CT: Computed Tomography, BAL: Bronchoalveolar Lavage, SPT: Skin Prick Test.

5. Treatment of *Alternaria* Allergy

Interventions for *Alternaria* spp. allergy require a multifaceted and individualized approach that includes environmental control strategies, pharmacological treatments, and AIT in selected cases. The primary goal is to reduce allergen burden and mitigate the associated inflammatory responses that manifest as AR, conjunctivitis, or asthma. Minimizing the exposure to fungal allergens is a cornerstone of management. This involves the identification and remediation of indoor sources of moisture and mold growth, ensuring adequate ventilation, repairing water damage, and maintaining indoor humidity below 50%. The use of dehumidifiers and high-efficiency particulate air (HEPA) filters may help reduce airborne fungal spore concentrations, especially in sensitized individuals [85–87].

The pharmacological management of fungal-induced AR and conjunctivitis does not differ substantially from the treatment protocols used for other aeroallergens, such as pollens, house dust mites, or animal dander. According to the Allergic Rhinitis and Its Impact on Asthma (ARIA) guidelines, intranasal corticosteroids are considered the first-line treatment because of their strong anti-inflammatory efficacy. In cases where symptom control remains inadequate, combination therapy may be warranted, incorporating second-generation oral antihistamines, intranasal antihistamines, typical antihistamines, or mast cell stabilizers when ocular involvement is present, topical antihistamines, or mast cell stabilizers [41,49]. In individuals sensitized to fungal allergens, including *Alternaria*, asthma management aligns with the stepwise pharmacological approach recommended by the Global Initiative for Asthma (GINA). Treatment is tailored to the level of symptom control and severity, beginning with the use of inhaled corticosteroids as foundational therapy. If control remains insufficient, escalation includes the addition of long-acting β2-agonists or leukotriene receptor antagonists, following GINA recommendations [51].

Allergen Immunotherapy to Alternaria

AIT is a disease-modifying treatment that involves the administration of increasing doses of specific allergens to induce immune tolerance [88,89]. Although specific data on its preventive role in *Alternaria* allergy are limited, the rising prevalence of sensitization in children and the typical progression from early exposure to rhinitis and eventually to asthma suggest that AIT could have a potential role in modifying the natural course of the disease and reducing the risk of long-term complications [90]. This fungus has been standardized over the past 35 years, and recombinant extracts are now utilized in clinical practice. Generally, immunotherapy with *A. alternata* extract has shown positive results, substantially reducing clinical manifestations and medication use compared to other models. Treatment tolerance is usually good, with minimal adverse reactions [90–95]. AIT for *A. alternata* involves subcutaneous immunotherapy (SCIT) and sublingual immunotherapy (SLIT).

Horst et al. conducted a double-blind, placebo-controlled (DBPC) clinical trial investigating the efficacy and safety of SCIT with a standardized *A. alternata* extract in patients with allergic rhinitis and/or asthma, including pediatric patients as young as 5 y (age range: 5–56 y). A total of 24 patients were enrolled, with 13 receiving active SCIT and 11 receiving the placebo. Treatment was administered using a rush protocol, followed by maintenance injections. Throughout the study, the patients in the SCIT group demonstrated substantial clinical improvements, including reduced symptom scores, decreased medication use, reduced skin reactivity to *Alternaria*, and increased tolerance to nasal allergen challenges. Immunologic responses include an increase in *Alternaria*-specific IgG levels. The treatment was generally well tolerated, although two mild asthma exacerbations occurred during the rush induction phase. These resolved without requiring discontinuation of therapy [96].

An RCT by Kuna et al. evaluated the efficacy and safety of SCIT with a standardized *A. alternata* extract in children and adolescents allergic to this mold. Fifty patients (ages 5–18 y) with *A. alternata*-induced AR and/or asthma were randomly assigned to receive either active treatment or placebo. After 3 y, the combined symptom medication scores decreased substantially by 38.7% in year two and 63.5% in year three ($p < 0.001$). This improvement was linked to a better quality of life and decreased sensitivity to the nasal allergen challenge. Mild side effects such as injection site edema were noted in seven patients [97]. The study by Kiliç et al. enrolled 16 children with bronchial asthma and *Alternaria* monosensitization, divided into an immunotherapy group (Group I, nine patients) and a control group (Group II, seven patients) [98]. One year after SCIT, Group I showed a substantial reduction in bronchial responsiveness to methacholine and *Alternaria* ($p = 0.03$, $p = 0.006$, respectively) compared to controls. Specific IgE levels were decreased in the immunotherapy group ($p = 0.001$). Following allergen provocation, sputum eosinophil counts were lower in the SIT group ($p = 0.011$), whereas sputum eosinophil cationic protein (ECP) levels did not change in the SIT group, but increased substantially in the control group.

An RCT by Tabar et al. evaluated the efficacy and safety of SCIT with two doses of Alt a 1, the major allergen of *A. alternata*, in adolescent and adult patients with rhinoconjunctivitis caused by *A. alternata* sensitization, with or without controlled asthma [99]. The active groups received either 0.2 μg or 0.37 μg of Alt a 1, administered subcutaneously, and the primary endpoint was the combined symptom and medication score. The treatment schedule included an induction phase with four weekly doses every 7 d, followed by one dose after 15 d, and a maintenance phase with one dose administered approximately every 30 d. Results showed substantial reductions in symptoms and medication use in the 0.37-μg group compared to the placebo after 12 months. Both the active groups demonstrated improved cutaneous reactivity, reduced IgE levels, and increased IgG4 levels. The safety profile was comparable across all groups with no serious adverse reactions [99].

To date, RCTs on the use of SLIT for *Alternaria* have been conducted predominantly in adults and have demonstrated substantial results for both AR and asthma [100,101].

Liu et al. reported the largest pediatric cohort treated with SCIT for *A. alternata*-induced respiratory allergies in China [102]. Of the 70 patients (aged 5–27 y), nearly half were children aged 5–11 y, and 31 received monotherapy with *A. alternata* extract. After at least 1 y of SCIT, the authors observed substantial clinical improvements, including reductions in total symptom scores (RTSS), medication use (RMS, CSMS), and enhanced asthma control (ACT). Additionally, spirometric parameters, such as FEV1%, MEF25, and PEF, improved substantially. Younger children (5–11 y) showed a better response to the combined symptom and medication scores than older patients. The therapy was well tolerated and no serious adverse events were reported [102] (Table 4).

Alternaria AIT faces challenges, such as inconsistent allergen dosages, adverse reactions, and prolonged treatment durations. The complexity of *A. alternata* allergenic proteins and the potential for adverse effects of native fungal extracts complicate treatment. Alternative strategies, such as hypoallergens or purified allergens (Alt a 1), show promise, but require further research to confirm their long-term safety and effectiveness. Research is increasingly focusing on *A. alternata* allergoids, which appear to offer safer and more stable alternatives to traditional immunotherapy, providing enhanced effectiveness and reducing the need for injections in polysensitized patients [103]. Brindisi et al. investigated the efficacy of SCIT using a polymerized Alt a 1 allergoid in children monosensitized to *A. alternata* with persistent AR and intermittent asthma [104]. A total of 42 children were enrolled, of whom 17 received active treatment and 25 continued symptomatic therapy. Various tests were conducted at the start (T0) and after 24 months (T1), including total IgE (tIgE), specific IgE (sIgE) for Alt a 1, nasal nitric oxide (nFeNO), nasal cytology, anterior active rhinomanometry, and spirometry. The results indicated that patients treated with allergoids showed substantial improvements, including a decrease in nFeNO, tIgE, and sIgE for Alt a 1, nasal eosinophil counts, and an increase in nasal airflow and FEV1. Specifically, there was a substantial reduction in allergic symptoms, with improvements observed both objectively and through laboratory measurements [104].

Future research should aim to enhance the efficacy of AIT by improving allergen standardization, optimizing treatment protocols, and identifying biomarkers that can predict treatment success. Given its potential to provide long-term relief and disease modification, AIT remains a crucial therapeutic option for *Alternaria*-induced allergic diseases in both.

Table 4. Clinical studies evaluating allergen immunotherapy (AIT) for *Alternaria alternata* in pediatric patients, either exclusively or as part of mixed-age cohorts that included children.

Study	Design & Participants	AIT Type	Main Findings	Safety Profile	Comment
Horst 1990 [96]	DBPC; 24 patients (5–56 yrs); 13 SCIT, 11 placebo	SCIT (standardized via RI)	↓ Symptoms and medication, skin reactivity; ↑ nasal challenge dose, specific IgG ($p < 0.001$)	2 mild asthma reactions during rush protocol.	Well-controlled DBPC study demonstrating both clinical and immunologic efficacy; limited by small sample and use of rush protocol, which may not reflect standard clinical practice.
Kuna 2011 [97]	RCT; 50 children/adolescents (5–18 yrs) with *A. alternata*-induced AR and/or asthma; placebo-controlled	SCIT (standardized extract)	↓ Symptoms: −38.7% (year 2), −63.5% (year 3); ↑ QoL; ↓ nasal allergen sensitivity	Mild (injection site oedema in seven pts).	Robust RCT with long-term follow-up demonstrating sustained clinical efficacy and improved quality of life; limited by small sample size and absence of mechanistic biomarker analysis.
Kiliç 2011 [98]	16 children with asthma and *Alternaria* mono-sensitization; Group I (9) SCIT, Group II (7) control	SCIT	↓ Bronchial reactivity; ↓ sIgE ($p = 0.001$); ↓ sputum eosinophils ($p = 0.011$); ↑ ECP in controls	Mild local reactions (injection site erythema and swelling in three patients); no systemic or severe adverse events reported.	Controlled prospective design; extensive clinical and immunologic endpoints (sIgE, ECP, sputum eosinophils, bronchial challenges); demonstrated early improvements in airway inflammation. Small sample size; short duration (1 year), not controlled-randomized study.
Tabar 2019 [99]	RCT; adolescents/adults with *Alternaria*-induced rhino-conjunctivitis ± asthma; 0.2 µg and 0.37 µg Alt a 1 vs. placebo	SCIT (Alt a 1)	0.37 µg group: ↓ symptoms/medication; ↓ IgE, ↑ IgG4; ↓ skin reactivity	The most common adverse events were local reactions at the injection site, which were mild and transient.	Well-designed RCT using a recombinant allergen with dose-response analysis; showed immunological and clinical benefits. Limited by short duration (12 months) and lack of long-term efficacy data.

Table 4. *Cont.*

Study	Design & Participants	AIT Type	Main Findings	Safety Profile	Comment
Liu 2024 [102]	31 subjects (mean age 12.03 ± 4.32; 42% 5–11 years) with perennial AR and/or asthma	SLIT (Alt a 1)	↓ Symptoms and meds; ↓ nasal eosinophils; ↑ nasal flow; effective even in polysensitized	Well tolerated; no serious effects.	Real-world pediatric data supporting SLIT efficacy in AR/asthma, even in polysensitized patients; limited by retrospective design, short follow-up (1 year), and lack of control group.
Brindisi 2023 [104]	42 children with AR ± asthma; 17 received polymerized Alt a 1 allergoid, 25 controls	SCIT (polymerized Alt a 1 allergoid)	↓ nFeNO, tIgE, sIgE; ↓ nasal eosinophils; ↑ airflow, FEV1; improved clinical/lab outcomes	No serious adverse effects; treatment was well tolerated without systemic reactions.	Prospective pediatric study showing clinical, functional, and immunologic improvements with polymerized Alt a 1 SCIT; limited by small sample size and lack of blinding.

Abbreviations: AIT = Allergen Immunotherapy; AR = Allergic Rhinitis; SCIT = Subcutaneous Immunotherapy; SLIT = Sublingual Immunotherapy; RCT = Randomized Controlled Trial; DBPC = Double-Blind Placebo-Controlled; QoL = Quality of Life; sIgE = Specific Immunoglobulin E; tIgE = Total Immunoglobulin E; IgG4 = Immunoglobulin G4; ECP = Eosinophil Cationic Protein; nFeNO = Nasal Fractional Exhaled Nitric Oxide; FEV1 = Forced Expiratory Volume in 1 Second; SPT = Skin Prick Test; RI = Rush Immunotherapy.

6. Conclusions

Molds, including *A. alternata*, represent a key component of human exposure and internal mycobiota, with sensitization prevalence influenced by geography and environmental exposure. *Alternaria alternata* is one of the most common mold allergens affecting both pediatric and adult populations. Although predominantly found in outdoor environments, it can colonize damp indoor settings, such as poorly ventilated buildings. Airborne spore concentrations, which are typically highest from May to November, are increasingly affected by climate change. Sixteen allergens were identified, of which Alt a 1 was the most clinically relevant. *Alternaria alternata* may also act as an adjuvant to enhance co-sensitization to other allergens. Asthma and allergic rhinitis are the most frequent clinical manifestations; however, diagnosis remains challenging due to allergen variability and limitations in diagnostic tools. Allergen immunotherapy via both sublingual and subcutaneous routes offers a targeted strategy for reducing symptoms and improving patient outcomes in both adults and children (Table 5).

Table 5. Overview of key characteristics of *Alternaria alternata* allergy.

Topic	Key Information
Habitat	Mainly outdoors; also indoors in damp, poorly ventilated spaces
Seasonal Presence	May–November; influenced by climate change
Sensitization Prevalence	Varies with environment and geography
Common Allergen	*Alternaria alternata*, especially Alt a 1
Immune Response	Activates epithelial cells and macrophages upon inhalation
Co-sensitization	Acts as an adjuvant enhancing other allergen responses (grass pollen, fruits)
Main Symptoms	Asthma and allergic rhinitis
Diagnosis	Clinical history, SPT, sIgE, Component-Resolved Diagnostics (CRD), nasal provocation test (key in uncertain cases)
Prevention	Minimize exposure through environmental control: reduce indoor humidity (<50%), ventilate damp spaces, eliminate mold-contaminated materials; avoid outdoor activities during peak spore seasons (dry, windy days).
Treatment	Intranasal corticosteroids, antihistamines for rhinitisInhaled corticosteroids, bronchodilators for asthma AIT

Author Contributions: Conceptualization, E.N.; methodology, E.N. and A.K.; resources, E.N. and A.K.; writing—original draft preparation, A.K.; writing—review and editing, M.G. (Mattia Giovannini), S.B., L.L., L.P., F.S., F.M., C.M., S.A., R.C., M.G. (Mariannita Gelsomino), L.C., M.M.d.G. and E.N.; supervision, E.N. All authors have read and agreed to the published version of the manuscript.

Funding: This research received no external funding.

Conflicts of Interest: MG reports personal fees from Sanofi, Thermo Fisher Scientific. The other authors declare no conflicts of interest.

Abbreviations

The following abbreviations are used in this manuscript:

IgE	Immunoglobulin E
AR	Allergic Rhinitis
AIT	Allergen Immunotherapy
EMA	European Medicines Agency
FDA	Food and Drug Administration
WHO	World Health Organization

IUIS	International Union of Immunological Societies
TLR	Toll-Like Receptor
TSLP	Thymic Stromal Lymphopoietin
IL	Interleukin
IFN-γ	Interferon gamma
TNF-α	Tumor Necrosis Factor alpha
PR5	Pathogenesis-related protein 5
FeNO	Fractional exhaled Nitric Oxide
ERMI	Environmental Relative Moldiness Index
ISAAC	International Study of Asthma and Allergies in Childhood
SPT	Skin Prick Test
sIgE	Specific Immunoglobulin E
CRD	Component-Resolved Diagnosis
AUC	Area Under the Curve
NPT	Nasal Provocation Test
NT	Nasal Testing
LAR	Local Allergic Rhinitis
NAR	Non-Allergic Rhinitis
AFRS	Allergic Fungal Rhinosinusitis
ABPM	Allergic Bronchopulmonary Mycosis
SAFS	Severe Asthma with Fungal Sensitization
ICS	Inhaled Corticosteroids
BAL	Bronchoalveolar Lavage
SCIT	Subcutaneous Immunotherapy
SLIT	Sublingual Immunotherapy
ECP	Eosinophil Cationic Protein
FEV1	Forced Expiratory Volume in 1 s
nFeNO	Nasal Fractional Exhaled Nitric Oxide

References

1. Fukutomi, Y.; Taniguchi, M. Sensitization to fungal allergens: Resolved and unresolved issues. *Allergol. Int. Off. J. Jpn. Soc. Allergol.* **2015**, *64*, 321–331. [CrossRef]
2. Vitte, J.; Michel, M.; Malinovschi, A.; Caminati, M.; Odebode, A.; Annesi-Maesano, I.; Caimmi, D.P.; Cassagne, C.; Demoly, P.; Heffler, E.; et al. Fungal exposome, human health, and unmet needs: A 2022 update with special focus on allergy. *Allergy* **2022**, *77*, 3199–3216. [CrossRef]
3. Agache, I.; Annesi-Maesano, I.; Cecchi, L.; Biagioni, B.; Chung, F.; D'Amato, G.; Damialis, A.; Del Giacco, S.; Dominguez Ortega, J.; Galán, C.; et al. EAACI Guidelines on Environmental Science for Allergy and Asthma-Recommendations on the Impact of Indoor Air Pollutants on the Risk of New-Onset Asthma and on Asthma-Related Outcomes. *Allergy* **2025**, *80*, 651–676. [CrossRef] [PubMed]
4. Sousa-Pinto, B.; Valiulis, A.; Melén, E.; Koppelman, G.H.; Papadopoulos, N.G.; Makela, M.; Haahtela, T.; Bonini, M.; Braido, F.; Brussino, L.; et al. Asthma and rhinitis control in adolescents and young adults: A real-world MASK-air study. *Pediatr. Allergy Immunol.* **2024**, *35*, e14080. [CrossRef] [PubMed]
5. Sousa-Pinto, B.; Costa, E.M.; Vieira, R.J.; Klimek, L.; Czarlewski, W.; Pfaar, O.; Bedbrook, A.; Amaral, R.; Brussino, L.; Kvedariene, V.; et al. Adherence to Treatment in Allergic Rhinitis During the Pollen Season in Europe: A MASK-air Study. *Clin. Exp. Allergy* **2025**, *55*, 226–238. [CrossRef]
6. Castagnoli, R.; Brambilla, I.; Giovannini, M.; Marseglia, G.L.; Licari, A. New approaches in childhood asthma treatment. *Curr. Opin. Allergy Clin. Immunol.* **2023**, *23*, 319–326. [CrossRef]
7. Abel-Fernández, E.; Martínez, M.J.; Galán, T.; Pineda, F. Going over Fungal Allergy: *Alternaria alternata* and Its Allergens. *J. Fungi* **2023**, *9*, 582. [CrossRef]
8. Hughes, K.M.; Price, D.; Torriero, A.A.J.; Symonds, M.R.E.; Suphioglu, C. Impact of Fungal Spores on Asthma Prevalence and Hospitalization. *Int. J. Mol. Sci.* **2022**, *23*, 4313. [CrossRef]
9. Krieger, J.; Jacobs, D.E.; Ashley, P.J.; Baeder, A.; Chew, G.L.; Dearborn, D.; Hynes, H.P.; Miller, J.D.; Morley, R.; Rabito, F.; et al. Housing interventions and control of asthma-related indoor biologic agents: A review of the evidence. *J. Public Health Manag. Pract.* **2010**, *16* (Suppl. 5), S11–S20. [CrossRef]

10. Eggleston, P.A. Environmental control for fungal allergen exposure. *Curr. Allergy Asthma Rep.* **2003**, *3*, 424–429. [CrossRef]
11. Kwong, K.; Robinson, M.; Sullivan, A.; Letovsky, S.; Liu, A.H.; Valcour, A. Fungal allergen sensitization: Prevalence, risk factors, and geographic variation in the United States. *J. Allergy Clin. Immunol.* **2023**, *152*, 1658–1668. [CrossRef]
12. Alvaro-Lozano, M.; Akdis, C.A.; Akdis, M.; Alviani, C.; Angier, E.; Arasi, S.; Arzt-Gradwohl, L.; Barber, D.; Bazire, R.; Cavkaytar, O.; et al. EAACI Allergen Immunotherapy User's Guide. *Pediatr. Allergy Immunol.* **2020**, *31* (Suppl. 25), 1–101. [CrossRef] [PubMed]
13. Lehmann, S.; Sprünken, A.; Wagner, N.; Tenbrock, K.; Ott, H. Clinical relevance of IgE-mediated sensitization against the moldMold *Alternaria alternata* in children with asthma. *Ther. Adv. Respir. Dis.* **2017**, *11*, 30–39. [CrossRef] [PubMed]
14. Gabriel, M.F.; Postigo, I.; Tomaz, C.T.; Martínez, J. *Alternaria alternata* allergens: Markers of exposure, phylogeny and risk of fungi-induced respiratory allergy. *Environ. Int.* **2016**, *89–90*, 71–80. [CrossRef] [PubMed]
15. Mari, A.; Schneider, P.; Wally, V.; Breitenbach, M.; Simon-Nobbe, B. Sensitization to fungi: Epidemiology, comparative skin tests, and IgE reactivity of fungal extracts. *Clin. Exp. Allergy J. Br. Soc. Allergy Clin. Immunol.* **2003**, *33*, 1429–1438. [CrossRef]
16. Heinrich, J.; Richter, K.; Frye, C.; Meyer, I.; Wölke, G.; Wjst, M.; Nowak, D.; Magnussen, H.; Wichmann, H.E. Die Europäische Studie zu Atemwegserkrankungen bei Erwachsenen (ECRHS)-Bisherige Ergebnisse und der Beitrag der beiden deutschen Studienzentren [European Community Respiratory Health Survey in Adults (ECRHS)]. *Pneumologie* **2002**, *56*, 297–303. [CrossRef]
17. Bousquet, P.J.; Hooper, R.; Kogevinas, M.; Jarvis, D.; Burney, P. Number of allergens to be tested to assess allergenic sensitization in epidemiologic studies: Results of the European Community Respiratory Health Survey I. *Clin. Exp. Allergy* **2007**, *37*, 780–787. [CrossRef]
18. Heinzerling, L.M.; Burbach, G.J.; Edenharter, G.; Bachert, C.; Bindslev-Jensen, C.; Bonini, S.; Bousquet, J.; Bousquet-Rouanet, L.; Bousquet, P.J.; Bresciani, M.; et al. GA(2)LEN skin test study I: GA(2)LEN harmonization of skin prick testing: Novel sensitization patterns for inhalant allergens in Europe. *Allergy* **2009**, *64*, 1498–1506. [CrossRef]
19. Corsico, R.; Cinti, B.; Feliziani, V.; Gallesio, M.T.; Liccardi, G.; Loreti, A.; Lugo, G.; Marcucci, F.; Marcer, G.; Meriggi, A.; et al. Prevalence of sensitization to *Alternaria* in allergic patients in Italy. *Ann. Allergy Asthma Immunol.* **1998**, *80*, 71–76. [CrossRef]
20. López Couso, V.P.; Tortajada-Girbés, M.; Rodriguez Gil, D.; Martínez Quesada, J.; Palacios Pelaez, R. Fungi Sensitization in Spain: Importance of the *Alternaria alternata* Species and Its Major Allergen Alt a 1 in the Allergenicity. *J. Fungi* **2021**, *7*, 631. [CrossRef]
21. Calderón-Llosa, O.M. Identificación y sensibilización a hongos ambientales en Lima, Perú [Identification and sensitization to environmental fungal spores in Lima City, Peru]. *Rev. Alerg. Mex.* **2024**, *71*, 82. [CrossRef] [PubMed]
22. Mvoundza Ndjindji, O.; Minto'o Rogombe, S.; Mougola Bissiengou, P.; Mveang-Nzoghe, A.; Leboueny, M.; Ouloungou Mbina Maloupazoa Siawaya, A.C.; KuissiKamgaing, E.; Ndeboko, B.; Ategbo, S.; Djoba Siawaya, J.F. Allergen sensitization and polysensitization pattern of adults and children in an urban Sub-Saharan African setting (Libreville, Gabon). *J. Allergy Clin. Immunol. Glob.* **2022**, *2*, 23–29. [CrossRef] [PubMed]
23. Mahboubi Oskouei, Y.; Farid Hosseini, R.; Ahanchian, H.; Jarahi, L.; Ariaee, N.; Jabbari Azad, F. Report of Common Aeroallergens among Allergic Patients in Northeastern Iran. *Iran. J. Otorhinolaryngol.* **2017**, *29*, 89–94. [PubMed]
24. Guan, K.; Liu, B.; Wang, M.; Li, Z.; Chang, C.; Cui, L.; Wang, R.Q.; Wen, L.P.; Leung, P.S.C.; Wei, J.F.; et al. Principles of Allergen Immunotherapy and Its Clinical Application in China: Contrasts and Comparisons with the USA. *Clin. Rev. Allergy Immunol.* **2019**, *57*, 128–143. [CrossRef]
25. Mazokha, K.S.; Manzhos, M.V.; Zhukova, N.N.; Makova, E.V.; Moiseeva, T.V. Sensitization to *Alternaria* in children in Samara. *Allergol. Immunol. Pediatr.* **2023**, *2*, 47–49. [CrossRef]
26. Fonseca-Guerra, I.R.; Beltrán Pineda, M.E.; Benavides Rozo, M.E. Characterization of *Alternaria alternata* and *Alternaria scrophulariae* Brown Spot in Colombian quinoa (*Chenopodium quinoa*). *J. Fungi* **2023**, *9*, 947. [CrossRef] [PubMed] [PubMed Central]
27. Thomma, B.P. *Alternaria* spp.: From general saprophyte to specific parasite. *Mol. Plant Pathol.* **2003**, *4*, 225–236. [CrossRef]
28. Kilic, M.; Ufuk Altintas, D.; Yilmaz, M.; Güneşer Kendirli, S.; Bingöl Karakoc, G.; Taskin, E.; Ceter, T.; Pinar, N.M. The effects of meteorological factors and *Alternaria* spore concentrations on children sensitised to *Alternaria*. *Allergol. et Immunopathol.* **2010**, *38*, 122–128. [CrossRef]
29. Lam, H.C.Y.; Anees-Hill, S.; Satchwell, J.; Symon, F.; Macintyre, H.; Pashley, C.H.; Marczylo, E.L.; Douglas, P.; Aldridge, S.; Hansell, A. Association between ambient temperature and common allergenic pollen and fungal spores: A 52-year analysis in central England, United Kingdom. *Sci. Total Environ.* **2024**, *906*, 167607. [CrossRef]
30. Forkel, S.; Beutner, C.; Schröder, S.S.; Bader, O.; Gupta, S.; Fuchs, T.; Schön, M.P.; Geier, J.; Buhl, T. Sensitization against Fungi in Patients with Airway Allergies over 20 Years in Germany. *Int. Arch. Allergy Immunol.* **2021**, *182*, 515–523. [CrossRef]
31. Choi, Y.J.; Lee, K.S.; Jeong, J.H.; Kim, K.; Yang, S.; Na, J.Y.; Hwang, J.K.; Choe, Y.; Kim, K.R.; Han, M.J.; et al. Annual Change in Fungal Concentrations and Allergic Sensitization Rates to *Alternaria* and *Cladosporium* in Korea During the Period 1998–2022. *Allergy Asthma Immunol. Res.* **2023**, *15*, 825–836. [CrossRef] [PubMed]
32. Fernández-Soto, R.; Navarrete-Rodríguez, E.M.; Del-Rio-Navarro, B.E.; Sienra-Monge, J.J.L.; Meneses-Sánchez, N.A.; Saucedo-Ramírez, O.J. Fungal Allergy: Pattern of sensitization over the past 11 years. *Allergol. Immunopathol.* **2018**, *46*, 557–564. [CrossRef] [PubMed]

33. Subri, M.S.M.; Arifin, K.; Sohaimin, M.F.A.M.; Abas, A. The parameter of the Sick Building Syndrome: A systematic literature review. *Heliyon* **2024**, *10*, e32431. [CrossRef] [PubMed]
34. O'Connor, G.T.; Walter, M.; Mitchell, H.; Kattan, M.; Morgan, W.J.; Gruchalla, R.S.; Pongracic, J.A.; Smartt, E.; Stout, J.W.; Evans, R.; et al. Airborne fungi in the homes of children with asthma in low-income urban communities: The Inner-City Asthma Study. *J. Allergy Clin. Immunol.* **2004**, *114*, 599–606. [CrossRef]
35. Soffer, N.; Green, B.J.; Acosta, L.; Divjan, A.; Sobek, E.; Lemons, A.R.; Rundle, A.G.; Jacobson, J.S.; Goldstein, I.F.; Miller, R.L.; et al. Alternaria is associated with asthma symptoms and exhaled NO among NYC children. *J. Allergy Clin. Immunol.* **2018**, *142*, 1366–1368.e10. [CrossRef]
36. Baxi, S.N.; Muilenberg, M.L.; Rogers, C.A.; Sheehan, W.J.; Gaffin, J.; Permaul, P.; Kopel, L.S.; Lai, P.S.; Lane, J.P.; Bailey, A.; et al. Exposures to molds in school classrooms of children with asthma. *Pediatr. Allergy Immunol.* **2013**, *24*, 697–703. [CrossRef]
37. International Union of Immunological Societies (IUIS) Allergen Nomenclature Sub-Committee. Allergen Nomenclature: *Alternaria alternata*. Available online: https://allergen.org/search.php?allergensource=Alternaria+alternata (accessed on 25 May 2025).
38. Allergome. Available online: http://www.allergome.org/ (accessed on 25 May 2025).
39. Strader, M.B.; Saha, A.L.; Fernandes, C.; Sharma, K.; Hadiwinarta, C.; Calheiros, D.; Conde-de-Oliveira, G.; Gonçalves, T.; Slater, J.E. Distinct proteomes and allergen profiles appear across the life-cycle stages of *Alternaria alternata*. *J. Allergy Clin. Immunol.* **2024**, *154*, 424–434. [CrossRef]
40. Arasi, S.; Barni, S.; Caminiti, L.; Castagnoli, R.; Giovannini, M.; Liotti, L.; Mastrorilli, C.; Mori, F.; Pecoraro, L.; Saretta, F.; et al. Latex Allergy in Children. *J. Clin. Med.* **2023**, *13*, 124. [CrossRef]
41. Rudert, A.; Portnoy, J. Mold allergy: Is it real and what do we do about it? *Expert Rev. Clin. Immunol.* **2017**, *13*, 823–835. [CrossRef]
42. Hernandez-Ramirez, G.; Barber, D.; Tome-Amat, J.; Garrido-Arandia, M.; Diaz-Perales, A. Alternaria as an Inducer of Allergic Sensitization. *J. Fungi* **2021**, *7*, 838. [CrossRef]
43. Rick, E.M.; Woolnough, K.; Pashley, C.H.; Wardlaw, A.J. Allergic Fungal Airway Disease. *J. Investig. Allergol. Clin. Immunol.* **2016**, *26*, 344–354. [CrossRef]
44. Percopo, C.M.; Ma, M.; Mai, E.; Redes, J.L.; Kraemer, L.S.; Minai, M.; Moore, I.N.; Druey, K.M.; Rosenberg, H. *Alternaria alternata* Accelerates Loss of Alveolar Macrophages and Promotes Lethal Influenza A Infection. *Viruses* **2020**, *12*, 946. [CrossRef]
45. Shin, S.H.; Ye, M.K.; Lee, D.W.; Chae, M.H.; Han, B.D. Nasal Epithelial Cells Activated with *Alternaria* and House Dust Mite Induce Not Only Th2 but Also Th1 Immune Responses. *Int. J. Mol. Sci.* **2020**, *21*, 2693. [CrossRef] [PubMed]
46. Liu, J.; Li, J.; Yin, J. Clinical relevance of *Alternaria alternata* sensitization in patients within type 2-high and type 2-low asthma. *Int. Immunopharmacol.* **2021**, *101 Pt A*, 108333. [CrossRef] [PubMed]
47. Wardlaw, A.J.; Rick, E.M.; Pur Ozyigit, L.; Scadding, A.; Gaillard, E.A.; Pashley, C.H. New Perspectives in the Diagnosis and Management of Allergic Fungal Airway Disease. *J. Asthma Allergy* **2021**, *14*, 557–573. [CrossRef] [PubMed]
48. Gómez-Casado, C.; Murua-García, A.; Garrido-Arandia, M.; Sánchez-Monge, R.; Barber, D.; Pacios, L.F.; Díaz-Perales, A. Alt a 1 from *Alternaria* interacts with PR5 thaumatin-like proteins. *FEBS Lett.* **2014**, *588*, 1501–1508. [CrossRef]
49. Bousquet, J.; Schünemann, H.J.; Togias, A.; Bachert, C.; Erhola, M.; Hellings, P.W.; Klimek, L.; Pfaar, O.; Wallace, D.; Ansotegui, I.; et al. Next-generation Allergic Rhinitis and Its Impact on Asthma (ARIA) guidelines for allergic rhinitis based on Grading of Recommendations Assessment, Development and Evaluation (GRADE) and real-world evidence. *J. Allergy Clin. Immunol.* **2020**, *145*, 70–80.e3. [CrossRef]
50. Asher, M.I.; García-Marcos, L.; Pearce, N.E.; Strachan, D.P. Trends in worldwide asthma prevalence. *Eur. Respir. J.* **2020**, *56*, 2002094. [CrossRef]
51. 2024 GINA Main Report Global Strategy for Asthma Management and Prevention. Available online: https://ginasthma.org/2024-report/ (accessed on 25 July 2025).
52. Novembre, E. Allergia all'Alternaria nel bambino: Aspetti clinici. *Medico e Bambino* **1991**, *7*, 29–30.
53. Cantani, A.; Ciaschi, V. Epidemiology of *Alternaria alternata* allergy: A prospective study in 6840 Italian asthmatic children. *Eur. Rev. Med. Pharmacol. Sci.* **2004**, *8*, 289–294.
54. Randriamanantany, Z.A.; Annesi-Maesano, I.; Moreau, D.; Raherison, C.; Charpin, D.; Kopferschmitt, C.; Lavaud, F.; Taytard, A.; De Blay, F.; Caillaud, D. Alternaria sensitization and allergic rhinitis with or without asthma in the French Six Cities study. *Allergy* **2010**, *65*, 368–375. [CrossRef] [PubMed]
55. Bush, R.K.; Prochnau, J.J. Alternaria-induced asthma. *J. Allergy Clin. Immunol.* **2004**, *113*, 227–234. [CrossRef] [PubMed]
56. Iossifova, Y.Y.; Reponen, T.; Ryan, P.H.; Levin, L.; Bernstein, D.I.; Lockey, J.E.; Hershey, G.K.; Villareal, M.; LeMasters, G. Mold exposure during infancy as a predictor of potential asthma development. *Ann. Allergy Asthma Immunol.* **2009**, *102*, 131–137. [CrossRef] [PubMed]
57. Portnoy, J.M.; Barnes, C.S.; Kennedy, K. Importance of mold allergy in asthma. *Curr. Allergy Asthma Rep.* **2008**, *8*, 71–78. [CrossRef]

58. Baxi, S.N.; Sheehan, W.J.; Sordillo, J.E.; Muilenberg, M.L.; Rogers, C.A.; Gaffin, J.M.; Permaul, P.; Lai, P.S.; Louisias, M.; Petty, C.R.; et al. Association between fungal spore exposure in inner-city schools and asthma morbidity. *Ann. Allergy Asthma Immunol. Off. Publ. Am. Coll. Allergy Asthma Immunol.* **2019**, *122*, 610–615.e1. [CrossRef]
59. Li, S.; Cao, S.; Duan, X.; Zhang, Y.; Gong, J.; Xu, X.; Guo, Q.; Meng, X.; Zhang, J. Household mold exposure in association with childhood asthma and AR in a northwestern city and a southern city of China. *J. Thorac. Dis.* **2022**, *14*, 1725–1737. [CrossRef]
60. Rosenbaum, P.F.; Crawford, J.A.; Anagnost, S.E.; Wang, C.J.; Hunt, A.; Anbar, R.D.; Hargrave, T.M.; Hall, E.G.; Liu, C.C.; Abraham, J.L. Indoor airborne fungi and wheeze in the first year of life among a cohort of infants at risk for asthma. *J. Expo Sci. Environ. Epidemiol.* **2010**, *20*, 503–515. [CrossRef]
61. Reponen, T.; Vesper, S.; Levin, L.; Johansson, E.; Ryan, P.; Burkle, J.; Grinshpun, S.A.; Zheng, S.; Bernstein, D.I.; Lockey, J.; et al. High environmental relative moldiness index during infancy as a predictor of asthma at 7 years of age. *Ann. Allergy Asthma Immunol.* **2011**, *107*, 120–126. [CrossRef]
62. Arshad, S.; Kurukulaaratchy, R.; Holloway, J.; Carra, S.; Ewart, S.; Karmaus, W.; Vijayanand, P.; Seumois, G.; Zhang, H. The association of *Alternaria* sensitization with asthma and AR in the Isle of Wight cohort from early childhood to adulthood. *J. Allergy Clin. Immunol.* **2024**, *153*, AB361. [CrossRef]
63. Serrano-Pariente, J.; Plaza, V. Near-fatal asthma: A heterogeneous clinical entity. *Curr. Opin. Allergy Clin. Immunol.* **2017**, *17*, 28–35. [CrossRef]
64. O'Hollaren, M.T.; Yunginger, J.W.; Offord, K.P.; Somers, M.J.; O'Connell, E.J.; Ballard, D.J.; Sachs, M.I. Exposure to an aeroallergen as a possible precipitating factor in respiratory arrest in young patients with asthma. *N. Engl. J. Med.* **1991**, *324*, 359–363. [CrossRef] [PubMed]
65. Kespohl, S.; Maryska, S.; Zahradnik, E.; Sander, I.; Brüning, T.; Raulf-Heimsoth, M. Biochemical and immunological analysis of moldMold skin prick test solution: Current status of standardization. *Clin. Exp. Allergy* **2013**, *43*, 1286–1296. [CrossRef] [PubMed]
66. Feo Brito, F.; Alonso, A.M.; Carnés, J.; Martín-Martín, R.; Fernández-Caldas, E.; Galindo, P.A.; Alfaya, T.; Amo-Salas, M. Correlation between, Alt a 1 levels and clinical symptoms in *Alternaria alternata*-monosensitized patients. *J. Investig. Allergol. Clin. Immunol.* **2012**, *22*, 154–159. [PubMed]
67. Hurraß, J.; Heinzow, B.; Walser-Reichenbach, S.; Aurbach, U.; Becker, S.; Bellmann, R.; Bergmann, K.C.; Cornely, O.A.; Engelhart, S.; Fischer, G.; et al. AWMF mold guideline "Medical clinical diagnostics for indoor mold exposure"—Update 2023 AWMF Register No. 161/001. *Allergol. Select.* **2024**, *8*, 90–198. [CrossRef]
68. Kespohl, S.; Maryska, S.; Bünger, J.; Hagemeyer, O.; Jakob, T.; Joest, M.; Knecht, R.; Koschel, D.; Kotschy-Lang, N.; Merget, R.; et al. How to diagnose mold allergy? Comparison of skin prick tests with specific IgE results. *Clin. Exp. Allergy* **2016**, *46*, 981–991. [CrossRef]
69. Fernández, C.; Bevilacqua, E.; Fernández, N.; Gajate, P.; de la Cámara, A.G.; Garcimartín, M.; Vives, R.; Rodríguez, J. Asthma related to *Alternaria* sensitization: An analysis of skin-test and serum-specific IgE efficiency based on the bronchial provocation test. *Clin. Exp. Allergy* **2011**, *41*, 649–656. [CrossRef]
70. Aden, E.; Weber, B.; Bossert, J.; Teppke, M.; Frank, E.; Wahl, R.; Fiebig, H.; Cromwell, O. Standardization of *Alternaria alternata*: Extraction and quantification of alt a 1 by using an mAb-based 2-site binding assay. *J. Allergy Clin. Immunol.* **1999**, *104*, 128–135. [CrossRef]
71. Sánchez, P.; Vélez-Del-Burgo, A.; Suñén, E.; Martínez, J.; Postigo, I. Fungal Allergen and Mold Allergy Diagnosis: Role and Relevance of *Alternaria alternata* Alt a 1 Protein Family. *J. Fungi* **2022**, *8*, 277. [CrossRef]
72. Nieto, M.; Lafuente, I.; Calderon, R.; Uixera, S.; Pina, R.; Calaforra, S.; Cortell, I.; Nieto, A.; Mazon, A. Component-resolved diagnosis: Performance of specific IgE to *Alternaria* compared to Alt a 1. *Pediatr. Allergy Immunol.* **2014**, *25*, 832–834. [CrossRef]
73. Krouse, J.H.; Shah, A.G.; Kerswill, K. Skin testing in predicting response to nasal provocation with alternaria. *Laryngoscope* **2004**, *114*, 1389–1393. [CrossRef]
74. Kupczyk, M.; Kaczmarek, J.; Kupryś, I.; Górski, P.; Kuna, P. The results of nasal provocation test do not correlate with the sIgE level, skin prick tests, and seasonal symptoms in children suffering from AR and/or asthma hypersensitive to *Alternaria tenuis*. *J. Allergy Clin. Immunol.* **2004**, *113*, S31. [CrossRef]
75. Fuiano, N.; Fusilli, S.; Incorvaia, C. A role for measurement of nasal IgE antibodies in diagnosis of *Alternaria*-induced rhinitis in children. *Allergol. Immunopathol.* **2012**, *40*, 71–74. [CrossRef] [PubMed]
76. Terada, T.; Kawata, R. Diagnosis and Treatment of Local AR. *Pathogens* **2022**, *11*, 80. [CrossRef] [PubMed]
77. Testera-Montes, A.; Eguiluz-Gracia, I.; Ariza Veguillaset, A.; Cassinello, M.S.; Torres, M.; Rondon Segovia, C. Clinical phenotype of local AR driven by *Alternaria alternata* allergen. *J. Allergy Clin. Immunol.* **2021**, *147*, AB238. [CrossRef]
78. Klimek, L.; Bardenhewer, C.; Spielhaupter, M.; Harai, C.; Becker, K.; Pfaar, O. Lokale allergische Rhinitis auf *Alternaria alternata*: Nachweis bei Patienten mit persistierender nasaler Symptomatik [Local AR to *Alternaria alternata*: Evidence for local IgE production exclusively in the nasal mucosa]. *HNO* **2015**, *63*, 364–372. [CrossRef]
79. Demirtürk, M.; Gelincik, A.; Ulusan, M.; Ertek, B.; Büyüköztürk, S.; Çolakoğlu, B. The importance of mold sensitivity in nonAR patients. *Int. Forum Allergy Rhinol.* **2016**, *6*, 716–721. [CrossRef] [PubMed]

80. Hoang, M.P.; Samuthpongtorn, J.; Chitsuthipakorn, W.; Seresirikachorn, K.; Snidvongs, K. Allergen-specific immunotherapy for local allergic rhinitis: A systematic review and meta-analysis. *Rhinology* **2022**, *60*, 11–19. [CrossRef]
81. Campo, P.; Canonica, G.W. Local Allergic Rhinitis. *J. Allergy Clin. Immunol. Pract.* **2024**, *12*, 1430–1433. [CrossRef]
82. Daniel, G.; Amedee, R.G. Allergic fungal rhinosinusitis: A review. *Ochsner J.* **2011**, *11*, 271–275.
83. Nakayama, T.; Miyata, J.; Inoue, N.; Ueki, S. Allergic fungal rhinosinusitis: What we can learn from allergic bronchopulmonary mycosis. *Allergol. Int.* **2023**, *72*, 521–529. [CrossRef]
84. Bush, A. Kids, Difficult Asthma and Fungus. *J. Fungi* **2020**, *6*, 55. [CrossRef] [PubMed]
85. Alaidroos, A.; Mosly, I. Preventing mold growth and maintaining acceptable indoor air quality for educational buildings operating with high mechanical ventilation rates in hot and humid climates. *Air Qual. Atmos. Health* **2023**, *16*, 341–361. [CrossRef]
86. Kim, S.H.; Ahn, G.R.; Son, S.Y.; Bae, G.N.; Yun, Y.H. Mold occurring on the air cleaner high-efficiency particulate air filters used in the houses of child patients with atopic dermatitis. *Mycobiology* **2014**, *42*, 286–290. [CrossRef]
87. Bernstein, J.A.; Levin, L.; Crandall, M.S.; Perez, A.; Lanphear, B. A pilot study to investigate the effects of combined dehumidification and HEPA filtration on dew point and airborne mold spore counts in day care centers. *Indoor Air* **2005**, *15*, 402–407. [CrossRef] [PubMed]
88. Sahiner, U.M.; Giovannini, M.; Escribese, M.M.; Paoletti, G.; Heffler, E.; Alvaro Lozano, M.; Barber, D.; Canonica, G.W.; Pfaar, O. Mechanisms of Allergen Immunotherapy and Potential Biomarkers for Clinical Evaluation. *J. Pers. Med.* **2023**, *13*, 845. [CrossRef]
89. Dramburg, S.; Hilger, C.; Santos, A.F.; de Las Vecillas, L.; Aalberse, R.C.; Acevedo, N.; Aglas, L.; Altmann, F.; Arruda, K.L.; Asero, R.; et al. EAACI Molecular Allergology User's Guide 2.0. *Pediatr. Allergy Immunol.* **2023**, *34* (Suppl. 28), e13854. [CrossRef]
90. Martínez-Cañavate Burgos, A.; Valenzuela-Soria, A.; Rojo-Hernández, A. Immunotherapy with *Alternaria alternata*: Present and future. *Allergol. Immunopathol.* **2007**, *35*, 259–263. [CrossRef]
91. Di Bona, D.; Albanesi, M.; Macchia, L. Is immunotherapy with fungal vaccines effective? *Curr. Opin. Allergy Clin. Immunol.* **2019**, *19*, 646–653. [CrossRef]
92. Di Bona, D.; Frisenda, F.; Albanesi, M.; Di Lorenzo, G.; Caiaffa, M.F.; Macchia, L. Efficacy and safety of allergen immunotherapy in patients with allergy to molds: A systematic review. *Clin. Exp. Allergy* **2018**, *48*, 1391–1401. [CrossRef]
93. Gazi, U.; Bahceciler, N.N. Immunotherapy against environmental fungi causing respiratory allergy. *J. Mycol. Med.* **2024**, *34*, 101517. [CrossRef] [PubMed]
94. Bozek, A.; Pyrkosz, K. Immunotherapy of mold allergy: A review. *Hum. Vacc. Immunother.* **2017**, *13*, 2397–2401. [CrossRef]
95. Coop, C.A. Immunotherapy for mold allergy. *Clin. Rev. Allergy Immunol.* **2014**, *47*, 289–298. [CrossRef] [PubMed]
96. Horst, M.; Hejjaoui, A.; Horst, V.; Michel, F.B.; Bousquet, J. Double-blind, placebo-controlled rush immunotherapy with a standardized *Alternaria* extract. *J. Allergy Clin. Immunol.* **1990**, *85*, 460–472. [CrossRef] [PubMed]
97. Kuna, P.; Kaczmarek, J.; Kupczyk, M. Efficacy and safety of immunotherapy for allergies to *Alternaria alternata* in children. *J. Allergy Clin. Immunol.* **2011**, *127*, 502–508.e5086. [CrossRef] [PubMed]
98. Kiliç, M.; Altintaş, D.U.; Yilmaz, M.; Bingöl-Karakoç, G.; Burgut, R.; Güneşer-Kendirli, S. Evaluation of efficacy of immunotherapy in children with asthma monosensitized to *Alternaria*. *Turk. J. Pediatr.* **2011**, *53*, 285–294.
99. Tabar, A.I.; Prieto, L.; Alba, P.; Nieto, A.; Rodríguez, M.; Torrecillas, M.; Huertas, B.; Gómez, E.; Fernández, F.J.; Blanca, M.; et al. Double-blind, randomized, placebo-controlled trial of allergen-specific immunotherapy with the major allergen Alt a 1. *J. Allergy Clin. Immunol.* **2019**, *144*, 216–223.e3. [CrossRef]
100. Cortellini, G.; Spadolini, I.; Patella, V.; Fabbri, E.; Santucci, A.; Severino, M.; Corvetta, A.; Canonica, G.W.; Passalacqua, G. Sublingual immunotherapy for *Alternaria*-induced allergic rhinitis: A randomized placebo-controlled trial. *Ann. Allergy Asthma Immunol.* **2010**, *105*, 382–386. [CrossRef]
101. Pozzan, M.; Milani, M. Efficacy of sublingual specific immunotherapy in patients with respiratory allergy to *Alternaria alternata*: A randomised, assessorblinded, patient-reported outcome, controlled 3-year trial. *Curr. Med. Res. Opin.* **2010**, *26*, 2801–2806. [CrossRef]
102. Liu, J.; Yin, J. A retrospective analysis of the clinical efficacy in patients treated with *Alternaria alternata* and *Dermatophagoides farinae* immunotherapy. *Front. Allergy* **2024**, *5*, 1453446. [CrossRef]
103. Abel-Fernandez, E.; Fernandez-Caldas, E.; Iborra, S. Characterisation of *Alternaria alternata* Allergoids: Evaluation of the Stability of Grass Pollen Allergen Extracts Mixed with *Alternaria alternata* Allergoids. *J. Fungi* **2025**, *11*, 181. [CrossRef]
104. Brindisi, G.; Gori, A.; Anania, C.; Martinelli, I.; Capponi, M.; De Castro, G.; Zicari, A.M. Subcutaneous Immunotherapy (SCIT) with the New Polymerized Molecular Allergoid Alt a1: A Pilot Study in Children with AR Sensitized to *Alternaria alternata*. *J. Clin. Med.* **2023**, *12*, 4327. [CrossRef]

medicina

MDPI

Article

Aeroallergen IgE-Reactivity Patterns and Respiratory Allergy in Children and Adults: A Retrospective Study in 1711 Patients from the Central Poland Urban Area

Barbara Majkowska-Wojciechowska *, Maciej Kulma and Marcin Kurowski *

Department of Immunology and Allergy, Medical University of Łódź, 90-419 Łódź, Poland
* Correspondence: barbara.majkowska-wojciechowska@umed.lodz.pl (B.M.-W.); marcin.kurowski@umed.lodz.pl (M.K.)

Abstract: *Background and Objectives*: Effects of allergen exposure may be modified through endogenous and exogenous factors, resulting in heterogeneity of clinical features, time course and intensity of symptoms of allergic disease. This creates challenges in allergy diagnosis and management, yet studies addressing the variability of allergen reactivity in relation to potential modifying factors are not numerous. The aim of the study was to retrospectively analyze the frequency and profile of reactivity to inhalant allergen extracts in patients followed in a single center in the years 2017–2020, in relation to sex, age, clinical symptoms and final clinical diagnosis. *Materials and Methods*: This is a retrospective analysis of skin prick test (SPT) results in 1711 outpatients, performed with dust mites, pollen (alder, hazel, birch, grasses, rye, mugwort), cat, dog and *Alternaria* allergens. Reactivity profiles were assessed in the entire population divided into sex and age subgroups. Relationships between SPT results, age, sex and clinical diagnosis were assessed using factor analysis. *Results*: The highest reactivity frequencies were found for grass (60.5%), rye (57.22%), birch (47.34%), alder (42.5%) and *Dermatophagoides pteronyssinus* mites (41.8%). Monovalent reactivity was found mainly to mugwort (3.2%, n = 55), followed by cat and mites allergens. Reactivity to ≥1 allergen was more frequent in males. The risk of allergic rhinitis (AR) was significantly higher in subjects allergic to grass, rye, hazel and alder pollen, as compared to subjects non-sensitized to these allergens. Reactivity to perennial allergens (dog, cat and dust mites) was significantly associated with asthma diagnosis. The risk of developing atopic dermatitis was significantly associated with reactivity to birch and alder pollen. *Conclusions*: SPTs are a valuable tool for assessing the occurrence of atopy and allergy. Reactivity to specific aeroallergens may be associated with increased probability of development of a given atopic condition. This warrants further studies regarding the interplay between possible modifiers of allergen exposure effects.

Keywords: aeroallergens; IgE-reactivity; allergen exposure; allergic diseases; allergy epidemiology; age differences; sex differences

1. Introduction

Allergies are common, non-infectious, chronic diseases affecting both children [1] and adults [2]. The growing number of respiratory diseases caused by inhaled allergens is a serious challenge for healthcare. Epidemiological studies indicate that about 40–50% of the world's population suffers from one or more allergic disease [3,4]. Among them, allergic rhinitis (AR) is most frequent and considered a global health problem. AR can co-occur with other allergic manifestations, e.g., asthma or conjunctivitis, thereby significantly influencing different aspects of the daily quality of life [5,6]. A considerable diagnostic challenge may be encountered in cases of IgE-reactivity and allergic inflammation limited to local nasal mucosa with no ascertainable IgE's, either in skin prick tests (SPTs) or in serum [7–9].

Multiple factors contributing to allergy pathogenesis and clearly differentiated clinical symptoms have already been identified. Although the relationship between allergic diseases and skin test results has already been investigated [10,11], in our opinion there is a lack of in-depth, detailed analyses of the number, spectrum and variability of sensitizing allergens and their relation to the sex and age of patients referred for allergy consultations. Therefore, we have decided to assess the distribution of the patterns of sensitizing allergens in the course of different allergic conditions. This cross-sectional, single-center study aimed to analyze the frequency of reactivity to allergens and its association with the presence of physician-diagnosed allergic disease in children and adults followed in an outpatient tertiary center.

The multinational 'GAN' Phase I study of the prevalence of rhinoconjunctivitis, asthma and eczema in children and adolescents in 25 countries showed a persistently high burden of these conditions and large differences in their prevalence between populations from different countries [12]. One of the most important risk factors for allergic rhinitis (AR) and asthma is IgE-dependent reactivity to one or more allergens [13].

Polish studies conducted in nine selected regions of the country indicate that the frequency of physician-diagnosed AR is 28.9%. The frequency of clinically confirmed asthma was 11.4% in children and 9.5% in adults [14]. In our previous study from Łódź and the Łódź Region (Central Poland), it was found that positive skin test results with at least one allergen from the standard airborne allergens panel were found in as many as 63.7% of urban children and 22.7% of children living in rural areas. At least one allergic disease was diagnosed in as many as 43.3% of urban children and 12.8% of rural children. Potential risk factors associated with the development of allergy differed significantly between urban and rural environments [15]. Clinical manifestations of allergy, their development, severity and progression result from the interplay of multiple factors, including maternal–fetal interactions, individual genetic and epigenetic status and environmental and ambient influence related to climate change, as well as dietary habits reflected in the microbiome [16–19].

Diagnosis of allergy is based on history taking, physical examination and diagnostic tests. During the diagnostic process, the use of appropriate tools to confirm IgE-dependent reactivity is necessary. Moreover, IgE-mediated reactivity results should be interpreted in the context of exposure to the presumed culprit allergen. Despite the broadening arsenal of molecular diagnostic tests, skin prick tests, which have a long history of utility in allergy practice, remain the core diagnostic tool in allergology, helpful in identifying environmental factors triggering allergy symptoms.

The use of standardized allergen extracts ensures reproducible results, as well as good specificity, sensitivity and low cost of testing. They also feature high safety with a low risk of systemic reactions. The results of skin tests usually show good correlation with the results of nasal, conjunctival, cutaneous, oral and bronchial provocations; however, in some cases discrepancies between symptoms' history and seasonal presentation and the results of specific IgE measurement may pose a diagnostic challenge, as observed during allergic IgE-mediated reaction limited to local mucosa without systemic involvement [7,20]. SPTs (together with serum-specific IgE and basophil activation tests) may also be considered one of the tools helpful in predicting the clinical reaction upon exposure to allergen, thus contributing to increased safety and efficacy of allergy diagnosis [21–24]. In addition, complete allergy diagnosis with the use of SPTs and specific IgE to allergen components can be valuable in predicting response to allergen immunotherapy as well as in assessment of the clinical significance of given allergen in eliciting clinical symptoms of allergy [25–31].

2. Materials and Methods

2.1. Study Design and Location

This study is a retrospective analysis of the frequency and distribution of IgE-dependent reactivity to allergens included into a standard panel of inhalant allergen extracts used for initial diagnostic assessment of patients referred to a tertiary outpatient allergy center in Poland. The center is affiliated with the University Hospital in the third largest city of Poland in terms of number of inhabitants located in the center of the country. The city area is 293.3 km^2 and the population, as of 30 June 2024, consisted of 645,700 inhabitants [32]. Data were further analyzed in relation to sex, age and final diagnoses, as established by an allergist and recorded in accordance with the ICD-10 classification [33]. The medical diagnoses considered in analyses included allergic rhinitis conjunctivitis, asthma, atopic dermatitis, chronic rhinitis, rhinopharyngitis, chronic sinusitis, nasal polyps, cough, urticaria, anaphylaxis and other unspecified. Data from patients with suspected allergies referred by primary physicians were screened for suitability. The analysis used data from the archived medical records of 1711 patients diagnosed and treated in the four-year period between 2017 and 2020. Patients attending the outpatient clinic were recruited, provided their respective medical records met the eligibility criteria, as listed below. No other specific selection criteria were employed. Criteria of data eligibility included detailed demographic description, complete description of symptoms' history and results of skin prick testing with airborne allergens panel (see below). Patients whose medical records were analyzed were permanent residents of the city of Łódź or its urban agglomeration.

2.2. Skin Prick Tests

The IgE-reactivity profile was determines by skin prick tests using an allergen kit from Allergopharma (Reinbek bei Hamburg, Germany). The test panel included the following eleven extracts of inhalant allergens: house dust mites *Dermatophagoides pteronyssinus* and *Dermatophagoides farinae*, alder (*Alnus glutinosa*), hazel (*Corylus avellana*), birch (*Betula verrucosa*), grasses mix (*Poaceae*), rye (*Secale cereale*), mugwort (*Artemisia vulgaris*), cat (*Felis domesticus*), dog (*Canis familiaris*) and *Alternaria alternata* mold spores, along with positive (histamine) and negative (diluent) controls.

Selection of the eleven allergen extracts included in the study was mainly driven by local aerobiology, previous studies and availability of extracts. This panel of allergens is commonly used—with small variations—in most allergy centers in our country as the first-line diagnostic tool in the assessment of patients with a suspected respiratory allergy.

The SPT procedure was performed in accordance with the established guidelines [34]. Histamine dihydrochloride (10 mg/mL) was used as the positive control and the solvent of the extracts was the negative control. Wheal size of 3 mm or greater than the negative control was considered positive, as it is commonly accepted in allergy diagnosis recommendations [35,36].

2.3. Statistical Methods

Allergic sensitization profiles were assessed in all subjects and further analyzed in subgroups created basing on sex and age. Wheal diameters in SPTs with each allergen were considered initial explained variables. They were subsequently reduced to four independent principal components using factor analysis.

These served as explanatory variables for testing within the gender and age of the participants. Two-way analysis of variance was used for this purpose.

Generalized methods (binomial distribution with a linking logit function) were used to assess the differences between proportions in the prevalence of allergic rhinitis and allergic asthma by gender and age categories of subjects.

Wherever there were more than two comparisons, an appropriate correction was applied (e.g., Benjamini–Hochberg corrects). However, all comparisons concerning proportions (chi-square and generalized linear/non-linear methods) in the binomial distribution are equivalent to testing proportions, so there is no need to test odds ratios (ORs). Odds ratios (ORs)—where applicable—were estimated with confidence intervals.

Factor analysis was used to reduce the number of variables. Principal components were selected as factors. Eleven dependent variables (positive SPTs) were reduced to four independent factors: PC1, PC2, PC3 and PC4. These factors replaced the variables with which they are most strongly related through factor loadings. Factors were named according to factor loading values ≥ 0.7. This method of variable reduction does not result in a loss of explained variability. Another advantage of principal components is that they are independent of each other, which cannot be said for the original variables.

Statistical significance was assumed at the level of $\alpha = 0.05$ and the confidence interval at the level of 0.95. In the case of more than two categories, the Benjamini–Hochberg post hoc test was performed using PQStat Software 2023 v1.8.6 (PQStat Software, Poznań, Poland). All other calculations were performed using Statistica 13.3 (StatSoft Polska, Kraków, Poland).

Chi-square tests were then performed between the disease entities determined by the allergists and the SPT results. Additionally, odds ratios with confidence intervals were calculated.

3. Results

3.1. Distribution of Sex and Age Groups

The studied population was characterized with the following sex and age distribution. Females accounted for 49% (n = 840) and males for 51% (n = 871) of patents. The mean age in the entire study group was 30.25 ± 6.95 years (age range: 2.57–86.42). The mean ages of males and females in the analyzed population were 27.90 ± 6.35 (age range: min.: 2.92; max.: 86.42) and 32.69 ± 17.2 (age range: min.: 2.57; max.: 77.97) years, respectively. Males were significantly more likely to be sensitized to grass pollen and house dust mites (Figure 1).

For further analysis, subjects were subdivided into three age subgroups, as presented in Table 1. The age distribution shows a predominance of patients aged 10 through 50 years, who constituted 74.81% of the group, followed by the age group 50 years and older, accounting for 14.1% of the studied population. Further details regarding the study group are provided in Table 1.

Table 1. Basic characteristics of the entire study group, as per division into age groups. SD, standard deviation.

	Group I <10 years	Group II ≥10–50 years	Group III >50 years
Number of subjects (n)	190	1280	241
Mean age ± SD	6.87 ± 2.0	28.11 ± 11.06	60.02 ± 6.65
Age range (years)	2.57–9.99	10.04–49.96	50.28–86.42
% of the total population	11.1%	74.81%	14.09%

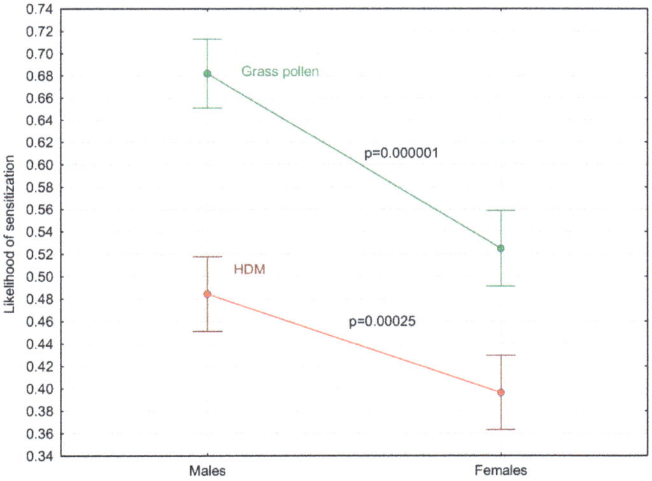

Figure 1. Sex differences in likelihood ratio of grass pollen reactivity and house dust mites reactivity in the entire study group. HDM, house dust mites.

3.2. Reactivity Profiles in the Entire Study Group

The highest IgE-reactivity frequencies were observed in cases of allergens of grass, rye, birch and alder pollen, and of *Dermatophagoides pteronyssinus* mite. The lowest frequencies of reactivity were found for allergens of dog and *Alternaria*. A detailed summary of the frequency of reactivity profiles and average wheal diameter are presented in Figure 2.

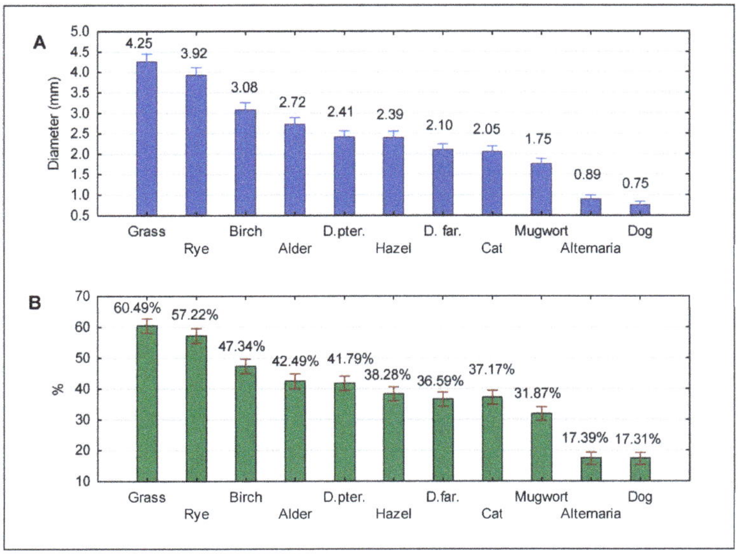

Figure 2. Panel (**A**) Diameters of wheal in skin prick tests with airborne allergens from the standard panel. Mean values (in mm) are shown as numerical values; 95% confidence intervals are indicated with whiskers. Panel (**B**) Frequency of positive skin prick test results with airborne allergens from the standard panel in the entire study group (n = 1711). D. pter., Dermatophagoides pteronyssinus; D. far., Dermatophagoides farinae.

Wheal diameters in SPTs were also higher with regard to allergens with which the SPT results were positive most frequently. In the entire study group, as shown in Figure 3, a significant positive correlation has been observed between the mean wheal diameter of positive SPTs with a given allergen extract and the percentage of positive SPT results with that allergen.

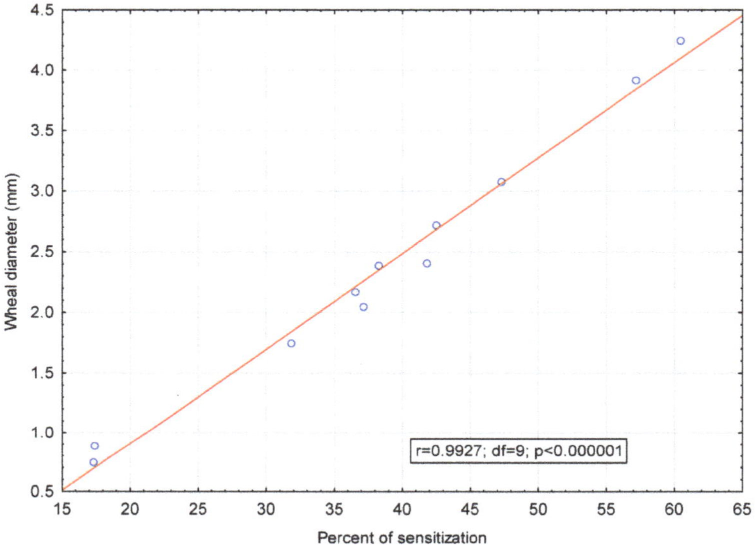

Figure 3. Results of the Pearson correlation between mean wheal diameter in skin prick tests with a given allergen in the entire study group (n = 1711) and percent of positive skin prick results with the same allergen ($r = 0.9927$, $r^2 = 0.9855$, $p < 0.000001$).

3.3. Monovalent and Polyvalent Reactivity

3.3.1. Monovalent Reactivity Profiles

Monovalent reactivity was found in 13.73% of the participants. As shown in Figure 4, the most common monovalent IgE-reactivity reactions in the entire study group were found in the following order: to mugwort pollen: 3.26% (n = 55) followed by cat allergens: 2.9% (n = 49) *D. pteronyssinus* mites. 1.84% (n = 31), grass pollen 1,48%, *Alternaria* 1,42%, birch pollen 1.12%, dog 0.95%, *D. farinae* mites 0,89% and alder pollen 0,006%. The number of monovalent reactivity was highest in age group II (10–50 years) and differed significantly from the remaining age groups (χ^2. = 52.5, df = 1, p = 0.000001, OR = 3.16 (2.29–4.36). Distribution of monovalent reactivity among age groups is presented in Table 2.

Table 2. Monovalent reactivity as per division into age groups.

	Number of Subjects with Monovalent Reactivity in a Given Group	Percentage of Subjects with Monovalent Reactivity in a Given Group
Group I <10 years (n = 190)	26	13.68%
Group II ≥10–50 years (n = 1280)	140	10.94%
Group III >50 years (n = 241)	69	28.63%
Total (n = 1711)	235	13.73%

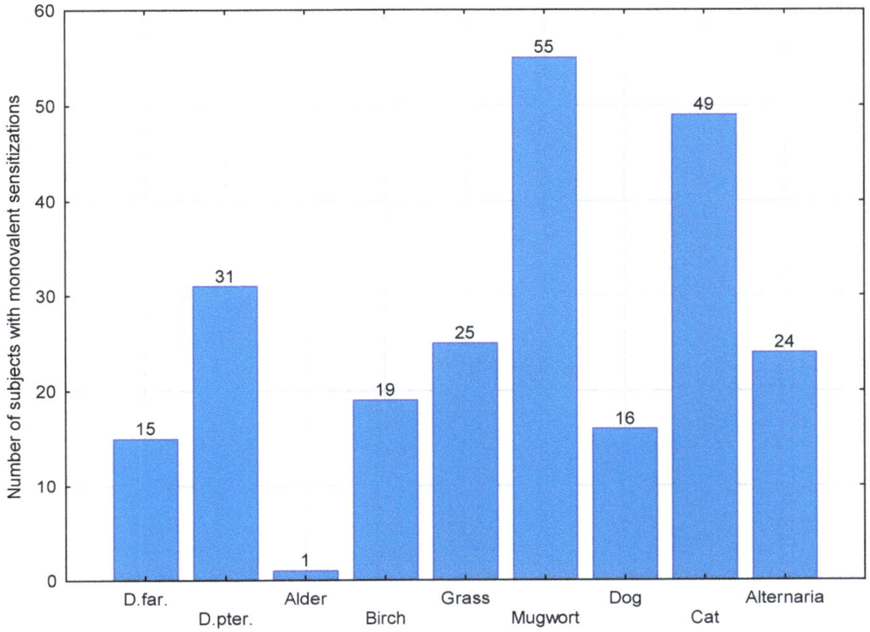

Figure 4. Distribution of the numbers of monovalent reactivity to airborne allergen extracts in the entire study group (n = 1711). No monovalent sensitization was observed in the case of rye pollen and hazel pollen. The percentage profiles is given in Section 3.3.1.

3.3.2. Polyvalent Reactivity Profiles

As many as 98.7% of the studied population had one or more positive SPT results. Polyvalent reactivity to two or more allergen extracts was found in 86% of subjects. Most often, in 17.8% of subjects, two positive SPT results were ascertained. Reactivity to all eleven allergen extracts was found in 1% of patients (Figure 5).

3.4. Factor Analysis

Data reduction using factor analysis allowed for the extraction of four principal components (factors) described below, which were considered as explained variables.

- Factor I was associated with positive SPT results to tree pollen extracts (alder, hazel, birch).
- Factor II characterized allergy to mites (Dermatophagoides pteronyssinus and Dermatophagoides farinae).
- Factor III was associated with allergies to grass pollen extracts: mix and rye.
- Factor IV determined allergies to animal allergens: dog and cat.

Sex and age were considered as explanatory variables.

The four independent principal components identified in the factor analysis allowed us to conclude that the wheal diameters for grass/cereals and mites were higher in men ($p < 0.0001$). For mites, the largest wheal diameter was obtained in age group II (10–50 years). It was significantly different from age group I (<10 years ($p = 0.0045$) and age group III (>50 years) ($p = 0.006$). The results of the factor analysis are presented in Table 3 and Figure 6.

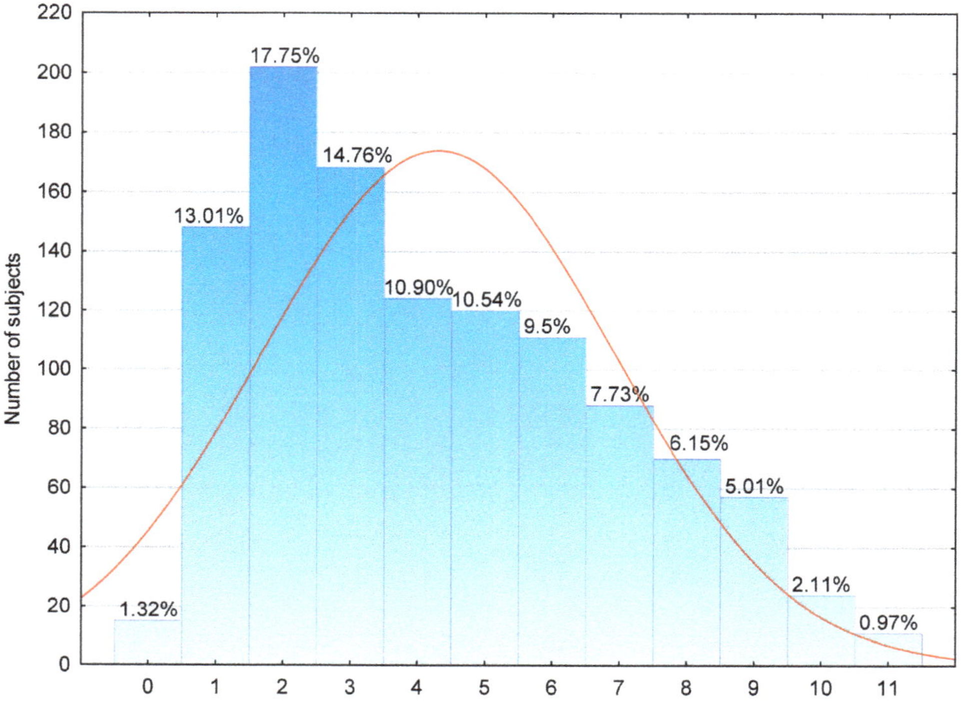

Figure 5. Distribution of the numbers of reactivity (lower X axis) in skin prick test panel in the entire group (n = 1711). Number of subjects with given number of reactivity is indicated on the Y axis with percentage of the total group indicated above each column.

Table 3. Results of the factor analysis of SPT positive results with regard to four principal components (as described in Section 2.3). SPT, skin prick test; PC, principal component.

	Variables	Factor Loadings Extraction Principal Components (PC). Marked Loadings > 0.7			
		PC1_Trees Pollen 1	PC2_ House Dust Mites 2	PC3_Grass Pollen 3	PC4_Pets 4
1.	*D. farinae*	−0.010730	**0.948330**	0.014072	0.080939
2.	*D. pteronyssinus*	−0.013067	**0.949340**	0.044677	0.050046
3.	Alder	**0.935816**	0.004489	0.190270	0.099719
4.	Hazel	**0.918262**	−0.010066	0.201667	0.092477
5.	Birch	**0.927786**	−0.014525	0.153930	0.102391
6.	Timothy	0.142750	−0.020950	**0.929728**	0.084068
7.	Rye	0.114222	−0.013704	**0.935631**	0.101022
8.	Mugwort	0.192302	0.069246	0.371463	0.048909
9.	Dog	0.142326	0.170201	0.021874	**0.715538**
10.	Cat	0.235508	0.186921	0.080663	**0.712500**
11.	*Alternaria*	−0.087785	−0.185442	0.122141	0.588676
	Explained variance	2.733860	1.904627	2.002449	1.423891
	Proportion of variance	0.248533	0.173148	0.182041	0.129445

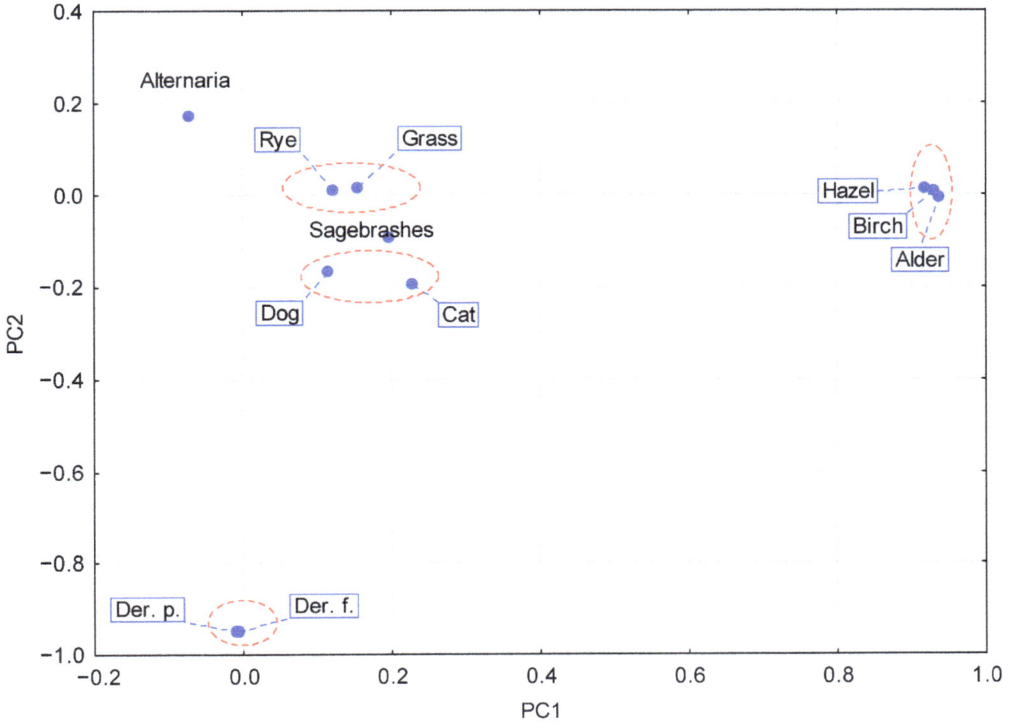

Figure 6. Graphical representation of the results from Table 3 for the first two factors PC1 and PC2, which explain the most variability. The charges marked with a dashed line characterize four distinct reactivity groups.

3.4.1. Testing of the Four Extracted Factors in Relation to Age, Sex and the Extracted Age Categories

Factor I—Allergy to Tree Pollen

The highest wheal diameters to tree pollen extracts were found in the age group 50+. They were significantly higher than in the youngest patients ($p = 0.0048$) than in the members of the age group 10–50 years ($p = 0.000003$). No significant differences were found in relation to the sex of the subjects (Figure S1).

Factor II—Allergy to House Dust Mites

For factor II, i.e., mite extracts, the highest reactivity rates were found in 10–50-year-olds. Statistically significant differences were noted with the youngest group ($p = 0.045$) and the oldest group ($p = 0.016$) (Figure S2A). Significantly higher values of wheal diameters were also noted in males (Figure S2B).

Factor III—Allergy to Grass and Rye Pollen

In cases of grass and rye pollen allergens, the highest value of wheal diameter was observed in age group II. Statistically significant differences occurred between all age categories: between category I and II ($p = 0.0004$); between II and III ($p = 0.00002$), and between I and III ($p = 0.0026$). Positive reactivity was significantly more frequent in men ($p > 0000001$) (Figure S3A,B).

Factor IV—Allergy to Pet Allergens

In cases of reactivity to pet allergens (dog/cat), the highest frequency was found for age category II (10–50-year-olds). Significant differences were obtained between age groups I and II, as well as II and III: $p = 0.023$ and $p = 0.019$, respectively. No significant differences were noted between the sexes (Figure S4).

3.5. Frequency of Clinical Diagnoses According to the ICD-10 Classification

From the archival patient charts, information was obtained that all patients included in the study were diagnosed with atopic diseases of atopic origin. These were allergic rhinitis, conjunctivitis, bronchial asthma and atopic dermatitis. Some patients were diagnosed with chronic rhinopharyngitis, chronic sinusitis, nasal polyps, cough, urticaria and other unspecified. The association of disease entities with the studied reactivity to specific inhalant allergens was estimated using the odds ratio (OR ± 95% CI). Detailed results are presented in Table S1.

3.6. Clinical Diagnoses in Relation to SPT Results

3.6.1. Allergic Rhinitis (AR)

In the study group, the chance of developing AR (J30) was more than three times higher in the case of grass allergy [OR = 3.24 (2.58–4.05), $p < 0.000001$] and more than two times with regard to rye, hazel and alder pollen allergens than in subjects without such reactivity.

It was found that the risk of allergic rhinitis had a significant relationship with reactivity to all extracts of inhalant allergens. It was most strongly associated with grass and rye pollen allergy, respectively, OR = 3.24 (2.58–4.05), $p = 0.000001$ and OR = 2.92 (2.33–3.65), $p = 0.000001$, followed by hazel pollen, OR = 2.26 (1.77–2.82), $p = 0.000001$, and alder, OR = 2.22 (1.75–2.82), $p = 0.000001$, as well as *Alternaria*, birch, cat and mites (Table S1). Regarding sex and age groups, AR diagnosis was significantly associated with male sex (Figure S5) and age group >50 years, as compared with the other age groups (Figure S6).

3.6.2. Asthma

The risk of developing asthma was associated to the highest extent with reactivity to allergens coming from dog (OR = 2.28 (1.75–2.98), $p < 0.000001$), cat (OR = 1.96 (1.60–2.41), $p < 0.000001$) and house dust mites (OR = 1.49 (1.21–1.82)). Regarding sex and age groups, asthma was significantly associated with female sex (Figure S5) and age groups 10–50 years and >50 years, as compared with the youngest group (Figure S6).

3.6.3. Other Atopic Conditions

The risk of the diagnosis of allergic conjunctivitis was associated with reactivity to hazel [OR = 1.86 (1.29–2.70); 0.0025], alder [OR = 1.86 (1.29–2.70)] and birch [OR = 1.54 (1.07–2.24)]. Regarding diagnosis of atopic dermatitis, its risk was highest in subject allergic to birch [(OR = 2.12 (1.36–3.25), $p < 0.001$) and alder (OR = 1.70 (1.11–2.60), $p = 0.014$)]. Negative associations between reactivity to different allergens and the risk of being diagnosed with a given condition were found with regard to chronic rhinopharyngitis (ICD-10: J31), chronic sinusitis (J32), nasal polyps (J33) and cough (R05). For example, in people with nasal polyps, the chance of being allergic to grasses was estimated to be four times lower than in people without polyps (Table S1). For ICD-10 codes, L50 (urticaria) and T78 (adverse effects, not elsewhere classified—which includes among others, anaphylactic shock, food hypersensitivity, different forms of angioedema and unspecified allergy), no significant associations were ascertained.

4. Discussion

In our retrospective study, we considered the results of skin prick tests and physicians' diagnoses in 1711 patients referred by primary physicians due to suspected immediate-type allergy. It should be emphasized and taken into account that these data come from a tertiary clinic and, as such, may overrepresent more severe allergy cases compared to the general population. In this analysis, we looked at the SPT results from different perspectives. Our cross-sectional studies, based on medical records, indicate that using SPTs is a valuable first-line approach in the assessment of subjects with suspected allergy to airborne allergens. According to Szmyd et al. [37], there are strong positive correlations between positive SPT results and serum-specific IgE concentrations, which allows for the diagnosis of inhalant allergy in 95% of cases. In addition, SPT results show good correlation with the results of nasal, conjunctival and other provocation tests [38].

In our group, the high prevalence of reactivity to pollen extracts, mainly grasses and rye, is quite surprising. In previous studies from our city and province, the highest frequency of reactivity was seen with regard to house dust mites, both in urban and rural pediatric populations. Similar results were also obtained by other researchers from our country. The highest prevalence of dust mite reactivity was found in studies of children and adults from the city of Krakow and among adult patients from the city of Bydgoszcz and the surrounding area [39,40]. Additionally, in patients with AD, the most common positive SPT result was observed during testing with *D. pteronyssinus* and *D. farinae*, while reactivity to grasses was the third most frequently ascertained [41]. It is suspected that such discrepancies result from differences in the recruitment of the studied groups. Diagnostic screening studies and epidemiological studies show, however, a high degree of repeatability [42].

The allergic reactivity profiles observed in this study indicate the greatest significance of grass pollen allergens in causing IgE-reactivity in the population of central Poland. These results are consistent with the results of the nationwide ECAP study conducted in the general population, where grass pollen allergens were shown to be the clinically most important group of aeroallergens in Poland. In the ECAP study, it was found that 21% of participants had positive SPTs to grass extracts, and 16% of them reported suggestive symptoms during the pollen season [43]. The *Poaceae* (grass) pollen seems to increase its expansiveness and is currently considered to be the leading biological pollutant in atmospheric air and the main cause of pollen allergy in Europe and the world [44,45]. The grass allergens described so far (13 groups) have been divided into water-insoluble ones, which seem to play a role in the centrally mediated inflammatory response, and water-soluble allergens, which are probably involved in the peripheral humoral response [46,47]. Pollen NADPH oxidase (which induces pollen tube growth) has also been shown to have a pro-inflammatory effect, independent of adaptive immune responses [48]. Animal studies have shown that activation of pollen NADPH affects the generation of reactive oxygen species and played an important role in the pathogenesis of allergy [49]. Additionally, air pollution and other biotic (e.g., microorganisms and viruses) and abiotic factors may influence pollen allergenicity. For example, they may contribute to oxidative stress, both to pollen and to human epithelial cells, which may promote allergy to grass and other plant pollen [50]. It has also been shown that pollen lipids can be internalized by dendritic cells presented by CD1 to NKT cells, which release IL-4 and promote the differentiation of Th0 lymphocytes into Th2 cells [51].

In addition, the allergen extracts used during SPTs contain proteins that have not yet been characterized, and so far we do not have the ability to assess their reactivity with IgE from patient sera. For example, recent proteomic analyses indicate the presence of up to 3000 newly identified proteins for each pollen taxon, which may contribute to their different allergenic potential [52].

4.1. Monovalent Reactivity

It is interesting that the most common monovalent reactivity was found to mugwort extract (*Artemisia*), with a general frequency of reactivity of 3.2% in the entire study group. Mugwort is a common plant in Poland, blooming from July to September, together with grasses and other weeds [53–56], which complicates management of allergy with reactivity to this taxon. The participation of mugwort pollen in the aeroplankton of the atmospheric air in our city has never been high during more than 20 years of pollen monitoring. Its influence on the development of IgE-reactivity has not been analyzed in more detail either. However, reports from Asian countries indicate that mugwort pollen allergens are considered clinically significant in the context of allergic disease development. For example, the frequency of reactivity to mugwort in northern China was estimated at 26–48% [57,58]. So far, seven potential mugwort pollen allergens with IgE binding ability have been identified [59]. The high cross-reactivity of mugwort allergens is also known. Available studies show that some allergen components of mugwort and ragweed may be mutually cross-reactive (e.g., Art v 1 with Amb a 4 and Art v 4 with Amb a 8) [60,61]. Aerobiological studies conducted in our city have indicated generally low exposure to ragweed pollen, which comes from long-distance transport, mainly from southern and eastern Europe, and showed that the pollen seasons for mugwort and ragweed are separated [55,62]. It may, therefore, be speculated that, in our region, reactivity to the Art v 1 mugwort pollen component can be a proverbial Trojan horse that would promote reactivity to the Amb a 4 ragweed pollen component.

In our population, we have identified a notable difference between the amount of monoreactivity to *D. farinae* and *D. pteronyssinus* mites. Considering the fact that allergens coming from these mites are highly cross-reactive, this difference may seem unexpected and discrepant. We can, however, speculate that it is associated with the influence of external factors (e.g., housing conditions and some biotic and abiotic indoor factors, including humidity, temperature and presence of microscopic fungi) upon the composition of the local acarofauna [63]. Our unpublished research shows that *D. pteronyssinus* is represented to a higher extent in the house dust samples collected in our city's apartments, compared to *D. farinae*. Other published data [64] show that in Poland, generally, older buildings and furnaces are more conducive to the presence of *D. pteronyssinus*, while new buildings with central heating systems are more favorable milieu for *D. farinae*. Nevertheless, in our city *D. pteronyssinus* mites were the dominant taxon. One may, therefore, assume that the rate of specific IgE-reactivity to either house dust mite can be associated with the level of exposure and reflect features of local acarofauna resulting from housing conditions and external modifying factors, as mentioned above.

Employing only skin prick testing to allergen extracts, and not the assessment of reactivity to allergen components, may be considered a limitation of the study. At the time when the patients had been assessed, component-resolved diagnostics was much less common and accessible in routine diagnostic management; therefore, the number of performed assessments of the levels of IgE specific to allergen components was not considerable and could not be subject to extensive analysis. Basing the assessment of mono- and polyreactivity solely on SPT positivity leaves out possible cross-reactivity between allergenic components belonging to the same groups and represented in different allergen sources, such as trees and furry animals. (e.g., PR-10, profilins, lipocalins). In this context, it should be taken into account that IgE-reactivity to alder and hazel allergen extracts may be in large part due to cross-reactivity of their allergens with birch allergens, whereas the majority of subjects apparently allergic to hazel and/or alder are, in fact, primarily reactive to birch pollen.

Cross-reactivity as a plausible explanation of apparent polysensitization to tree allergens is further supported by significant gamma-correlations between the compared frequencies of positive SPTs to alder and hazel, alder and birch and birch and hazel pollen ($p < 0.00001$). However, with regard to mugwort pollen, a very weak correlation was found between the number of positive SPTs with mugwort and the number of positive SPT results with all of the trees present in the allergens panel. Results of the additional gamma-correlation analysis between positive SPTs with extracts of potentially cross-reactive allergen sources are presented in the Supplementary Material as Table S2.

This issue requires a broadened and deepened separate analysis. Considering this, patient diagnostics should be enriched with an assessment of clinical significance, molecular studies and determination of possible cross-reactions.

4.2. Reactivity and Age

The division into three age groups made in this study showed heterogeneity in the allergy profiles. Surprisingly, the identification of three age clusters showed that in subjects aged over 50, the highest frequencies of allergies to grass and rye were observed. This is difficult to explain using known immunological mechanisms. Several studies show that in senior age groups a progressive loss of the ability to respond to antigen stimulation as well as immune dysfunction are observed [65,66].

4.3. Atopy and Sex

In our study, the frequency of one or more positive SPT responses was higher among males compared to females in each decade of life. This contrast suggests that factors other than type I hypersensitivity reactions are responsible for the differences. Numerous scientific studies have analyzed multidimensional immunological and inflammatory mechanisms. Sex differences can manifest themselves at different levels, mainly genetic, anatomical and endocrine. Many researchers emphasize that sex hormones, such as estrogen and testosterone, can affect respiratory diseases [67,68], but their effects are multifactorial, e.g., dependent on age, menopause, obesity, stage of the menstrual cycle, etc. It is known that sex hormones mediate cellular and humoral immune pathways and may partially explain the increased frequency of inflammation in women compared to men. Studies indicate that estrogen may contribute to airway inflammation in women with asthma, while testosterone may have a protective effect in men [69].

In the National Health and Nutrition Examination Survey (NHANES), serum testosterone levels were found to be inversely associated with the risk of developing current asthma in both sexes [70]. In males, it was reported that each 1-unit increase in testosterone levels reduced the odds of developing asthma by 11%. In general, testosterone in men may reduce Th2 airway inflammation by reducing IL-13 expression and eosinophil infiltration in the airways [71].

4.4. SPT Results and Allergic Diseases

It should be emphasized that reactivity to hazel, alder and birch pollen is positively associated with conjunctivitis. In the context of newer studies, the eye cannot be neglected or omitted in the context of allergic diseases and conjunctival symptoms, as a complication of allergic rhinitis should be given more recognition. It was found that proteases from hazel and birch pollen, as well as the grains of other taxa, can induce both IgE-dependent and IgE-independent reactions [72]. They can contribute to the decomposition of tear fluid proteins and damage to the epithelial cells, in particular in polluted urban environments [73].

It is believed that the development of allergies may be influenced by various exogenous—mainly environmental—factors, e.g., progressive urbanization, lifestyle changes, increased exposure to air pollution and allergens [74]. Our previous studies show that exposure to pollen seems to be of particular importance in already sensitized subjects. However, it must be underlined that clinical symptoms mainly occur when the level of exposure exceeds the individual threshold level. Additional factors may also contribute to the development of allergy symptoms. For example, Olivieri et al. [75] showed interactions between atopy, seasonal exposure to pollen, and FeNO, total IgE and FEV1/FVC levels, which were of a dose-response nature.

Our studies show that the risk of allergic rhinitis, conjunctivitis and atopic eczema was strongly associated with reactivity to pollen of locally flowering plants. Although seasonal exposure to birch pollen in our region is almost twice as high, but shorter in duration than grass pollen (unpublished data), grass and rye allergens turned out to be the most aggressive, more often promoting allergy symptoms in our group.

In parallel to diagnostic and epidemiological studies, our center conducts aerobiological studies in the city center. The main grass pollen season in Poland lasts about 80–90 days between the end of May, throughout June until mid-July. Data from the years 2003–2024 indicate a significant increase in grass pollen concentrations over a more than twenty-year period ($p = 0.045$; $r^2 = 0.186$; unpublished data), while birch pollen concentrations show two-year fluctuations, but without a significant increase in concentrations over the last 22 seasons.

A recent study by Klangkalya et al. [76] indicated that, in children, only the cut-off value of the wheal in SPTs of 6.6 mm provided 100% specificity for predicting AR induced by HDM. However, in our work, the wheal size criterion of the positive SPT result was assumed at $\geq$3 mm. Perhaps in future studies different values may be used as criteria for analyses.

It should again be emphasized that the risk of developing allergies depends on many factors, including genetic, epigenetic, prenatal, perinatal and environmental ones, and their mutual interactions [15,77]. Growing up in a polluted urban environment confers an increased risk of developing allergies in early childhood. In our previous studies, differences in the frequency of allergies in children were found depending on the region of residence within the same city. They were significantly higher in the downtown district compared to districts located far from the city center [78]. Similar findings, i.e., differences in pediatric asthma incidence between districts of the same town differing in terms of proximity to industrial facilities, have recently been described in another region of Poland [79].

In addition, the results of the study by Stelmach et al. [80], conducted in our city among children living in an orphanage, indicated a low frequency of atopy (12.5% positive SPT) and atopic diseases. For example, seasonal allergic rhinitis was found in only 2.5% (3 out of 120) of children. Similarly, in children living in foster care homes the presence of atopic diseases was observed in 11.3%, which is almost half as many as in the control population, in children living with their parents (26%), despite the fact that all children came from the same area of the city. The authors suggest that exceptionally difficult living conditions and multiple infections in early childhood may lead to lower reactivity in later life [81].

In our study, we have not addressed or interpreted the data on symptoms occurring upon exposure to allergens. Similarly, the severity of symptoms of allergic disease has not been interpreted in the exposure or SPT result context. This study focused on the association between IgE-reactivity and the presence of diagnosis of given condition, as per available medical records. Such an approach, i.e., based on the presence of given diagnosis in medical records, always bears the possibility of bias or error. However, retrospective data from large populations are likely to be recorded in a non-standardized manner, unless a uniform scheme of their collection is established beforehand. This was not the case here, which should be considered as a factor influencing further clinical interpretation of these data.

5. Conclusions

Our study is representative of the urban population of central Poland and offers a platform for the assessment of the relationships between IgE-reactivity and allergic disease. Identification of sensitizing allergens, i.e., exposure risk factors for the development of symptoms, is crucial for allergy diagnostics. Reactivity profiles determined using a basic panel of skin tests may vary depending on sex, age groups and individual disease entities of allergic origin. The results of our study can serve as an objective reference to the frequency of allergen occurrence in the urban environment in central Poland, but also in similar climate and geographical conditions. Accurate diagnosis combined with optimal therapy requires the use of appropriate tests confirming allergen reactivity and obtaining detailed information on exposure to the presumed culprit allergen.

The results of this study can, therefore, be summarized in the following main points:

- According to the results of SPTs, the most important sensitizing allergens in allergic subjects in central Poland were the pollen from grass (60.5%), rye (57.22%) and birch (47.34%).
- The most common monovalent reactivity found was that to mugwort pollen.
- The frequency of one or more positive SPT results was higher among males.
- The age distribution shows the highest reactivity of allergies in the age group 10–50 years, with male predominance
- In patients with clinically diagnosed AR, the probability of developing symptoms was higher in those sensitized to grass pollen, rye, alder, hazel, *Alternaria*, birch, cat, *D. pteronyssinus* and *D. farinae* allergens.
- Higher odds of developing asthma were associated with positive SPT results with dog, cat and dust mite allergens.
- Higher odds of developing atopic dermatitis were associated with positive SPT results with birch and alder pollen allergens.
- Higher odds of developing allergic conjunctivitis were associated with positive SPT results with alder, hazel and birch pollen allergens.

Due to the high prevalence of allergic diseases in Poland and worldwide, there is an urgent need to study the spectra of reactivity and their relationship with allergy. Identification of the most frequent reactivity profiles associated with target-organ manifestations of allergic disease in a given geographical area may provide valuable descriptive data with regard to a description of clinical phenotypes of allergy. Trends in the prevalence of reactivity to specific allergens depending on age and physician-diagnosed allergic disease in Poland have rarely been studied in both children and adults. Our research focuses on the reactivity profiles in individual allergic diseases, as well as age- and sex-related differences in patients diagnosed and treated in an outpatient allergy clinic. In this context, it adds to the current state of knowledge on the epidemiology and distribution of reactivity to the most common airborne allergens in Central Europe. Further studies in this geographical area are needed in order to cover a broader spectrum of reactivity and to analyze possible variations and fluctuations in allergen reactivity profiles over longer periods. This aspect of studies on allergen reactivity profiles deserves particular recognition in the light of climate changes, which may affect the extent and patterns of exposure to seasonal airborne allergens. We can foresee that climate change-associated shifts in the IgE-reactivity profile extended over longer periods may incur modifications in recommended immunotherapy schemes and enforce changes in routine diagnostic work-up with regard to allergen reactivity assessed through SPT and serum-specific IgE concentrations.

Supplementary Materials: The following supporting information can be downloaded at: https://www.mdpi.com/article/10.3390/medicina61091676/s1, Figure S1. Comparison of variance in mean wheal size between age categories with regard to tree (birch, hazel, alder) pollen allergens sensitization (Factor I). * p = 0.0048; ** p = 0.00003. Figure S2. Comparison of variance in mean wheal size in SPTs with house dust mites (*D. pteronyssinus*, *D. farinae*) allergens between age groups (panel A) and sexes (panel B); * p = 0.045; ** p = 0.016; *** p = 0.00008. Figure S3. Comparison of variance in mean wheal size in SPT with grass pollen allergens between age groups (panel A) and sexes (panel B); * p = 0.026; ** p = 0.0004; *** p = 0.00002; **** p = 0.00000005. Figure S4. Comparison of variance in mean wheal size in SPTs with cat and dog allergens (Factor IV) between age groups. * p = 0.023; ** p = 0.019. Figure S5: Differences between proportions in the prevalence of allergic rhinitis and asthma by sex categories of subjects. Figure S6. Differences between proportions in the prevalence of allergic rhinitis and asthma by age categories of subjects. Table S1. Associations between physician-diagnosed allergic/atopic conditions (as retrieved from archival patients' charts) and allergic sensitization ascertained by skin prick tests (SPTs). Table S2. Gamma correlations for compared frequencies of positive SPT results (positive result defined as a wheal $\geq$3 mm diameter).

Author Contributions: Conceptualization, B.M.-W. and M.K. (Maciej Kulma); methodology, B.M.-W.; formal analysis, B.M.-W.; investigation, B.M.-W.; data curation, B.M.-W., M.K. (Maciej Kulma) and M.K. (Marcin Kurowski); writing—original draft preparation, B.M.-W. and M.K. (Maciej Kulma); writing—review and editing, B.M.-W. and M.K. (Marcin Kurowski); supervision, B.M.-W.; All authors have read and agreed to the published version of the manuscript.

Funding: This research received no external funding.

Institutional Review Board Statement: In accordance with the following laws of the Republic of Poland, (1) Act on the Profession of Medical Doctor and Dentist announced 5 December 1996 (Journal of Laws of the Republic of Poland 2024 no. 1287); (2) Regulation of the Minister of Health of 26 January 2023, on the Bioethics Committee and the Appeals Bioethics Committee 1996 (Journal of Laws of the Republic of Poland 2023 no. 218), retrospective studies of past medical records are not considered medical experiments involving human subjects and, as such, do not require assessment and approval from the bioethics committee. Approval for the analysis of retrospective patient data was obtained from the university hospital management, as per internal procedures.

Informed Consent Statement: Not applicable.

Data Availability Statement: The data presented in this study are available upon reasonable request from the corresponding author (B.M.-W.).

Acknowledgments: The authors would like to acknowledge Zbigniew Wojciechowski for his contribution and help with statistical analysis of data.

Conflicts of Interest: The authors declare no conflicts of interest.

Abbreviations

The following abbreviations are used in this manuscript:

SPT	Skin prick test
AR	Allergic rhinitis
ICD-10	International Statistical Classification of Diseases and Related Health Problems, Tenth Revision

NADPH	Nicotinamide Adenine Dinucleotide Phosphate
OR	Odds ratio
CI	Confidence interval
IL	Interleukin
HDM	House dust mite(s)
FeNO	Fractional exhaled nitric oxide
FEV1	Forced expiratory volume in one second
FVC	Forced vital capacity

References

1. Rezwan, T.; Perez, M.; Jacobs, S.; Shafik, J.; Mitchell, W.B.; Conrad, L.A.; Soshnick, S.H. Correlation between Total IgE Level and Asthma Symptom Severity in Hospitalized Children. *J. Allergy Clin. Immunol. Glob.* **2025**, *4*, 100452. [CrossRef]
2. Scelo, G.; Torres-Duque, C.A.; Maspero, J.; Tran, T.N.; Murray, R.; Martin, N.; Menzies-Gow, A.N.; Hew, M.; Peters, M.J.; Gibson, P.G.; et al. Analysis of Comorbidities and Multimorbidity in Adult Patients in the International Severe Asthma Registry. *Ann. Allergy Asthma Immunol.* **2024**, *132*, 42–53. [CrossRef]
3. Wang, H.; Li, X.-B.; Chu, X.-J.; Cao, N.-W.; Wu, H.; Huang, R.-G.; Li, B.-Z.; Ye, D.-Q. Ambient Air Pollutants Increase the Risk of Immunoglobulin E–Mediated Allergic Diseases: A Systematic Review and Meta-Analysis. *Environ. Sci. Pollut. Res.* **2022**, *29*, 49534–49552. [CrossRef]
4. Guo, Y.; Cai, S.; Deng, J.; Li, J.; Qiu, L.; Sun, Q.; Cui, Y.; Li, L.; Yu, L.; Yin, H.; et al. Trends and Hotspots of Acupuncture for Allergic Rhinitis: A Bibliometric Analysis from 2002 to 2022. *Complement. Ther. Med.* **2023**, *78*, 102984. [CrossRef]
5. Cingi, C.; Gevaert, P.; Mösges, R.; Rondon, C.; Hox, V.; Rudenko, M.; Muluk, N.B.; Scadding, G.; Manole, F.; Hupin, C.; et al. Multi-Morbidities of Allergic Rhinitis in Adults: European Academy of Allergy and Clinical Immunology Task Force Report. *Clin. Transl. Allergy* **2017**, *7*, 17. [CrossRef]
6. Seys, S.F.; Quirce, S.; Agache, I.; Akdis, C.A.; Alvaro-Lozano, M.; Antolín-Amérigo, D.; Bjermer, L.; Bobolea, I.; Bonini, M.; Bossios, A.; et al. Severe Asthma: Entering an Era of New Concepts and Emerging Therapies: Highlights of the 4th International Severe Asthma Forum, Madrid, 2018. *Allergy* **2019**, *74*, 2244–2248. [CrossRef] [PubMed]
7. Mortada, M.M.; Kurowski, M. Challenges in Local Allergic Rhinitis Diagnosis, Management, and Research: Current Concepts and Future Perspectives. *Medicina* **2023**, *59*, 929. [CrossRef]
8. Krzych-Fałta, E.; Wojas, O. Local Allergic Rhinitis or Local Allergic Conjunctivitis? *Alergol. Pol. Pol. J. Allergol.* **2023**, *10*, 310–314. [CrossRef]
9. Berghi, O.; Dumitru, M.; Cergan, R.; Musat, G.; Serboiu, C.; Vrinceanu, D. Local Allergic Rhinitis—A Challenge for Allergology and Otorhinolaryngology Cooperation (Scoping Review). *Life* **2024**, *14*, 965. [CrossRef] [PubMed]
10. Testera-Montes, A.; Jurado, R.; Salas, M.; Eguiluz-Gracia, I.; Mayorga, C. Diagnostic Tools in Allergic Rhinitis. *Front. Allergy* **2021**, *2*, 721851. [CrossRef]
11. Riggioni, C.; Ricci, C.; Moya, B.; Wong, D.; Van Goor, E.; Bartha, I.; Buyuktiryaki, B.; Giovannini, M.; Jayasinghe, S.; Jaumdally, H.; et al. Systematic Review and Meta-analyses on the Accuracy of Diagnostic Tests for IgE-mediated Food Allergy. *Allergy* **2024**, *79*, 324–352. [CrossRef]
12. García-Marcos, L.; Asher, M.I.; Pearce, N.; Ellwood, E.; Bissell, K.; Chiang, C.-Y.; El Sony, A.; Ellwood, P.; Marks, G.B.; Mortimer, K.; et al. The Burden of Asthma, Hay Fever and Eczema in Children in 25 Countries: GAN Phase I Study. *Eur. Respir. J.* **2022**, *60*, 2102866. [CrossRef] [PubMed]
13. Romano, M.R.; James, S.; Farrington, E.; Perry, R.; Elliott, L. The Impact of Perennial Allergic Rhinitis with/without Allergic Asthma on Sleep, Work and Activity Level. *Allergy Asthma Clin. Immunol.* **2019**, *15*, 81. [CrossRef]
14. Krzych-Fałta, E.; Wojas, O.; Raciborski, F.; Furmańczyk, K.; Chrzanowska, M.; Samoliński, B.; Lipiec, A.; Piekarska, B.; Gujski, M. Specificity and Sensitivity of Questionnaires in the Diagnosis of Allergic Diseases. *Adv. Dermatol. Allergol.* **2024**, *41*, 594–603. [CrossRef]
15. Majkowska-Wojciechowska, B.; Pełka, J.; Korzon, L.; Kozłowska, A.; Kaczała, M.; Jarzebska, M.; Gwardys, T.; Kowalski, M.L. Prevalence of Allergy, Patterns of Allergic Sensitization and Allergy Risk Factors in Rural and Urban Children. *Allergy* **2007**, *62*, 1044–1050. [CrossRef] [PubMed]
16. Pereira, R.N.; Rodrigues, R.M.; Madalena, D.A.; Vicente, A. Tackling Food Allergens—The Role of Food Processing on Proteins' Allergenicity. In *Advances in Food and Nutrition Research*; Elsevier: Amsterdam, The Netherlands, 2023; Volume 106, pp. 317–351. ISBN 978-0-443-19304-0.
17. Aldakheel, F.M. Allergic Diseases: A Comprehensive Review on Risk Factors, Immunological Mechanisms, Link with COVID-19, Potential Treatments, and Role of Allergen Bioinformatics. *Int. J. Environ. Res. Public Health* **2021**, *18*, 12105. [CrossRef] [PubMed]

18. Finn, P.W.; Perkins, D.L. Born to Wheeze or Learned When We Were Young: Maternal and Environmental Factors Influence Atopic Risk. *Trans. Am. Clin. Climatol. Assoc.* **2023**, *133*, 181–192.
19. Fujimura, K.E.; Sitarik, A.R.; Havstad, S.; Lin, D.L.; Levan, S.; Fadrosh, D.; Panzer, A.R.; LaMere, B.; Rackaityte, E.; Lukacs, N.W.; et al. Neonatal Gut Microbiota Associates with Childhood Multisensitized Atopy and T Cell Differentiation. *Nat. Med.* **2016**, *22*, 1187–1191. [CrossRef]
20. Wang, H.; Jiang, X.; Zhang, P.; Li, Y.; Wang, Y.; Li, X. Allergen-Specific IgE in the Tear Fluid of Chinese Patients with Common Allergic Conjunctivitis in Autumn and Winter. *Int. Ophthalmol.* **2023**, *43*, 4541–4549. [CrossRef]
21. Satnarine, T.; Makkoukdji, N.; Pundit, V.; Vignau, A.; Sharma, P.; Warren, D.; Kleiner, G.; Gans, M. Peanut Allergy Diagnosis: Current Practices, Emerging Technologies, and Future Directions. *Allergies* **2025**, *5*, 4. [CrossRef]
22. Haidar, L.; Bănărescu, C.F.; Uța, C.; Moldovan, S.I.; Zimbru, E.-L.; Zimbru, R.-I.; Ciurariu, E.; Georgescu, M.; Panaitescu, C. Pollen–Food Allergy Syndrome: Allergens, Clinical Insights, Diagnostic and Therapeutic Challenges. *Appl. Sci.* **2024**, *15*, 66. [CrossRef]
23. Gawryjołek, J.; Krogulska, A. Diagnostics of Peanut Allergy—Part I. *Alergol. Pol. Pol. J. Allergol.* **2022**, *9*, 160–169. [CrossRef]
24. Krupka Olek, M.; Bożek, A.; Foks Ciekalska, A.; Grzanka, A.; Kawczyk-Krupka, A. Assessment of Hypersensitivity to House Dust Mites in Selected Skin Diseases Using the Basophil Activation Test: A Preliminary Study. *Medicina* **2024**, *60*, 1608. [CrossRef] [PubMed]
25. Izmailovich, M.; Semenova, Y.; Abdushukurova, G.; Mukhamejanova, A.; Dyussupova, A.; Faizova, R.; Gazaliyeva, M.; Akhvlediani, L.; Glushkova, N.; Kalmakhanov, S.; et al. Molecular Aspects of Allergen-Specific Immunotherapy in Patients with Seasonal Allergic Rhinitis. *Cells* **2023**, *12*, 383. [CrossRef] [PubMed]
26. Połomska, J.; Dydak, P.; Sozańska, B.; Sikorska-Szaflik, H. Peanut Allergy and Component-Resolved Diagnostics Possibilities—What Are the Benefits? *Nutrients* **2023**, *15*, 5132. [CrossRef] [PubMed]
27. Wąsik, J.; Likońska, A.; Kurowski, M. IgE-Mediated Allergy and Asymptomatic Sensitization to Cannabis Allergens—Review of Current Knowledge and Presentation of Six Cases. *Medicina* **2024**, *60*, 954. [CrossRef]
28. Jankowski, W.; Przychodniak, D.; Kurowski, M. LTP Syndrome and Edible Insect Allergy in a Patient with Recurrent Anaphylaxis Incidents. *Alergol. Pol. Pol. J. Allergol.* **2024**, *12*, 138–139. [CrossRef]
29. Zhang, J.; Tang, Y.; Yang, D.; Yu, J. Investigating Allergen-Specific IgE Distribution and Correlations in Chronic Urticaria: A Retrospective Study in Shanghai, China. *Eur. J. Med. Res.* **2025**, *30*, 182. [CrossRef]
30. Liu, M.; Liu, L.; Qi, W.; Zheng, X.; Chen, J.; Yao, J.; Li, Y.; Lin, J.; Li, X.; Hu, X.; et al. Interpreting Epidemiologic Distribution of Total and Specific IgE Levels for Food Allergy in Southern China from 2004 to 2023: Understanding the Mechanisms and Focusing on Prevention. *BMC Public Health* **2024**, *24*, 3022. [CrossRef]
31. Wang, J.; Xu, B.; Jia, X.; He, Y.; Jia, B.; Li, J.; Xu, M. Predictive Value of Der p 2-Specific IgE for Subcutaneous Immunotherapy in Children with Allergic Rhinitis. *Sci. Rep.* **2024**, *14*, 25467. [CrossRef]
32. Łódź Raport o Stanie Miasta. BS_p25_120_20250530. PDF. Available online: https://bip.uml.lodz.pl/ (accessed on 7 September 2025).
33. World Health Organization. International Statistical Classification of Diseases and Related Health Problems 10th Revision 2019. World Health Organization: Geneva, Switzerland, 2019.
34. Bousquet, J.; Heinzerling, L.; Bachert, C.; Papadopoulos, N.G.; Bousquet, P.J.; Burney, P.G.; Canonica, G.W.; Carlsen, K.H.; Cox, L.; Haahtela, T.; et al. Practical Guide to Skin Prick Tests in Allergy to Aeroallergens. *Allergy* **2012**, *67*, 18–24. [CrossRef] [PubMed]
35. Wallace, D.V.; Bahna, S.L.; Goldstein, S.; Hamilton, R.G.; Cohn, J.R. American Academy of Allergy, Asthma & Immunology Work Group Report: Allergy Diagnosis in Clinical Practice. *J. Allergy Clin. Immunol.* **2007**, *120*, 967–969. [CrossRef] [PubMed]
36. Kowalski, M.L.; Ansotegui, I.; Aberer, W.; Al-Ahmad, M.; Akdis, M.; Ballmer-Weber, B.K.; Beyer, K.; Blanca, M.; Brown, S.; Bunnag, C.; et al. Risk and Safety Requirements for Diagnostic and Therapeutic Procedures in Allergology: World Allergy Organization Statement. *World Allergy Organ. J.* **2016**, *9*, 33. [CrossRef] [PubMed]
37. Szmyd, B.; Biedrzycka, M.; Rogut, M.; Daszkiewicz, G.; Hałucha, J.; Kaszkowiak, M.; Kowalski, M.L.; Kurowski, M. Assessment of Skin Prick Tests and sIgE Measurement Performance in the Diagnosis of Food and Inhalat Allergy. *Alerg. Astma Immunol.* **2020**, *25*, 104–110. (In Polish)
38. Ansotegui, I.J.; Melioli, G.; Canonica, G.W.; Caraballo, L.; Villa, E.; Ebisawa, M.; Passalacqua, G.; Savi, E.; Ebo, D.; Gómez, R.M.; et al. IgE Allergy Diagnostics and Other Relevant Tests in Allergy, a World Allergy Organization Position Paper. *World Allergy Organ. J.* **2020**, *13*, 100080. [CrossRef]
39. Czarnobilska, E.; Klimaszewska-Rembiasz, M.; Gaweł, B.; Obtułowicz, A. Prevalence of Allergic Diseases in Primary School Children in Cracow and Surroundings—An Attempt to Define Main Risk Factors. *Przegląd Lekarski* **2002**, *59*, 422–426. (In Polish)
40. Wojciechowska, M.; Hnatyszyn-Dzikowska, A.; Bartuzi, Z. Sensitization to Haptens, Inhalant and Food Allergensamong Patients Diagnosed for Contact Allergy. *Alerg. Astma Immunol.* **2016**, *21*, 110–120. (In Polish)

41. Sybilski, A.J.; Raciborski, F.; Lipiec, A.; Tomaszewska, A.; Lusawa, A.; Samel-Kowalik, P.; Walkiewicz, A.; Krzych-Fałta, E.; Samoliński, B. Epidemiology of Atopic Dermatitis in Poland According to the Epidemiology of Allergic Disorders in Poland (ECAP) Study. *J. Dermatol.* **2015**, *42*, 140–147. [CrossRef]
42. Antico, A.; Lima, G.; Arisi, M.; Ostan, A.; Morrica, B. Assay of Prick Test Inoculum Volume. II. Average Values and Individual Variability. *Ann. Allergy Asthma Immunol.* **2000**, *85*, 145–149. [CrossRef]
43. Samoliński, B.; Raciborski, F.; Lipiec, A.; Tomaszewska, A.; Krzych-Fałta, E.; Samel-Kowalik, P.; Walkiewicz, A.; Lusawa, A.; Borowicz, J.; Komorowski, J.; et al. Epidemiology of allergic diseases in Poland. *Alergol. Pol. Pol. J. Allergol.* **2014**, *1*, 10–18. (In Polish) [CrossRef]
44. Worm, M.; Lee, H.; Kostev, K. Prevalence and Treatment Profile of Patients with Grass Pollen and House Dust Mite Allergy. *JDDG J. Dtsch. Dermatol. Ges.* **2013**, *11*, 653–661. [CrossRef] [PubMed]
45. García-Mozo, H. Poaceae Pollen as the Leading Aeroallergen Worldwide: A Review. *Allergy* **2017**, *72*, 1849–1858. [CrossRef]
46. Dramburg, S.; Hilger, C.; Santos, A.F.; de Las Vecillas, L.; Aalberse, R.C.; Acevedo, N.; Aglas, L.; Altmann, F.; Arruda, K.L.; Asero, R.; et al. EAACI Molecular Allergology User's Guide 2.0. *Pediatr. Allergy Immunol.* **2023**, *34* (Suppl. 28), e13854. [CrossRef] [PubMed]
47. Abou Chakra, O.R.; Sutra, J.-P.; Poncet, P.; Lacroix, G.; Sénéchal, H. Key Role of Water-Insoluble Allergens of Pollen Cytoplasmic Granules in Biased Allergic Response in a Rat Model. *World Allergy Organ. J.* **2011**, *4*, 4–12. [CrossRef] [PubMed]
48. Dharajiya, N.; Boldogh, I.; Cardenas, V.; Sur, S. Role of Pollen NAD(P)H Oxidase in Allergic Inflammation. *Curr. Opin. Allergy Clin. Immunol.* **2008**, *8*, 57–62. [CrossRef]
49. Wang, X.-L.; Takai, T.; Kamijo, S.; Gunawan, H.; Ogawa, H.; Okumura, K. NADPH Oxidase Activity in Allergenic Pollen Grains of Different Plant Species. *Biochem. Biophys. Res. Commun.* **2009**, *387*, 430–434. [CrossRef]
50. Visez, N.; De Nadaï, P.; Choël, M.; Farah, J.; Hamzé, M.; Sénéchal, H.; Pauwels, M.; Frérot, H.; Thibaudon, M.; Poncet, P. Biochemical Composition of Phleum Pratense Pollen Grains: A Review. *Mol. Immunol.* **2021**, *136*, 98–109. [CrossRef]
51. Raith, M.; Swoboda, I. Birch Pollen—The Unpleasant Herald of Spring. *Front. Allergy* **2023**, *4*, 1181675. [CrossRef]
52. Darnhofer, B.; Tomin, T.; Liesinger, L.; Schittmayer, M.; Tomazic, P.V.; Birner-Gruenberger, R. Comparative Proteomics of Common Allergenic Tree Pollens of Birch, Alder, and Hazel. *Allergy* **2021**, *76*, 1743–1753. [CrossRef]
53. Rapiejko, J.; Puc, M.; Piotrowska-Weryszko, K.; Myszkowska, D.; Chodkowski, J.; Malkiewicz, M.; Jurkiewicz, D.; Siergiejko, G.; Chłopek, K.; Lipiec, A. Analysis of Artemisia Pollen Season in Selected Cities of Poland in 2022. *Alergoprofil* **2023**, *19*, 13–19. [CrossRef]
54. Majkowska–Wojciechowska, B.; Balwierz, Z.; Kowalski, M. Pollen Counts Analysis in the Atmosphere of Lodz (Poland) during Vegetation in 2008. *Alerg. Astma Immunol.* **2008**, *13*, 250–263.
55. Majkowska-Wojciechowska, B.; Balwierz, Z.; Kowalski, M.L. Changes in the Concentration of Pollen over an 11-Year Period in a Polish Urban Environment. *Acta Agrobot.* **2016**, *69*, 1–11. [CrossRef]
56. Majkowska-Wojciechowska, B.; Balwierz, Z.; Kowalski, M. Pollen and Spores of Microscopic Fungi in Atmospheric Air Lodz in 2013. *Alerg. Astma Immunol.* **2015**, *20*, 192–198. (In Polish)
57. Ma, T.; Wang, H.; Chen, Y.; Zhuang, Y.; Shi, H.; Yu, R.; Guo, M.; Yin, J.; Wang, X. Sensitization Spectrum of Inhaled Allergens in Outpatients in Beijing Area. *Chin. J. Allergy Clin Immunol.* **2021**, *15*, 136–143. (In Chinese)
58. Yu, Y.; Yan, X.; Wang, L.; Dong, L.; Song, D.; Liu, J.; Gao, X. Investigation and Analysis of Inhalant Allergens in Patients with Allergic Rhinitis in Yinchuan, China. *Int. Arch. Allergy Immunol.* **2024**, *186*, 445–453. [CrossRef]
59. Wang, M.; Ma, J.; Yang, Z.; Wang, W.; Sa, Y.; Ma, F.; Zhang, W.; He, X.; Chen, G.; Ma, X. Immunoproteomic Analysis and Identification of Possible Allergenic Proteins in Artemisia Annua Pollen. *Int. Immunopharmacol.* **2025**, *146*, 113837. [CrossRef]
60. Asero, R. Is the Strange Case of Mugwort Sensitivity in Ragweed-Allergic Subjects Coming Eventually to a Solution? *Eur. Ann. Allergy Clin. Immunol.* **2011**, *43*, 67–68.
61. Pablos, I.; Eichhorn, S.; Machado, Y.; Briza, P.; Neunkirchner, A.; Jahn-Schmid, B.; Wildner, S.; Soh, W.T.; Ebner, C.; Park, J.-W.; et al. Distinct Epitope Structures of Defensin-like Proteins Linked to Proline-rich Regions Give Rise to Differences in Their Allergenic Activity. *Allergy* **2018**, *73*, 431–441. [CrossRef]
62. Stępalska, D.; Myszkowska, D.; Piotrowicz, K.; Kluska, K.; Chłopek, K.; Grewling, Ł.; Lafférsová, J.; Majkowska-Wojciechowska, B.; Malkiewicz, M.; Piotrowska-Weryszko, K.; et al. High Ambrosia Pollen Concentrations in Poland Respecting the Long Distance Transport (LDT). *Sci. Total Environ.* **2020**, *736*, 139615. [CrossRef]
63. Bergmann, K.-C. Biology of House Dust Mites and Storage Mites. *Allergo J. Int.* **2022**, *31*, 272–278. [CrossRef]
64. Solarz, K. Risk of Exposure to House Dust Pyroglyphid Mites in Poland. *Ann. Agric. Environ. Med. AAEM* **2001**, *8*, 11–24.
65. Lee, K.-A.; Flores, R.R.; Jang, I.H.; Saathoff, A.; Robbins, P.D. Immune Senescence, Immunosenescence and Aging. *Front. Aging* **2022**, *3*, 900028. [CrossRef]

66. Ventura, M.T.; Scichilone, N.; Paganelli, R.; Minciullo, P.L.; Patella, V.; Bonini, M.; Passalacqua, G.; Lombardi, C.; Simioni, L.; Ridolo, E.; et al. Allergic Diseases in the Elderly: Biological Characteristics and Main Immunological and Non-Immunological Mechanisms. *Clin. Mol. Allergy* **2017**, *15*, 2. [CrossRef] [PubMed]
67. Warren, K.J.; Deering-Rice, C.; Huecksteadt, T.; Trivedi, S.; Venosa, A.; Reilly, C.; Sanders, K.; Clayton, F.; Wyatt, T.A.; Poole, J.A.; et al. Steady-State Estradiol Triggers a Unique Innate Immune Response to Allergen Resulting in Increased Airway Resistance. *Biol. Sex Differ.* **2023**, *14*, 2. [CrossRef] [PubMed]
68. Harvey, B.J.; McElvaney, N.G. Sex Differences in Airway Disease: Estrogen and Airway Surface Liquid Dynamics. *Biol. Sex Differ.* **2024**, *15*, 56. [CrossRef] [PubMed]
69. Cephus, J.-Y.; Stier, M.T.; Fuseini, H.; Yung, J.A.; Toki, S.; Bloodworth, M.H.; Zhou, W.; Goleniewska, K.; Zhang, J.; Garon, S.L.; et al. Testosterone Attenuates Group 2 Innate Lymphoid Cell-Mediated Airway Inflammation. *Cell Rep.* **2017**, *21*, 2487–2499. [CrossRef]
70. Han, Y.-Y.; Yan, Q.; Yang, G.; Chen, W.; Forno, E.; Celedon, J.C. Serum Free Testosterone and Asthma, Asthma Hospitalisations and Lung Function in British Adults. *Thorax* **2020**, *75*, 849–854. [CrossRef]
71. Trivedi, S.; Deering-Rice, C.E.; Aamodt, S.E.; Huecksteadt, T.P.; Myers, E.J.; Sanders, K.A.; Paine, R.; Warren, K.J. Progesterone Amplifies Allergic Inflammation and Airway Pathology in Association with Higher Lung ILC2 Responses. *Am. J. Physiol.-Lung Cell. Mol. Physiol.* **2024**, *327*, L65–L78. [CrossRef]
72. Dou, X.; Zhang, W.; Zhang, X. Exploring the Immunological Underpinnings of Allergic Conjunctivitis: The Role of CD4 + T Cells and SLAM Expression in Ocular Surface Disease. *Int. Ophthalmol.* **2025**, *45*, 77. [CrossRef]
73. Rabensteiner, D.F.; Rabensteiner, J.; Horwath-Winter, J.; Lang-Loidolt, D.; Wedrich, A.; Heidinger, A.; Schwantzer, G.; Schmut, O. Extracts of Different Pollen Species and Their Effect on Human Tear Fluid and an Epithelial Cell Line. *Cutan. Ocul. Toxicol.* **2019**, *38*, 93–103. [CrossRef]
74. Montoro, J.; Antolín-Amérigo, D.; Izquierdo-Domínguez, A.; Zapata, J.; García-Gallardo, M.; González, R.; Armentia, A.; Rondón, C.; Fernández, M.; Pedrero, S.; et al. Climate Change–Associated Environmental Factors and Pollutants: Impact on Allergic Diseases, Epidemiology, Severity, and Health Care Burden. *J. Investig. Allergy Clin. Immunol.* **2025**, *35*, 240–250. [CrossRef]
75. Olivieri, M.; Marchetti, P.; Murgia, N.; Nicolis, M.; Torroni, L.; Spiteri, G.; Ferrari, M.; Marcon, A.; Verlato, G. Natural Pollen Exposure Increases in a Dose-dependent Way Fraction of Exhaled Nitric Oxide (FeNO) Levels in Patients Sensitized to One or More Pollen Species. *Clin. Transl. Allergy* **2022**, *12*, e12096. [CrossRef] [PubMed]
76. Klangkalya, N.; Watcharoot, K.; Adithep, S.; Potjanee, K.; Wanlapa, J.; Wiparat, M. Skin Prick Test and Serum Specific IgE in Predicting Dust Mite-Induced Allergic Rhinitis Diagnosed from Nasal Provocation Test in Chronic Rhinitis Children. *Asian Pac. J. Allergy Immunol.* **2025**, *42*, 354–360. [CrossRef]
77. Kurowski, M.; Majkowska-Wojciechowska, B.; Wardzyńska, A.; Kowalski, M.L. Associations of Allergic Sensitization and Clinical Phenotypes with Innate Immune Response Genes Polymorphisms Are Modified by House Dust Mite Allergen Exposure. *Arch. Med. Sci.* **2011**, *6*, 1029–1036. [CrossRef]
78. Majkowska-Wojciechowska, B.; Laskowska, B.; Wojciechowski, Z.; Kowlaski, M. Występowanie Alergii Wśród Dzieci Łódzkich Szkół Podstawowych: Związek z Warunkami Środowiska Domowego i Szkolnego. *Alerg. Astma Immunol.* **2000**, *5*, 115–122.
79. Góra, D.J.; Kupiec, J. Analysis of the Incidence of Asthma among Pupils of Primary Schools in Bielsko-Biala Located in Areas with Various Degrees of Industrialization. *Alergol. Pol. Pol. J. Allergol.* **2024**, *11*, 211–216. [CrossRef]
80. Stelmach, I.; Smejda, K.; Kaczmarek, J.; Stelmach, W.; Kuna, P. Prevalence of Atopy and Atopic Diseases in Children Living in an Orphanage in Lodz Area Pilot Study. *Pol. Merkur. Lekarski* **2006**, *20*, 531–534. (In Polish)
81. Stelmach, I.; Smejda, K.; Jerzynska, J.; Stelmach, W.; Majak, P.; Stelmach, P.; Kuna, P. Decreased Markers of Atopy in Children with Presumed Early Exposure to Allergens, Unhygienic Conditions, and Infections. *Ann. Allergy Asthma Immunol.* **2007**, *99*, 170–177. [CrossRef]

MDPI AG
Grosspeteranlage 5
4052 Basel
Switzerland
Tel.: +41 61 683 77 34

Medicina Editorial Office
E-mail: medicina@mdpi.com
www.mdpi.com/journal/medicina